T0211347

Establishing Preventive Services

Issues in Children's and Families' Lives
AN ANNUAL BOOK SERIES

Senior Series Editor

Thomas P. Gullotta, *Child and Family Agency of Southeastern Connecticut*

Editors

Gerald R. Adams, *University of Guelph, Ontario, Canada*

Bruce A. Ryan, *University of Guelph, Ontario, Canada*

Robert L. Hampton, *University of Maryland, College Park*

Roger P. Weissberg, *University of Illinois at Chicago, Illinois*

Drawing upon the resources of Child and Family Agency of Southeastern Connecticut, one of this nation's leading family service agencies, Issues in Children's and Families' Lives is designed to focus attention on the pressing social problems facing children and their families today. Each volume in this series will analyze, integrate, and critique the clinical and research literature on children and their families as it relates to a particular theme. Believing that integrated multidisciplinary approaches offer greater opportunities for program success, volume contributors will reflect the research and clinical knowledge base of the many different disciplines that are committed to enhancing the physical, social, and emotional health of children and their families. Intended for graduate and professional audiences, chapters will be written by scholars and practitioners who will encourage readers to apply their practice skills and intellect to reducing the suffering of children and their families in the society in which those families live and work.

Healthy Children 2010

*E*stablishing
*P*reventive
*S*ervices

Editors

Roger P. Weissberg
Thomas P. Gullotta
Robert L. Hampton
Bruce A. Ryan
Gerald R. Adams

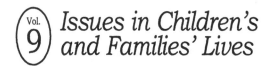

Vol.
9

*Issues in Children's
and Families' Lives*

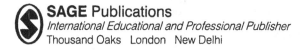

SAGE Publications
International Educational and Professional Publisher
Thousand Oaks London New Delhi

For information:

SAGE Publications, Inc.
2455 Teller Road
Thousand Oaks, California 91320
E-mail: order@sagepub.com

SAGE Publications Ltd.
6 Bonhill Street
London EC2A 4PU
United Kingdom

SAGE Publications India Pvt. Ltd.
M-32 Market
Greater Kailash I
New Delhi 110 048 India

Library of Congress Cataloging-in-Publication Data
Main entry under title:
Healthy children 2010: **ESTABLISHING PREVENTIVE SERVICES**/edited by
    Roger P. Weissberg . . . [et al.].
        p.   cm.—(Issues in children's and families' lives; v. 9)
    Includes bibliographical references and index.
    ISBN 0-7619-1089-1 (cloth).—ISBN 0-7619-1090-5 (pbk.)
    1. Preventive health services for children—United States.
I. Weissberg, Roger P., 1951-   . II. Series.
RJ102.E826   1997   97-4687
362.1'9892'000973—dc21

This book is printed on acid-free paper.

97 98 99 00 01 02 03 10 9 8 7 6 5 4 3 2 1

Acquiring Editor: C. Deborah Laughton
Editorial Assistant: Eileen Carr
Production Editor: Astrid Virding
Production Assistant: Denise Santoyo
Book Designer/Typesetter: Marion Warren
Cover Designer: Lesa Valdez
Print Buyer: Anna Chin

To two terrific children, Elizabeth and Ted.
Elizabeth will be 23 and Ted will be 20 in 2010.
May you each have a happy, healthy
childhood and adolescence.

To Stephanie Wright,
my loving wife, and partner,
who does so much to keep our family happy and healthy.

To Irving B. Harris,
a remarkable individual who cares about children
in jeopardy and breaking the cycle of poverty through
effective, innovative preventive services.

Contents

Foreword

$E_{stablishing}$ *Preventive Services* and its companion volume *Enhancing Children's Wellness* accompany the 4th National Hartman Conference occurring in 1997. These volumes conclude a 12 month period of publishing activity in the **Issues in Children's and Families' Lives** book series that can only be described as frantic. Over the last 12 months, we have published four important volumes focused on turning the promise of health promotion and illness prevention into reality.

Roughly 12 months ago, I had the honor of editing Martin Bloom's (1996) seminal volume *Primary Prevention Practices*. In that work Bloom lucidly explains prevention's paradigm illustrating its principles with numerous practical examples drawn from across the life span. A few months later *Primary Prevention Works* was published (Albee & Gullotta, 1997). This volume reflected not only on the recent tumultuous history of prevention in the United States but, using the National Mental Health Association's Lela Rowland award recipients as examples, provided readers with numerous proven programs of cost effective interventions that promote health and reduce the risk of illness.

Joining these works are now two additional volumes, *Enhancing Children's Wellness* and *Establishing Preventive Services* both edited by Roger Weissberg and his colleagues (Weissberg, Gullotta, Hampton, Ryan, & Adams, 1997). The first, *Enhancing Children's Wellness,* examines the health status of young people against criteria established in the *Healthy People 2000*. In a number of critical areas like substance abuse, depression, and suicide, it details the continuing risks that face youth and offers concrete actions that must be taken to reduce those risks and strengthen young people's resiliency to those risks.

The second, *Establishing Preventive Services,* is an ideal companion volume not only to *Enhancing Children's Wellness* but to the two earlier books. Its distinguished contributing scholars succinctly identify barriers to improving the health status of children and note opportunities for either removing or reducing those negating forces. In studying their contributions, I was struck by the observation that there is a critical difference between an ideal locale for preventive interventions and the practices that actually take place in those settings. Judging effectiveness requires an understanding of the lessons taught. I learned that even in ideal settings with good practices that a change in community leadership can have devastating consequences on program effectiveness. It was a sobering reminder of the frailness with which all of us in the helping professions daily live with—regardless of practice focus or discipline. And I came to appreciate that even in ideal supportive settings with good practices, the manner, way, and force in which those interventions are administered have significant effects on outcome. Like our colleagues who have developed new effective medicines to cure stubborn diseases, preventionists experience disappointment and frustration when a proven intervention is misused and then wrongly accused of being ineffective.

I commend this volume to social science professionals, policy makers, and students to study its lessons of triumph and failure. I urge you to apply its knowledge to your own practice and to join us as together we push, pull, and drag this nation's policies and behavior toward better health.

—Thomas P. Gullotta
Senior Series Editor

References

Albee, G. W., & Gullotta, T. P. (1997). *Primary prevention works.* Thousand Oaks, CA: Sage.

Bloom, M. (1996). *Primary prevention practices.* Thousand Oaks, CA: Sage.

U.S. Department of Health and Human Services (1991). *Healthy people 2000: National health promotion and disease prevention objectives.* Washington, DC: U.S. Government Printing Office.

Acknowledgments

W̱e begin by acknowledging the outstanding authors who contributed high-quality chapters to this volume. At the outset, my coeditors and I invited top scholars and leaders in the fields of health promotion and preventive mental health. These authors are distinguished both for the scientific rigor of their work and the creative ways in which they conceptualize, design, implement, evaluate, and disseminate innovative programs for children and youth.

Several organizations and individuals have generously provided financial and intellectual support for our efforts to disseminate information about ways to establish effective preventive services for children. We acknowledge the NIMH Prevention Research Branch and Office on AIDS for funding the University of Illinois at Chicago (UIC) Prevention Research Training Program in Urban Children's Mental Health and AIDS Prevention (1-T32-MH19933), and we are especially grateful to Eve Moscicki, Peter Muehrer, Leonard Mitnick, and Doreen Spilton-Koretz for their support. We also thank the Irving B. Harris Grandchildren Charity Trust, the Ounce of Prevention Fund (especially Harriet Meyer and Portia Kennel), the University of Illinois at Chicago Great Cities Program, and the Office of Educational Research and Improvement of the U.S. Department of Education through a grant to the Mid-Atlantic Laboratory for Student Success at the Temple University Center for Research in Human Development and Education. These sources of support allow my colleagues, students, and myself to develop and evaluate innovative school and community health enhancement and preventive services.

I also appreciate the support of the Surdna Foundation, the Fetzer Institute, the University of Illinois at Chicago, Daniel Goleman,

Eileen Growald, Robert Sherman, Timothy Shriver, David Sluyter, Serita Winthrop, and colleagues from the Collaborative for the Advancement of Social and Emotional Learning (CASEL). Recently, I became Executive Director of CASEL and I am delighted about the constructive, leading role that CASEL is playing to support the dissemination of effective school-based preventive services.

I appreciate my friendship and many collaborations with Tom Gullotta, Senior Editor of the series Issues in Children's and Families' Lives and a coeditor on this volume. He is a delight to work with because he is energetic, optimistic, savvy, and has a fine sense of humor; he cares about children and families and works hard to improve the quality of services they receive. I also express my appreciation to Carol Bartels Kuster, my colleague, coauthor, and collaborator, who has effectively supported efforts to bring this project to closure.

One goal of this volume is to foster high-quality implementation and widespread dissemination of effective preventive services for children by raising awareness about innovative family-, school-, and community-based strategies. It becomes more possible to enhance positive youth development when concerned individuals work together to share their collective wisdom, energy, and commitment. We thank C. Deborah Laughton, Eileen Carr, Kate Peterson, and the fine people at Sage for their support in publishing this volume and affording us the opportunity to share information about state-of-the-art preventive services.

—Roger P. Weissberg
University of Illinois at Chicago

CHAPTER 1

Introduction and Overview: Prevention Services—From Optimistic Promise to Widespread, Effective Practice

ROGER P. WEISSBERG

CAROL BARTELS KUSTER

THOMAS P. GULLOTTA

There is tremendous optimism and enthusiasm for the promise of prevention. Although there have been tangible accomplishments—especially during the past two decades—in prevention research and practice, there is also the realistic recognition that much remains to be achieved (Institute of Medicine, 1994; Weissberg & Greenberg, 1997). The chapters in this book elaborate on three central themes regarding future efforts to establish effective, enduring prevention services for our nation's children and youth. First, scientists, practitioners, and policymakers must collaborate to diversify the portfolio of coordinated family-, school-, and community-based prevention services and strategies (see Chapters 2 to 6). Second, rigorous evaluations of prevention programs are critical both to document their efficacy and to identify ways to improve their quality (see Chapter 7). Third, because the positive effect of well-conceptualized and well-designed prevention programs is diminished when they are ineffectively conducted, it is important to attend to implementation quality—especially as programs are disseminated on a widespread basis (see Chapters 8 and 9).

1

Concurrently with this volume, Sage has published Volume 8, *Healthy Children 2010: Enhancing Children's Wellness* (Weissberg, Gullotta, Hampton, Ryan, & Adams, 1997). *Enhancing Children's Wellness* presents recommendations to improve children's health status by the year 2010 in the following categorical areas: drug abuse (Dusenbury & Falco, 1997); high-risk sexual behavior, sexually transmitted diseases, and pregnancy (Sagrestano & Paikoff, 1997); violence (Murray, Guerra, & Williams, 1997); depression (Compas, Connor, & Wadsworth, 1997); suicide (Kalafat, 1997); nutrition (Perry, Lytle, & Story, 1997); unintentional injuries (Tuchfarber, Zins, & Jason, 1997); and academic performance (Hawkins, 1997).

The authors in *Enhancing Children's Wellness* provided integrative analyses of the latest research-based prevention and health promotion practices in their categorical topic area. Beyond that, they reinforced several themes highlighted in the book's first two chapters that reviewed common findings across multiple domains of problem behavior (Dryfoos, 1997; Weissberg & Kuster, 1997). First, these social, emotional, and behavioral problems often co-occur in the same individuals. Second, common family-, school-, and community-based risk and protective factors influence the development of varied social and health problems. Third, as Dryfoos (1997) concluded, we need to move beyond short-term categorical prevention efforts to comprehensive, multiyear approaches that address the social and psychological environment that gives rise to these problems. In this way we can affect tangibly the large numbers of young people experiencing social and health problems.

The current volume, *Healthy Children 2010: Establishing Preventive Services,* provides strategies to establish and successfully implement coordinated, effective prevention services in key socializing settings that powerfully affect the growth and development of children. Emphasizing developmentally and contextually appropriate prevention service delivery models, the authors identify state-of-the-art, empirically based strategies to strengthen the environments in which children develop.

Chapters 2 to 6 review ways to strengthen the family, child care systems, early childhood education, school-based mental health service delivery and primary prevention approaches, community-based mental health programming, and school-based health services. Programs with strong conceptualization, design, and implementation have potential to enhance children's social, emotional, and physical wellness, thereby reducing the incidence of problems across multiple domains (Weissberg & Greenberg, 1997). Chapter 7 reminds us of the importance of theory-guided evaluation to clarify the process of program implementation, the extent of program outcomes, and the factors that enhance or diminish program effects. Chapters 8 and 9 emphasize that quality of program implementation is a critical mediator of potential program impact, and these chapters highlight strategies to disseminate programs broadly while maintaining their efficacy.

Why *Healthy People 2010* Objectives Must Become a National Priority

As the year 2010 approaches, there is growing national concern about the large number of young people who engage in risk behaviors for negative social, emotional, and physical health outcomes such as drug abuse, teen pregnancy, AIDS, delinquency, depression, school dropout, and suicide (U.S. Department of Health and Human Services, Public Health Service [DHHS], 1991). Dryfoos (1990) estimated that 25% of American youth engage in multiple social and health risk behaviors, and an additional 25% experiment with some risk behaviors. The remaining 50%, who currently do not engage in such behavior, may nonetheless need effective education and consistent support to avoid such involvement. More recently, Dryfoos (1997) estimated that 30% of 14- to 17-year-olds engage in multiple problem behaviors that place them at high risk of extremely negative consequences, and about 35% are experimenting with various risky activities that jeopardize their futures.

Today's young people face greater risks to their current and future health and social development than ever before (Carnegie Council on Adolescent Development, 1995). American children and youth are smoking, drinking, having sex, committing violence, and becoming involved with gangs at younger and younger ages (National Commission on the Role of the School and the Community in Improving Adolescent Health, 1990). The social and health problems of America's children and youth are caused, to a large extent, by significant changes that have occurred in families, schools, neighborhoods, and the media during the past few decades. Major social-environmental changes include dramatic alterations in family composition and stability, the breakdown of traditional neighborhoods and extended families, reduced amounts of meaningful and supportive personal contact between young people and positive adult role models, the proliferation of media messages that positively portray health-damaging behavior, and changing demographics resulting in increasing numbers of economically and educationally disadvantaged young people entering school (DHHS, 1996; National Commission on Children, 1991; Zill & Nord, 1994).

Changes in societal conditions and the changing behavior of our young people have prompted widespread calls for innovative family-, school-, and community-based prevention and health promotion approaches to address students' health and social needs (Carnegie Council on Adolescent Development, 1995; National Commission on the Role of the School and the Community in Improving Adolescent Health, 1990; Report of the National Mental Health Association Commission on the Prevention of Mental-Emotional Disabilities, 1986). In assessing the current functioning of children and their families, Dryfoos (1994) concluded that (a) a substantial percentage of young people will fail to grow into healthy, productive adults unless there are major changes in the way they are nurtured and educated; (b) although families and schools traditionally carried out the responsibilities for raising and educating children, they require transformation to fulfill these obligations more effectively; and (c) we need new types of community resources and services to support the development of children into responsible, healthy, fully contributing members of society.

The Role of *Healthy People 2010* in Establishing Effective Prevention Services for Young People

In 1979, the surgeon general published *Healthy People* (U.S. Department of Health, Education, and Welfare, Public Health Service, 1979), which summarized the nation's health accomplishments since 1900. *Healthy People* contended that further improvements in the health of Americans would require the widespread implementation of effective health promotion and disease prevention strategies. In spite of considerable enthusiasm for the concept of prevention at the federal level during the 1970s, most professionals readily acknowledged the gap between prevention's potential and concrete record of performance. For example, in the foreword to *Primary Prevention: An Idea Whose Time Has Come,* Bertram Brown, then director of the National Institute of Mental Health, commented, "The lack of a sophisticated and comprehensive primary prevention program in mental health stands today as a major barrier between our present knowledge and resources and the goals this country has established for its mental health system" (1977, p. iii). Similarly, Emory Cowen (1977, p. 1) in "Baby-Steps Toward Primary Prevention" wrote:

> Kelly (1975) opened the First Vermont Conference on Primary Prevention with these words: "In my opinion, the topic of primary prevention is a most exciting and overdue challenge for psychology!" (p. 1). From the spinal cord—mine and others—the reaction to that statement is "Right on!" But, once past the initial surge of effusion and mutual backslapping often associated with the consensual validation of mushy abstract terms, several vexing facts surface: (a) agreeing with those words is a lot easier than doing decent primary prevention, [and] (b) however much the concept is pedestalized, it has, so far, done remarkably little to advance mental health.

The publication of *Healthy People* in 1979 and the *Report of the Task Panel on Prevention* (1978) marked a period of increased activity in prevention research and practice. A decade later, when the Office of Disease Prevention and Health Promotion (ODPHP) coordinated a broad-based national effort to develop a second report, *Healthy People 2000: National Health Promotion and Disease Prevention Objectives* (DHHS, 1991), there was a growing research and practice literature on which to base recommendations for prevention and health promotion services. *Healthy People 2000* defined three overarching goals: to increase health across the life span, to reduce health disparities among Americans, and to achieve access to preventive services for all Americans.

Healthy People 2000 identified more than 300 health objectives, organized into 22 priority areas, to be accomplished by the year 2000. These objectives have guided health promotion and disease prevention policies and programs at the federal, state, and local levels during the 1990s. The objectives were divided into three types (DHHS, 1991, p. 90):

1. Health status objectives to reduce death, disease, and disability
2. Risk reduction objectives to reduce the prevalence of risks to health or to increase behaviors known to reduce risk
3. Services and protection objectives to increase comprehensiveness, accessibility, and/or quality of preventive services and preventive interventions

It is the last set, the services and protection objectives, that is the focal point for this volume.

As comprehensive as *Healthy People 2000* is, the services and protection objectives do not go far enough toward addressing the needs of young people (American Medical Association, Department of Adolescent Health, 1990). One goal of this volume is to fill this gap through elaboration of salient threats to children's well-being and identification of promising preventive services. Our hope is that the ideas contained herein will contribute to the national discussion for *Healthy People 2010*. In this book and in its companion volume, *Healthy Children 2010: Enhancing Children's Wellness* (Weissberg et al., 1997), we strongly recommend that *Healthy People 2010* increase the number, specificity, and accuracy of child-focused service, prevention, and protection objectives related to children's mental health as well as their physical health and social functioning.

Establishing effective preventive services is a crucial aspect of changing the life course for those children at risk of failure. Investigators have developed several classification models for prevention (Cowen, 1983; Institute of Medicine, 1994). The most common terminology historically used for public health and preventive mental health includes the terms *primary prevention* and *secondary prevention* (Cowen, 1983). Primary prevention is dually focused on forestalling the development of psychological problems and enhancing people's psychosocial competence and health (Cowen, 1983). Primary prevention programs reduce the incidence of problems through group- or population-oriented interventions, rather than targeting individuals who exhibit behavioral and emotional symptoms. They focus on well-functioning groups of people or those who, because of environmental circumstances or life events, are epidemiologically at risk for adverse psychological outcomes. Such programs are provided within the context of mainstream institutions, settings, and social policies rather than through specialized services for those manifesting psychological, social, or physical problems. In addition, primary prevention programs should be theoretically and empirically based, using information about risk and protective processes to increase the intervention's promise of promoting positive behavioral outcomes. Secondary prevention programs seek to reduce the prevalence or to lower the rates of established cases of disorder or illness in the population. They reduce the duration of a disorder through early case finding combined with prompt and effective intervention. One pathway to secondary prevention involves identifying behavioral or emotional symptoms of dysfunction early in someone's development and providing treatment to reduce the potential for later, more severe psychopathology. For our purposes, *establishing preventive services* involves both primary and secondary preventive services for mental, social, and physical health problems.

The Appendix lists all 46 *Healthy People 2000* services and protection objectives for children. These objectives focus primarily on five main topic areas:

1. Quality school health education
2. School readiness
3. Maternal and infant health
4. Primary care providers
5. State and federal policies

Although these objectives are positive steps, other crucial areas of need are sorely neglected. Some of the most notable gaps include (a) a lack of mental health service objectives (only Objective 6.14 begins to address this need); (b) a lack of attention to school-based prevention other than health education (e.g., school-based health clinics and primary preventive services such as screenings are not mentioned); (c) a lack of services to families (only Objectives 14.11-14.16 regarding maternal and infant health and Objective

7.15 regarding housing for battered women and their children address aspects of family life); and (d) a lack of comprehensive program strategies to enhance preschool children's readiness to succeed in school. We will elaborate on two issues to illustrate the type of critical thinking we hope will prevail as children's prevention service objectives for *Healthy People 2010* are established.

For example, Objective 6.3 in the Mental Health and Mental Disorders section recommends: "Reduce to less than 10 percent the prevalence of mental disorders among children and adolescents" (p. 211). The target for this objective was based, in part, on an inaccurate baseline estimate that 12% of young people under age 18 have mental disorders. The *Healthy People 2000: Midcourse Review and 1995 Revisions* (DHHS, 1995) changed Objective 6.3 as follows: "Reduce to less than 17 percent the prevalence of mental disorders among children and adolescents" (p. 191), based on an estimated baseline that actually 20% of young people have diagnosable mental disorders. Given the large numbers of young people experiencing mental health problems, it is striking that *Healthy People 2000* provides only one child-focused, secondary prevention services and protection objective (6.14), which states:

> Increase to at least 75 percent the proportion of providers of primary care for children who include assessment of cognitive, emotional, and parent-child functioning with appropriate counseling, referral, and follow up, in their clinical practice. (p. 219)

There are many other secondary and primary prevention services that could be recommended involving innovative family-, school-, and community-based preventive and competence enhancement programs. Chapters 2 to 6 of this volume present many promising directions.

Objective 8.4 provides another illustration that there is considerable room for improvement in describing issues related to implementation and evaluation of primary prevention programs. Specifically, Objective 8.4 recommends that the nation: "Increase to at least 75 percent the proportion of the Nation's elementary and secondary schools that provide planned and sequential kindergarten through 12th grade quality school health education" (p. 255). Beyond this core objective, there are many supplementary objectives encouraging—in the context of quality school health education—a focus on nutrition; alcohol, tobacco, and other drugs; conflict resolution; injury prevention and control; HIV; and sexually transmitted diseases (McGinnis & DeGraw, 1991). Although we applaud this set of objectives, we note that according to the definition of quality school health education used in the *Healthy People 2000 Review, 1995-96* (National Center for Health Statistics, 1996), only 2.3% of schools actually provided all recommended components of quality school health education. Furthermore, concern has been expressed about emphasizing the inclusion of certain components in health education, such as conflict resolution, because current research has not documented the efficacy of this violence prevention approach (Murray et al., 1997).

Obviously, the well-being of young people requires and deserves greater attention from policymakers, service providers, and prevention researchers (Fleming, 1996). The intent of this volume is to spark discussion and debate among these groups about the most promising solutions and most effective methods for meeting these needs. This volume emphasizes the important contributions of various systems such as families, early childhood education, health clinics, and schools to the well-being of children. We suggest that the social, emotional, and physical needs of children and adolescents are best met through multiple and, ideally, coordinated systems. Furthermore, ensuring that we are using our best and most effective initiatives requires empirical program evaluation, strong implementation practices, and skilled dissemination efforts. We have encouraged the authors to elaborate on these concepts and to provide concrete objectives based on empirical research and field experience.

Summary of Chapters

Chapter 2:
Policy Efforts to Enhance Child and Family Life: Goals for 2010 (Edward F. Zigler and Matia Finn-Stevenson)

Edward Zigler and Matia Finn-Stevenson present cogent arguments for integrating developmental research and social policy to improve the family life of children. After reviewing data about the changing conditions of family life and the powerful deleterious effects that stressful family circumstances have on children's mental health, they offer creative, family-centered recommendations for developing effective and family-friendly policy. The authors emphasize the importance of ensuring that our knowledge about effective programs is used and that workable, empirically based solutions to our pressing social problems are implemented through translation into public policy. They also draw attention to the need for family support services, an area sorely neglected in *Healthy People 2000*. Zigler and Finn-Stevenson use the issues of lack of quality child care and the effects of divorce as illustrations to describe obstacles in translating research into policy and offer suggestions for researchers, service providers, and policymakers to improve their collaborative efforts to make good social policy and program decisions.

Zigler and Finn-Stevenson describe their innovative School of the 21st Century, which calls for developing a more effective child care system within the already established educational system. The components in this model include parent education and support, including home visitations, from birth to age 3; all-day, year-round child care for 3- to 5-year-olds; before- and after-school and vacation care for children up to age 12; and health and nutrition education for parents and family day care providers. They contend that the School of the 21st Century can cost-effectively enhance coordination and resource sharing among existing school and community programs such as Head Start, other preschool and after-school services, and programs for children with special needs. The authors conclude with two major preventive service objectives for *Healthy People 2010*. The first is that all children would have access to good-quality child care; the second is that provisions be made to increase the availability of support services to families. In addition to being important in their own right, increasing preventive services in these areas would help the nation meet other health objectives such as reducing drug use (Dusenbury & Falco, 1997) or mental disorders (Compas et al., 1997; Kalafat, 1997) among children and youth. Currently, more than 400 schools in 13 states have implemented the School of the 21st Century. Greatly expanding that number by the year 2010 would foster improved health among young people well into the 21st century.

Chapter 3:
Defining and Implementing School Readiness:
Challenges for Families, Early Care and Education, and
Schools (Sharon L. Kagan and Michelle J. Neuman)

With the exception of maternal/infant health objectives, *Healthy People 2000* has only one service recommendation for children under age 5—Objective 8.3 states:

> Achieve for all disadvantaged children and children with disabilities access to high quality and developmentally appropriate preschool programs that help prepare children for school, thereby improving their prospects with regard to school performance, problem behaviors, and mental and physical health. (p. 254)

In their scholarly and visionary chapter, Sharon Kagan and Michelle Neuman challenge framers of *Healthy People 2010* to go beyond the limited recommendations for preschool children and families presented in *Healthy People 2000*. They stress the importance of understanding school readiness not simply as a child's readiness to learn or to benefit from formal schooling but also as family, school, and community readiness to meet the needs of each child. The authors offer a broad definition of *readiness* at the child level including five dimensions: physical health and motor development, social and emotional development, approaches toward learning, language usage, and general knowledge. Similar to Zigler and Finn-Stevenson, they emphasize the primary importance of families in shaping children's early development and learning.

Kagan and Neuman discuss parents' role in collaborating effectively with schools and communities to enhance their children's positive growth. They emphasize the need to establish early child care and family support systems that assist the development of families as a whole, as a normalized part of our social fabric, much as free public education has become a normalized social institution. From this perspective, readiness is not the burden of individual children (e.g., to know their numbers or ABCs) but is the shared responsibility of parents, schools, and communities. Kagan and Neuman contend that *Healthy People 2010* has the opportunity to focus more attention on the needs of young children by establishing more, specific objectives that support readiness. They frame their prevention-service goals around three core messages: (a) conceptualize readiness as children's readiness, family readiness, school readiness, and community readiness; (b) generate adequate assessment systems for children, schools, and communities; and (c) consider children and families holistically. By building from the blueprints offered in Chapters 2 and 3, the authors of *Healthy People 2010* will be more likely to establish comprehensive, coordinated systems to affect tangibly children's growth and development during their important early years.

Chapter 4:
Schools and the Enhancement of Children's Wellness:
Some Opportunities and Some Limiting Factors
(Emory L. Cowen)

Currently, there are too many children who experience social, emotional, and physical health problems, and there are not sufficient resources and personnel available to address these needs. Given the gap between the large number of children who require help and the limited services available, Emory Cowen asks, "What useful roles can schools play as part of a concerted social effort targeted to the enhancement of children's wellness?" (p. 98). He describes a variety of prevention methods including early detection and treatment programs for children showing beginning signs of maladjustment, establishing health promotion curricula, engineering health-enhancing school and class environments, and developing coordinated outreach systems to families and community settings. His vision requires a shift in focus from schools as "problem containers" to schools as "skill enhancers."

Cowen describes four decades of the Primary Mental Health Project (PMHP), an innovative, internationally renowned, secondary prevention, service-delivery model for the early detection and prevention of school maladjustment (Cowen, Hightower, Pedro-Carroll, Work, Wyman, & Haffey, 1996). PMHP has four structural components: (a) a focus on primary-grade children; (b) systematic screening for the early identification of children experiencing school maladjustment; (c) employing carefully selected, trained and supervised nonprofessional counselor assistants to provide direct individual or small-group services to high-risk children; and (d) changing professional roles of school mental health professionals to reduce their direct service delivery in favor of increased participation in early screening, the training and supervision of counselor assistants, and consultation with teachers and other school personnel about cost-effective intervention strategies. PMHP is currently in more than 700 school districts nationally and exponentially increases the effective, helping services that schools can provide. As the authors of *Healthy People 2010* consider options for expanding the number of mental health services and protection objectives, increasing the number of schools that provide high-quality early detection and secondary prevention services for children should be given high priority.

The important secondary prevention service contributions of PMHP notwithstanding, Cowen also champions the critical importance of school-based primary prevention programming in addressing the question, "What could schools do to optimize the wellness and school adaptation of *all* children from the start, beyond targeting programs to the identifiable fraction at risk?" (p. 103). He identifies three core roles for school mental health professionals: (a) diagnosis and treatment for children with serious problems; (b) early detection and secondary prevention for at-risk children; and (c) primary prevention with emphases on competence promotion, the modification of class and school environments, and school-family-community partnerships to enhance wellness. He calls for major changes in the preparation and training of educators and mental health personnel laying the foundation for increased allocation of efforts to primary prevention and wellness enhancement service delivery.

Chapter 5:
Mental Health Services for Children and Adolescents (Mary Jane Rotheram-Borus)

As mentioned previously, only one *Healthy People 2000* objective (6.14) targets children's mental health needs. Although Objective 6.14 expresses a worthy goal, it does not begin to address the full spectrum of children's mental health needs, nor does it acknowledge the importance of other nonclinical or nonmedical service providers in identifying and treating children's mental health problems. The true scope of problems experienced by children and the type and number of services involved are far larger and more complex than this service objective recognizes. Mary Jane Rotheram-Borus notes that "children with mental health problems are more likely to present in special education, foster care, primary health care, the juvenile justice system, and substance abuse treatment than in the mental health system" (p. 127). Furthermore, the needs, service pathways, and outcomes experienced by children depend in large part on structural characteristics of their communities (e.g., policy, financing, organization) as well as personal characteristics of the children and their families (e.g., age, gender, ethnicity, income). She outlines a theoretical model of factors that influence children's needs, access to and use of services, and treatment outcomes. This comprehensive model can help to frame future service objectives for meeting children's mental health needs.

In her review of the current state of service delivery to children, Rotheram-Borus elucidates the deleterious effects of the lack of coordination across programs and underscores the need for a more integrated approach. Troubled youth frequently have not just one problem, but many. Yet a lack of service coordination often means that although these youngsters may receive services of some sort, these services likely treat only parts of their problems. For example, juvenile justice may treat a youngster's violent behaviors, special education treats the learning disability, and a substance abuse treatment program handles the drug addiction. Furthermore, current social policies promote "sector shifting"; that is, the burden of care may be shifted from one agency to another based on cost, not on treatment needs. Thus, the type of care received may be based more on which agency can pick up the tab and less on what services are really needed. Such a disjointed and haphazard approach is neither economical nor optimally effective.

Rotheram-Borus recommends three central strategies in setting appropriate goals for 2010: (a) establish goals for communities, rather than the nation; (b) create a national surveillance system to monitor annually the implementation of the goals; and (c) link funding to the delivery of community-level outcomes to provide incentive and resources for communities to improve their delivery system. These strategies, combined with greater attention to issues of access and dissemination of effective programs will enhance the likelihood of meeting children's mental health needs.

Chapter 6:
Improving Access to Health Care:
School-Based Health Centers (Shauna L. Dowden, Richard D. Calvert, Lisa Davis, and Thomas P. Gullotta)

The most frequently cited services and protection objective for children in *Healthy People 2000* invokes quality school health education (Objective 8.4). Many other objectives recommend particular components of school curricula that are ideally part of such a comprehensive educational program (see the Appendix). Although health education is an important part of attempts to reduce levels of risk among youth (Weissberg & Elias, 1993), it is not sufficient to meet the pressing health needs of many children. As several authors in this volume make clear, structural issues such as a lack of access to quality medical, mental, and social service programs as well as individual issues such as income and ethnicity interfere with healthy development, regardless of the amount of health education a child receives. Given the rising levels of drug and alcohol use, risky sexual behavior, and violence among youth, it is clear that many of the physical and emotional needs of children are not being met under the current patchwork of programs (described previously by Rotheram-Borus) designed to address isolated risk factors or problems. Finding workable solutions to these problems requires innovative use of current resources (e.g., schools) and development of new methods of service delivery.

In this chapter, Dowden and colleagues offer just such an imaginative and innovative comprehensive service delivery model. Their school-based alternative provides many potential benefits such as accessibility and economy without sacrificing quality and provision of service. In fact, their approach enhances service provision, particularly preventive care, to children and families. In many cases, the school-based health center may be a child or parent's only link to health care providers. Furthermore, housing medical, dental, and mental health services within a child's school greatly increases the likelihood of service integration and organization. Although, to date, there have been few evaluation studies on the effectiveness of such an approach, these authors provide a clear rationale and concrete recommendations based on their own experiences in Connecticut.

Chapter 7:
Evaluation of Prevention Programs for Children
(Ernest Valente, Jr. and Kenneth A. Dodge)

The Institute of Medicine (1994) contends:

> There could be no wiser investment in our country than a commitment to foster the prevention of mental disorders and the promotion of mental health through rigorous research with the highest of methodological standards. Such a commitment would yield the potential for healthier lives for countless individuals and the general advancement of the nation's well-being. (p. 550)

Ernest Valente and Ken Dodge build and elaborate on this theme in their chapter by reviewing cutting-edge efforts in program evaluation and providing a set of comprehensive guidelines for evaluators. Good evaluation is important not only as a "score card" of progress but also for the generation of new theoretical understanding, better implementation practices, and improved dissemination of effective programs.

The Institute of Medicine (1994) identifies a five-stage sequence for prevention research: (a) identify a problem, review epidemiological data to determine its extent, and collaborate with communities to determine their level of concern about it; (b) identify risk and protect factors for the problem to understand its development; (c) design and conduct pilot efficacy trials and confirmatory replication trials to prevent the problem; (d) design, implement, and analyze large-scale preventive interventions; and (e) facilitate the dissemination, adoption, and ongoing evaluation of programs into community service settings. Valente and Dodge focus primarily on the formal evaluation of large-scale preventive interventions promoting positive mental health in young people—that is, the fourth stage in this sequence—but their detailed commentary has implications for all five stages. The program evaluation practices they endorse will (a) advance our theoretical understanding of how problem behaviors develop in young people, (b) measure and clarify the extent and quality of program implementation, (c) identify the most effective interventions to ensure that public health prevention efforts have maximum effect, (d) provide a base for more effective program dissemination, and (e) accurately document both the successes and limitations of preventive interventions with the goal of improving their quality over time. It is the widespread dissemination of effective prevention programs and strategies that will meaningfully enhance wellness and reduce problem behaviors among young people in future years.

Chapter 8:
Making Prevention Work (Denise C. Gottfredson, Carolyn M. Fink, Stacy Skroban, and Gary D. Gottfredson)

A fundamental premise of this volume is that preventive efforts are necessary to reduce risk factors and promote protective factors. However, not every prevention effort is created (or implemented) equal. The past few decades have seen a proliferation of prevention programs addressing a vast array of risk factors; some successfully, others not. In their chapter, Denise Gottfredson and colleagues explore some reasons why many school-based programs fail to achieve their goals. Interweaving relevant research findings in the prevention literature with observations based on their own experiences with a failed school-based prevention program, the authors summarize characteristics of programs and schools where innovative efforts are unlikely to succeed. For example, lack of technical training and ongoing support for implementation, the perception that the program is imposed by "outsiders" to the community or school, lack of leadership by key personnel within the school or school district, and general organizational incapacity greatly impair effective implementation of even the best programs. They emphasize that meeting the *Healthy People 2000* goal of providing quality school health education will require not only the development of good programs but also equally good program implementation skills. Their analysis of their own efforts to implement a comprehensive school-based health education program is a first step toward identifying common barriers to implementation and to reminding us that even the "best laid plans" require continuing attention and refinement.

Chapter 9:
Reinterpreting Dissemination of Prevention Programs as Widespread Implementation With Effectiveness and Fidelity (Maurice J. Elias)

Although the importance of program dissemination is frequently acknowledged among program developers and evaluators, it is rarely a priority. Similarly, *Healthy People 2000* does not set goals or make recommendations for program dissemination—this aspect of service provision is routinely ignored. Demonstration programs and pilot projects, even good ones, often "wither on the vine" due to a lack of incentive or ability to disseminate. Maurice Elias provides a thoughtful analysis of dissemination issues that reveals their true importance for building prevention efforts that work.

Elias's focus is on ensuring that what we know works gets implemented in more than just the demonstration setting—that is, widespread implementation. He encourages us to consider the sources of energy and direction in getting good programs running—local people and initiative. His advice echoes that of Gottfredson and colleagues, that outsiders rarely create positive lasting change for communities. Although we can and should export programs that work, we must simultaneously respect the need for local citizens to create something that will work in their setting. Without the drive and enthusiasm of this next level of implementers, new programs are unlikely to flourish. In this sense, adhering strictly to what worked elsewhere may be less important than assisting communities to revise programs to meet their own unique needs. Elias makes the important point that a sense of ownership and contribution to the intervention is important not only for adults but also for the targeted children. Programs that involve their target audience in the intervention design are more likely to set appropriate and meaningful goals and thus are more likely to flourish than those that adhere to rigid criteria—that is, fidelity. Services and protection objectives for 2010 would do well to include incentives and goals for widespread implementation of effective and meaningful interventions.

Conclusions

A bare-bones list of recommendations culled from these chapters can hardly do justice to the depth and richness of ideas presented here. However, given the importance of these topics in addressing the health needs of children, we feel it appropriate to reiterate some of the most promising directions to pursue:

1. Improve accessibility of quality early childhood care and education through the development of an adequately funded infrastructure of services.

2. Use schools as the foundation for the provision of comprehensive services to children and parents, beginning in infancy and continuing until adulthood.

3. Encourage the development of school-family and school-community partnerships that target the welfare of all children.

4. Prepare educators to also be action researchers in their own schools, systematically assessing what works and what does not in their locations.

5. Encourage communities to set goals for themselves rather than attempt to set and reach national goals. Funding can be linked to attainment of community-level goals and administered through a national monitoring system.

6. An increase in the strength and quality of prevention programs, not simply the quantity, is crucial, particularly for those children most in need. Research on implementation and evaluation practices are necessary to ensure the delivery of quality programs.

Overall, the central message of this volume is the importance of striving to achieve a better balance of support systems that can improve children's health. This necessitates a much broader conceptualization of prevention and preventive services than that found in *Healthy People 2000*. It expands the circle of influence beyond just schools and primary care physicians to include roles for families, preschools, health clinics, youth clubs, businesses, communities, and policymakers—all of whom are essential players in improving services to children.

APPENDIX

Healthy People 2000 Services
and Protection Objectives for Children

I. Quality School Health Education and Related Services

1.8 Increase to at least 50 percent the proportion of children and adolescents in 1st through 12th grade who participate in daily school physical education.

1.9 Increase to at least 50 percent the proportion of school physical education class time that students spend being physically active, preferably engaged in lifetime physical activities.

2.17 Increase to at least 90 percent the proportion of school lunch and breakfast services and child care food services with menus that are consistent with the nutrition principles in the Dietary Guidelines for America.

2.19 Increase to at least 75 percent the proportion of the Nation's schools that provide nutrition education from preschool through 12th grade, preferably as part of quality school health education.

3.10 Establish tobacco-free environments and include tobacco use prevention in the curricula of all elementary, middle, and secondary schools, preferably as part of quality school health education.

4.13 Provide to children in all school districts and private schools primary and secondary school educational programs on alcohol and other drugs, preferably as part of quality school health education.

5.8 Increase to at least 85 percent the proportion of people aged 10 through 18 who have discussed human sexuality, including values surrounding sexuality, with their parents and/or have received information through another parentally endorsed source, such as youth, school, or religious programs.

7.16 Increase to at least 50 percent the proportion of elementary and secondary schools that teach nonviolent conflict resolution skills, preferably as a part of quality school health education.

8.4   Increase to at least 75 percent the proportion of the Nation's elementary and secondary schools that provide planned and sequential kindergarten through 12th grade quality school health education.

8.9   Increase to at least 75 percent the proportion of people aged 10 and older who have discussed issues related to nutrition, physical activity, sexual behavior, tobacco, alcohol, other drugs, or safety with family members on at least one occasion during the preceding month.

9.18 Provide academic instruction on injury prevention and control, preferably as part of quality school health education, in at least 50 percent of public school systems (Grades K through 12).

18.10 Increase to at least 95 percent the proportion of schools that have age-appropriate HIV education curricula for students in 4th through 12th grade, preferably as part of quality school health education.

19.12 Include instruction in sexually transmitted disease transmission prevention in the curricula of all middle and secondary schools, preferably as part of quality school health education.

II. School Readiness

8.3   Achieve for all disadvantaged children and children with disabilities access to high-quality and developmentally appropriate preschool programs that help prepare children for school, thereby improving their prospects with regard to school performance, problem behaviors, and mental and physical health.

III. Maternal and Infant Health

14.11 Increase to at least 90 percent the proportion of all pregnant women who receive prenatal care in the first trimester of pregnancy.

14.12 Increase to at least 60 percent the proportion of primary care providers who provide age-appropriate preconception care and counseling.

14.13 Increase to at least 60 percent the proportion of women enrolled in prenatal care who are offered screening and counseling on prenatal detection of fetal abnormalities.

14.14 Increase to at least 90 percent the proportion of pregnant women and infants who receive risk-appropriate care.

14.15 Increase to at least 95 percent the proportion of newborns screened by State-sponsored programs for genetic disorders and other disabling conditions and to 90 percent the proportion of newborns testing positive for disease who receive appropriate treatment.

14.16 Increase to at least 90 percent the proportion of babies aged 18 months and younger who receive recommended primary care services at the appropriate intervals.

17.15 Increase to at least 80 percent the proportion of providers of primary care for children who routinely refer or screen infants and children for impairments of vision, hearing, speech and language, and assess other developmental milestones as part of well-child care.

17.16 Reduce the average age at which children with significant hearing impairment are identified to no more than 12 months.

21.2 Increase to at least 50 percent the proportion of people who have received, as a minimum within the appropriate interval, all of the screening and immunization services and at least one of the counseling services appropriate for their age and gender as recommended by the U.S. Preventive Services Task Force.

IV. Primary Care Providers

5.9 Increase to at least 90 percent the proportion of pregnancy counselors who offer positive, accurate information about adoption to their unmarried patients with unintended pregnancies.

5.10 Increase to at least 60 percent the proportion of primary care providers who provide age-appropriate preconception care and counseling.

6.14 Increase to at least 75 percent the proportion of providers of primary care for children who include assessment of cognitive, emotional, and parent-child functioning, with appropriate counseling, referral, and follow up, in their clinical practices.

7.12 Extend protocols for routinely identifying, treating, and properly referring suicide attempters, victims of sexual assault, and victims of spouse, elder, and child abuse to at least 90 percent of hospital emergency departments.

7.15 Reduce to less than 10 percent the proportion of battered women and their children turned away from emergency housing due to lack of space.

9.21 Increase to at least 50 percent the proportion of primary care providers who routinely provide age-appropriate counseling on safety precautions to prevent unintentional injury.

13.12 Increase to at least 90 percent the proportion of all children entering school programs for the first time who have received an oral health screening, referral, and follow up for necessary diagnostic, preventive, and treatment services.

V. State and Federal Policies

3.13 Enact and enforce in 50 States laws prohibiting the sale and distribution of tobacco products to youth younger than age 19.

3.14 Increase to 50 the number of States with plans to reduce tobacco use, especially among youth.

3.15 Eliminate or severely restrict all forms of tobacco product advertising and promotion to which youth younger than age 18 are likely to be exposed.

4.16 Increase to 50 the number of States that have enacted and enforce policies, beyond those in existence in 1989, to reduce access to alcoholic beverages by minors.

4.17 Increase to at least 20 the number of States that have enacted statutes to restrict promotion of alcoholic beverages that is focused principally on young audiences.

4.18 Extend to 50 States legal blood alcohol concentration tolerance levels of .04 percent for motor vehicle drivers aged 21 and older and .00 percent for those younger than age 21.

7.13 Extend to at least 45 States implementation of unexplained child death review systems.

7.14 Increase to at least 30 the number of States in which at least 50 percent of children identified as neglected or physically or sexually abused receive physical and mental evaluation with appropriate follow up as a means of breaking the intergenerational cycle of abuse.

9.14 Extend to 50 States laws requiring safety belt and motorcycle helmet use for all ages.

9.15 Enact in 50 States laws requiring that new handguns be designed to minimize the likelihood of discharge by children.

9.19 Extend requirements for the use of effective head, face, eye, and mouth protection to all organizations, agencies, and institutions sponsoring sporting and recreation events that pose risk of injury.

13.15 Increase to at least 40 the number of States that have an effective system for recording and referring infants with cleft lips and/or palates to craniofacial anomaly teams.

17.20 Increase to 50 the number of States that have service systems for children with or at risk of chronic and disabling conditions, as required by Public Law 101-239.

20.13 Expand immunization laws for schools, preschools, and day care settings to all States for all antigens.

20.15 Improve financing and delivery of immunizations for children and adults so that virtually no American has a financial barrier to receiving recommended immunizations.

21.4 Improve financing and delivery of clinical preventive services so that virtually no American has a financial barrier to receiving, at a minimum, the screening, counseling, and immunization services recommended by the U.S. Preventive Services Task Force.

References

American Medical Association, Department of Adolescent Health. (1990). *Healthy youth 2000: National health promotion and disease prevention objectives for adolescents.* Chicago: Author.

Brown, B. S. (1977). Foreword. In D. C. Klein & S. E. Goldstone (Eds.), *Primary prevention: An idea whose time has come* (pp. iii-iv). (DHEW Publication No. PHS 77-447). Washington, DC: U.S. Government Printing Office.

Carnegie Council on Adolescent Development. (1995). *Great transitions: Preparing adolescents for a new century/Concluding report of the Carnegie Council on Adolescent Development.* New York: Carnegie Corporation of New York.

Compas, B., Connor, J., & Wadsworth, M. (1997). Prevention of depression. In R. P. Weissberg, T. P. Gullotta, R. L. Hampton, B. A. Ryan, & G. R. Adams (Eds.),

Healthy children 2010: Enhancing children's wellness (pp. 129-174). Thousand Oaks, CA: Sage.

Cowen, E. L. (1977). Baby-steps toward primary prevention. *American Journal of Community Psychology, 5,* 1-22.

Cowen, E. L. (1983). Primary prevention in mental health: Past, present, and future. In R. D. Felner, L. A. Jason, J. N. Moritsugu, & S. S. Farber (Eds.), *Preventive psychology: Theory, research, and practice* (pp. 11-25). New York: Pergamon.

Cowen, E. L., Hightower, A. D., Pedro-Carroll, J. L., Work, W. C., Wyman, P. A., & Haffey, W. G. (1996). *School-based prevention of children at risk: The Primary Mental Health Project.* Washington, DC: American Psychological Association.

Dryfoos, J. G. (1990). *Adolescents at risk: Prevalence and prevention.* New York: Oxford University Press.

Dryfoos, J. G. (1994). *Full-service schools: A revolution in health and social services for children, youth, and families.* San Francisco: Jossey-Bass.

Dryfoos, J. G. (1997). The prevalence of problem behaviors: Implications for programs. In R. P. Weissberg, T. P. Gullotta, R. L. Hampton, B. A. Ryan, & G. R. Adams (Eds.), *Healthy children 2010: Enhancing children's wellness* (pp. 17-46). Thousand Oaks, CA: Sage.

Dusenbury, L. A., & Falco, M. (1997). School-based drug abuse prevention strategies: From research to policy and practice. In R. P. Weissberg, T. P. Gullotta, R. L. Hampton, B. A. Ryan, & G. R. Adams (Eds.), *Healthy children 2010: Enhancing children's wellness* (pp. 47-75). Thousand Oaks, CA: Sage.

Fleming, M. (1996). *Healthy youth 2000: A mid-decade review.* Chicago: American Medical Association, Department of Adolescent Health.

Hawkins, J. D. (1997). Academic performance and school success: Sources and consequences. In R. P. Weissberg, T. P. Gullotta, R. L. Hampton, B. A. Ryan, & G. R. Adams (Eds.), *Healthy children 2010: Enhancing children's wellness* (pp. 278-305). Thousand Oaks, CA: Sage.

Institute of Medicine. (1994). *Reducing risks for mental disorders: Frontiers for preventive intervention research.* Washington, DC: National Academy Press.

Kalafat, J. (1997). Prevention of youth suicide. In R. P. Weissberg, T. P. Gullotta, R. L. Hampton, B. A. Ryan, & G. R. Adams (Eds.), *Healthy children 2010: Enhancing children's wellness* (pp. 175-213). Thousand Oaks, CA: Sage.

Kelly, J. G. (1975, June). *The search for ideas and deeds that work.* Keynote address at Vermont Conference on the Primary Prevention of Psychopathology, Burlington, VT.

McGinnis, J. M., & DeGraw, C. (1991). Healthy schools 2000: Creating partnerships for the decade. *Journal of School Health, 61,* 292-297.

Murray, M. E., Guerra, N., Williams, K. R. (1997). Violence prevention for the 21st century. In R. P. Weissberg, T. P. Gullotta, R. L. Hampton, B. A. Ryan, & G. R. Adams (Eds.), *Healthy children 2010: Enhancing children's wellness* (pp. 105-128). Thousand Oaks, CA: Sage.

National Center for Health Statistics. (1996). *Healthy people 2000 review, 1995-96.* Hyattsville, MD: Public Health Service.

National Commission on Children. (1991). *Beyond rhetoric: A new American agenda for children and families.* Washington, DC: U.S. Government Printing Office.

National Commission on the Role of the School and the Community in Improving Adolescent Health. (1990). *Code Blue: Uniting for healthier youth.* Alexandria, VA: National Association of State Boards of Education.

Perry, C. L., Lytle, L. A., & Story, M. (1997). Promoting healthy dietary behaviors. In R. P. Weissberg, T. P. Gullotta, R. L. Hampton, B. A. Ryan, & G. R. Adams (Eds.), *Healthy children 2010: Enhancing children's wellness* (pp. 214-249). Thousand Oaks, CA: Sage.

Report of the National Mental Health Association Commission on the Prevention of Mental-Emotional Disabilities. (1986). *The prevention of mental-emotional disabilities.* Alexandria, VA: National Mental Health Association.

Report of the Task Panel on Prevention. (1978). *Task panel reports submitted to the President's Commission on Mental Health* (Vol. 4, pp. 1822-1863). Washington, DC: U.S. Government Printing Office.

Sagrestano, L. M., & Paikoff, R. L. (1997). Preventing high-risk sexual behavior, sexually transmitted diseases, and pregnancy among adolescents. In R. P. Weissberg, T. P. Gullotta, R. L. Hampton, B. A. Ryan, & G. R. Adams (Eds.), *Healthy children 2010: Enhancing children's wellness* (pp. 76-104). Thousand Oaks, CA: Sage.

Tuchfarber, B., Zins, J. E., & Jason, L. A. (1997). Prevention and control of injuries. In R. P. Weissberg, T. P. Gullotta, R. L. Hampton, B. A. Ryan, & G. R. Adams (Eds.), *Healthy children 2010: Enhancing children's wellness* (pp. 250-277). Thousand Oaks, CA: Sage.

U.S. Department of Health, Education, and Welfare, Public Health Service. (1979). *Healthy people: The surgeon general's report on health promotion and disease prevention* (DHEW Publication No. PHS 79-55071). Washington, DC: U.S. Government Printing Office.

U.S. Department of Health and Human Services, Public Health Service. (1991). *Healthy people 2000: National health promotion and disease prevention objectives* (DHHS Publication No. PHS 91-50212). Washington, DC: U.S. Government Printing Office.

U.S. Department of Health and Human Services, Public Health Service (1995). *Healthy people 2000: Midcourse review and 1995 revisions.* Washington, DC: U.S. Government Printing Office.

U.S. Department of Health and Human Services, Public Health Service. (1996). *Trends in the well-being of America's children and youth: 1996.* Washington, DC: Author.

Weissberg, R. P., & Elias, M. J. (1993). Enhancing young people's social competence and health behavior: An important challenge for educators, scientists, policy makers, and funders. *Applied & Preventive Psychology: Current Scientific Perspectives, 3,* 179-190.

Weissberg, R. P., & Greenberg, M. T. (1997). School and community competence-enhancement and prevention programs. In W. Damon (Series Ed.) & I. E. Sigel & K. A. Renninger (Vol. Eds.). *Handbook of child psychology: Vol 4. Child psychology in practice* (5th ed.). New York: John Wiley.

Weissberg, R. P., & Kuster, C. B. (1997). Introduction and overview: Let's make "Healthy Children 2010" a national priority. In R. P. Weissberg, T. P. Gullotta, R. L. Hampton, B. A. Ryan, & G. R. Adams (Eds.), *Healthy children 2010: Enhancing children's wellness* (pp. 1-16). Thousand Oaks, CA: Sage.

Zill, N., & Nord, C. W. (1994). *Running in place: How American families are faring in a changing economy and an individualistic society.* Washington, DC: Child Trends.

CHAPTER 2

Policy Efforts to Enhance Child and Family Life: Goals for 2010

EDWARD F. ZIGLER
MATIA FINN-STEVENSON

The importance of integrating developmental research and social policy is becoming increasingly evident as educators as well as researchers and clinicians in psychology and other related disciplines focus on ways to address the needs of children and families. Concern for the well-being of children is not new. During the past 30 years in particular, but even earlier as well, children have been cited as a neglected group, and numerous study panels have called for greater recognition of the problems they face (e.g., Joint Commission on Mental Health of Children, 1969; National Commission on Children, 1990; President's Commission on Mental Health, 1978; Select Panel for the Promotion of Child Health, 1981). As we near the beginning of the 21st century, the concern for children and families has taken on a sense of urgency. Many researchers are actively monitoring the well-being of children and directing their work toward the understanding of how social problems contribute to mental dysfunction as well as to finding ways to enhance child and family life.

In this chapter, we discuss these developments, focusing not only on the possibilities but also on the challenges inherent in bridging the disparate worlds of research and social policy. We provide several examples of the opportunities that now exist for researchers and service providers to contribute to the development of programs and policies for children and families. We note that their effectiveness in this regard is dependent on a thorough knowledge of the developmental research as well as their familiarity and understanding of the social policy process and their ability to work with policymakers.

Background

The interest in social policy among professionals in disciplines related to child and family life can be traced to a number of developments, a major one of these being the implementation during the 1960s and 1970s of federally sponsored social programs such as Project Head Start (Zigler & Muenchow, 1992; Zigler & Styfco, 1993; Zigler & Valentine, 1979). The growth in the number of such programs, as well as the funds made available for them, enabled developmental psychologists and professionals from other disciplines to apply their knowledge and training to such areas as program development and evaluation, which had not previously received their attention (Phillips, 1987; Salkind, 1983; Takanishi, DeLeon, & Pallak, 1983). In another development, new lines of research led to the appreciation that children do not develop in a vacuum. They grow up within the social context and are influenced by various aspects of their immediate environment as well as by the more remote social institutions such as the school, neighborhood, the workplace, government, and the mass media (Bronfenbrenner, 1979). This realization gave impetus to ecological studies and the compilation of information on children's behavior, achievement, and physical and mental health (Miringoff, 1993; Zill, Sigal, & Brim, 1983). *Healthy People 2000* and its offshoot, *Healthier Youth by the Year 2000,* are examples of such projects, focusing not only on the identification of objectives to promote the health and well-being of children and youth but also on the compilation of data to help ascertain the most pressing of problems faced by children and their families.

Scope of the Problem

On the basis of the information made available through such efforts, it has become apparent that an ever-growing number of children and adolescents in the United States face serious problems. *Healthy People 2000,* in its *Midcourse Review and 1995 Revisions* (U.S. Department of Health and Human Services, Public Health Service [DHHS], 1995), cites some progress that has been made in recent years in such areas as infant mortality rates, but notes also that much more needs to be done to address unintentional injuries, homicides, and suicides among children and youth, as well as other problems such as teen pregnancy and substance abuse. Other reports, such as *The Index of Social Health* (Miringoff, 1993), document the fact that although in other countries there has been significant progress in meeting the needs of children in such areas as health, education, social welfare, and economic well-being, the social health of children in the United States has declined, with children being much worse off today than they were in the 1980s.

Of particular concern is the growing incidence of mental health problems among children and youth. A committee of the Institute of Medicine (1989), convened at the request of the National Institute of Mental Health (NIMH), studied the mental health status of children and adolescents in the United States. It found that at least 12% of children under age 18 (7.5 million children) have a diagnosable mental illness and that many other children exhibit broader indicators of dysfunction, including substance abuse, teen pregnancy, and school dropout, which the committee defined as consequences of or risk factors for developing mental disorders. Kazdin (1993), in a review of recent epidemiological studies, indicates that the problem is larger in scope. He estimates that 17%-22% or approximately 11 to 14 million children under age 18 suffer developmental, emotional, and behavioral problems.

The fact that so many children are affected by mental disorders suggests that the problem is widespread nationally. The fiscal costs of this problem to society are difficult to estimate, in part because mental health disorders often occur in conjunction with other problems such as substance abuse, making it hard to separate the costs of treatment associated with each disorder. However, studies that are available suggest that the costs of childhood mental disorders are staggering. Rice, Kelman, and Dunmeyer (1990), for example, found that treatment services for mentally ill children aged 14 and under exceed $1.5 billion a year, a figure also cited by *Healthy People 2000* (DHHS, 1991). Others suggest that the costs are much higher; besides treatment costs, there are indirect costs and costs for nonhealth services, which are borne by families, the schools, the juvenile justice system, and other social institutions (Office of Technology Assessment, 1986). Mental health disorders in children are not only costly, they also place an emotional burden on individuals, families, and society at large.

Contributing Factors

Perhaps even more significant than the findings on the prevalence and cost of childhood mental disorders are the findings on the factors that contribute to the development of such disorders. More research is needed to unravel the causes and determinants of mental health problems among children and adolescents. However, the available evidence suggests that biological, psychological, social, and environmental factors are implicated as causal agents. In some cases, an interaction between these factors exacerbates children's vulnerability to mental disorders. Among an increasing number of children, social and environmental risk factors are involved in the onset of mental dysfunction (Tuma, 1989). Included among these are risk factors that are all too common among children growing up today: prolonged separations between the parent and child (Tennant, 1988), physical or sexual abuse (Allen & Oliver, 1982; Kashani, Beck, & Hoepper, 1987), poverty (Garmezy, 1985; Rutter, 1976), marital discord (Wallerstein, 1988), instability in the family environment (Rutter, 1987), and a variety of other stressors related to family life (American Psychiatric Association, 1987; Institute of Medicine, 1989; Tuma, 1989). A child experiencing such stressful conditions may suffer emotional distress and/or behavioral disturbances for a relatively short period of time (Rutter, 1983), but sometimes and among some children, there are long-term, serious consequences. Whereas children who experience one of the above risk factors may not be any more likely to suffer serious consequences than children with no risk factors, the more risks or stressors that are present in children's lives, the greater the probability of long-term damaging outcomes (Rutter, 1980).

It is also noted that some of the above risk factors compound other problems that, when they occur in isolation, may have no negative effects. For example, some infants experience central nervous system difficulties. These may be overcome if the infants

are reared in stable and supportive environments but are exacerbated if they are raised in unstable, poor education, low-income,
or otherwise stressful family environments (Sameroff, Seifer, &
Zax, 1987). Likewise, premature low birth weight babies, who are
more vulnerable to environmental insufficiencies than are full-term
babies, may experience developmental problems if they are reared
by unresponsive adults but may suffer no negative consequences if
they receive appropriate care.

Changes in Family Life. These research findings have important
implications because many children today face potentially damaging experiences that stem from difficult conditions in family life
(Tuma, 1989). During the past 30 years, our society has undergone
economic and social changes that have transformed the structure
of the family and the roles and responsibilities of men and women.
These changes have made child rearing a more challenging task than
it had been in the past and have created stressful conditions for
children and adults.

One of the changes affecting family life has been the increased
fragmentation and isolation of the family. This is especially evident
in high rates of divorce among families with children, as we discuss
later in the chapter. It is also evident in the growth in the number
of single-parent families. Single-parent families are generally
characterized by female heads of household, poverty, and the
presence of young children (Burns & Scott, 1994; U.S. Bureau of
the Census, 1988). Currently, one of every four children in the
United States lives in a single-parent family, and among African
Americans, the numbers are one of every two children (National
Center for Children in Poverty, 1993). A related change in family
life is the isolation and lack of social support that many families are
experiencing. This has occurred in part because people move frequently in search of employment and often they do not remain in
any one place long enough to establish close relationships
(Gormley, 1995; National Commission on Children, 1990). As a
result, many families no longer live near or have access to the
support and assistance of friends and relatives. Referred to by some
as a decrease in "social capital" (Coleman, 1987), the lack of social
support is notable, because having access to a support system often
mediates the negative consequences of stress (Garmezy, 1985;
Gore, 1980).

Many families, especially those with young children, are also experiencing serious economic difficulties, and many of them live in poverty. In part, this is due to the increase in single-parent families. Other contributing factors are cuts in public assistance and a scarcity of well-paying jobs, which have led to a decline in the real value of family income (Children's Defense Fund, 1993). This is emphasized in a recent report (Women's Bureau, 1994) that indicates in 71% of two-parent families, both parents have to work just to meet the family's basic needs. Among single-parent families, the parent's need to work is even more acute because, often, the one parent is sole supporter of the children (National Commission on Children, 1990).

The decline in real income and the increase in the number of families in poverty affect adults and children. For children, the consequences are particularly serious because a significant percentage of families in poverty are those with young children. According to the U.S. Bureau of the Census (1988), the poverty rate of young families has almost doubled between 1968 and 1988 and continues to be a major problem in the 1990s (National Center for Children in Poverty, 1993).

The ramifications of living in poverty are numerous and include assaults on children's physical and mental health (Huston, McLoyd, & Garcia-Coll, 1994). Margolis and Farran (1985) found that in many families, a drop in income leads to poor health care for the children. Klerman (1991) found that poor families have no access to health care and that other conditions associated with poverty, such as lack of money to spend on health-promoting activities, hunger, and lack of transportation and adequate housing further exacerbate the problem. The result: Poor children experience more health problems and have a higher mortality rate.

There is also a powerful albeit indirect link between poverty and mental health disorders (McLeod & Shanahan, 1993), leading to the conclusion that poverty is one of the major risk factors in such disorders (Albee, 1986; Rutter, 1976). Although at one time mental dysfunction, low achievement, and other problems associated with poverty were discussed in terms of assumed negative traits of poor children, researchers now realize that the major sources of psychopathology associated with poverty stem from environmental stresses and feelings of powerlessness and frustration (Albee, 1986). It is further noted that among poor families, there is a high incidence of poor prenatal care, low birth weight, and malnutrition (Brown, Gershoff, & Cook, 1992), which are known to contribute to children's vulnerabilities to environmental stress (DHHS, 1991; Institute of Medicine, 1989).

Need for Policies to Enhance Child and Family Life: Contributions From Research

The stressful conditions noted above are just a few examples of the changed circumstances under which many children live. Other potentially damaging conditions are discussed later in the chapter. Although the majority of families are affected by these changes in family life, social policies in the United States have not kept pace with societal changes. Our society is, as a result, in a state of disequilibrium wherein social policies are not in synchrony with the realities of family life (Hoffman, 1989).

It is this disequilibrium that is creating difficulties for families. Admittedly, not all mental health and other problems children experience stem from such difficulties. There are other contributing factors, some of which are elaborated on elsewhere in this book. However, the stressful conditions under which many children live place a burden on children's ability to cope with the demands of school, the family, and relationships with peers.

The problems that emanate from the changing conditions of family life touch on economic realities, traditions, and institutional structures, to name just a few aspects, so solutions may come about slowly (Zeitlin, 1989). Nevertheless, professionals in disciplines related to children's development can contribute to the enhancement of family life in several ways.

Monitoring the Status of Children and Families

One such contribution may be the monitoring of the needs of children and families and the services available to meet these needs. The importance of this activity is illustrated in the *Healthy People 2000* project and other similar efforts, which provide useful information on the basis of which policy decisions may be made and actions taken on behalf of children and families. In *Healthy People*

2000, for example, the focus is on the identification of specific goals that help shape the research agenda, training activities, and the provision of services designed to address needs. Similar activities are undertaken by other organizations. The National Center for Children in Poverty (1995), for example, examined how various states are promoting the healthy development of children, finding that eight states have developed exemplary strategies and that several others have made significant investments in programs designed to meet the needs of children and families. This kind of service-tracking study is a useful indicator of state commitment to addressing the needs of children and may be used to spur action in other states as well.

At times, monitoring activities illuminate systemic changes that may be necessary. Knitzer (1993), in her description of the Children's Defense Fund's analysis of children's mental health problems and services, notes that the study "highlighted systemic problems and underscored the need to invent a children's mental health system that would be more responsive to the children and families using it" (p. 9). Such study can lead to the implementation of changes. However, this is not always the case. Thompson and Wilcox (1995), in their analysis of federal support for child maltreatment research, noted that despite the importance of research to provide greater understanding of this social issue, as well as the increase in public awareness of the scope of the problem of child abuse and neglect, federal support for research and demonstration studies in the area has actually waned in recent years. Thus, it is evident that awareness of the problem and the identification of the needs of children are, in and of themselves, not always sufficient, but they are necessary first steps in the policy process.

Use of Research

Child and family life may also be enhanced if we direct attention to the study of children's responses to various conditions under which they live. This focus on research is important. It can provide an understanding of how children are affected by different conditions and of why some children are able to cope with difficulties in their lives whereas other children succumb (Garmezy, 1985). The research can also illuminate the ways children cope with problems so that we can devise useful strategies for intervention and prevention. Although there are many examples of how scientific research can be a constructive force in the policy process, given the limited scope of this chapter, we will discuss studies and policy responses to only two societal changes that have had a profound effect on family life: maternal employment and divorce.

Maternal Employment

Maternal employment has had a profound effect not only on family life but on society in general. This phenomenon, related in large part to the economic hardships faced by many families as well as to other societal changes, is especially apparent among women who have young children. For women with school-age children, full-time employment has been relatively common for about two decades, but even among these women, there has been an increase in employment, with upward of 75% (up from 65% in 1965) of such mothers now working out of the home (Bureau of Labor Statistics, 1992). In 1950, the percentage of women with children under age 6 who were working out of the home was 11.9%; by 1987, it had grown to 56.8%, and in 1992, it was 58% (Bureau of Labor Statistics, 1992).

The increase in the number of working mothers has been especially significant among those with infants. In 1987, 31% of women with infants a year old and under were working, and today 54% of them are in the workforce, with many of them returning to work within a few weeks of the birth of the baby. It is projected that 93% of working women of childbearing age will become pregnant during this decade, so the number of mothers with infants returning to work will increase (Hofferth & Wissoker, 1992).

The research on the effects of maternal employment on children indicates that in and of itself maternal employment is not necessarily associated with negative or positive effects on children (Greenberger & Bronfenbrenner, 1989; Hoffman, 1989). Rather, parental attitudes to the mother's employment are more significant in their effects on children than is the mother's employment status (Hoffman, 1986, 1989).

But researchers point out that although maternal employment appears to be benign in its effects on children, in many dual-worker families both the parents and the children experience an inordinate amount of stress. The stress stems from the fact that although women have assumed new roles within the workplace, they have not abdicated their traditional responsibilities to family life and child rearing. This has resulted in role conflict and guilt among mothers in particular (Hoffman, 1989; Moen & Dempster, 1987), as well as changes in lifestyle and difficulties that permeate the whole family system. Studies have found that close to 40% of employed parents, both women and men, indicate that they experience severe conflict, guilt, and stress (Friedman, 1987). For children, this state of affairs means that not only do they have less time with their parents, but they are also affected by the fact that their parents are under stress from trying to do too much.

Not only families but also other institutions are affected by the increase in women's participation in the out-of-home labor force. Employers, anxious about worker productivity, are concerned about women who are juggling work and family responsibilities, and some employers are also beginning to realize that they may be losing valued female employees when child rearing conflicts with full-time work. Other institutions, such as the school, have to implement changes to accommodate the needs of children not only during school hours but also before and after school (Zigler, 1987, 1989). Additionally, changes have occurred in some professions that were previously associated with flexible work schedules that enabled mothers to work and at the same time rear their children. Teachers, for example, are finding that they have to extend their workday and thus disrupt their own family life because many of their students' parents are working and unavailable for parent conferences and other school events during the day (Zeitlin, 1989).

Increased Demand for Child Care. Although there are several difficulties associated with women's participation in the labor force, none are as significant as the unprecedented demand for child care services. Today, child care is one of the most widely recognized social problems. Virtually everyone, from working parents to chief executives of major corporations, is discussing the lack of good-quality, affordable child care services. Two pieces of legislation have been enacted to address the issue. One is the 1988 Family Support Act, which, as part of an effort to reform welfare, includes child care assistance for women in school or training or who work. The other is the 1990 Child Care and Development Block Grant, which, among other provisions, provides child care subsidies to low-income families. Although these pieces of legislation may be considered a step in the right direction, there is just too little money involved (Children's Defense Fund, 1994a, 1994b), so they may be considered, at best, only a partial solution to the problem (Zigler & Finn-Stevenson, 1996).

The recent attention to the child care issue is not surprising, given the increase in the number of infants and children who need child care. However, it belies the fact that the child care problem is hardly new; it has been a major social problem for nearly three decades. At the 1970 White House Conference on Children, the need for child care services was noted as the number one priority for the nation to address. At the time, Congress passed the Child Development Act, which would have enabled the country to begin to build a child care system. However, two obstacles—ideological arguments against the use of child care and the lack of public awareness of the need for child care services—stood in the way of policy action on the issue, and the bill was vetoed by President Nixon (Nelson, 1982). As a result, the problem exacerbated, reaching crisis proportions before finally attracting national recognition.

At the heart of the issue is the fact that child care continues to be regarded as an individual family problem to be addressed by parents. This is evident in the fact that the majority of businesses do not make provisions to ease the stresses associated with balancing work and family life and that despite the enactment of the family support legislation and the Child Care and Development Block Grant, we are still far short of having a comprehensive solution to the problem.

In an attempt to address the problem, it is important to identify its various parts, because no society acts until it has a sense of the immediacy, magnitude, and nature of the problem (Zigler & Finn, 1981). One aspect of the child care problem is the high cost of services. This is a major concern for parents, many of whom choose a child care facility solely on the basis of cost. This point is made by Hofferth and Wissoker (1992), who found that parents often switch facilities if the price increases. Precise data on what families spend on child care are not available, but it is indicated that parents pay anywhere between $1,500 and $10,000 a year, depending on the quality of care and the age of the children involved. It is estimated that full-time child care for preschoolers costs an average of $3,000 a year, and that for infants the costs can exceed $9,600 a year. With the cost of care being so prohibitive, it is not surprising that it is one of the major factors in choosing child care.

The high cost of care is significant in part because child care costs are a major expenditure for families, and the amount of money families spend on child care is directly related to their income. Low-income families spend less on child care in absolute terms than do higher-income families, but the proportion of the family budget that is taken up by child care costs is greater among low-income families, who have to allocate as much as 25% to 30% of their earnings to child care (Friedman, 1987).

When parents select a child care setting, they are paying for an environment where a significant portion of the child rearing will occur. With children spending their entire day, every day in child care, this environment affects the child's course of development. If the quality of the environment falls below a certain level, the child's optimal development will be compromised.

Although mental health professionals are contributing in various ways to efforts to address the child care problem, especially significant have been the research studies undertaken to identify the factors associated with good-quality child care. Knowledge of such factors is important in the policy arena. For example, standards of quality and their expression in state licensing codes governing the operation of child care facilities are attempts to objectively define a basic minimum to ensure the well-being of children. But even this minimum is often not attained in the regulations in some states and there are no consistent standards of quality to which all states must adhere. In states where standards are considered good, the average quality of centers seem to be good as well (Helburn et al., 1995), but this is of little comfort given the fact that the standards in many states leave much to be desired.

In defining quality, a distinction is made between a child care environment that is nurturant and one that is merely custodial. In a nurturant environment, where children are given opportunities for play and social interactions and where providers interact with children and attend to their individual needs, providers are often trained in child development and are able to provide developmentally appropriate care. This is an environment, in short, that is conducive to optimal development and learning. In a custodial setting, or poor-quality environment, minimal attention is paid to the children, who are often left wandering aimlessly around the room or watching television.

In such environments, there are often too many children for any one caregiver to care for, and the children are placed in large groups thus receiving little if any adult attention.

The research has shown that good-quality child care is determined by several factors: group size, staff to child ratios appropriate for the age of the children, and providers and administrators who are trained in child development or a related field (Bredekamp, 1987; Hayes, Palmer, & Zaslow, 1990; Helburn et al., 1995). In terms of provider training in particular, it was found that providers who are trained in child development are more likely than those not receiving such training to be sensitive and responsive to the individual needs of the children and knowledgeable about creating an environment that is conducive to optimal growth and development (Roupp, Travers, Glantz, & Coelen, 1979). Continuity of care, that is, care by the same providers over time, is also an important determinant of quality (Phillips, 1987, 1995), and this assumes more importance with infants and very young children, who need to get to know and become familiar with the routines of caregivers to develop a sense of trust and security. In facilities of poor quality, staff turnover is over 40% (Whitebook, Howes, & Phillips, 1990). Many providers stay on the job for less than 6 months, then move on to other jobs. Multiple changes in providers or in child care arrangements created by staff turnover have been found to have a negative effect on children, resulting in insecure attachment to the mother (Hayes et al., 1990).

Although we know the determinants of good-quality care, the majority of children in the United States receive poor-quality care whether they are in child care centers, family day care homes, or in the care of relatives. Several national studies attest to this fact. One of the studies, known as the Child Care Staffing Study (Whitebook et al., 1990), found that in over half of the centers studied, the quality was poor, providers lacked training and were not adequately paid, and annual employee turnover was so high that it gave cause for concern, because infants and young children need continuity of care. In another national study, this one on children in family day care homes and the care of relatives, only 9% of such settings were rated as being of good quality, meaning that they offered care that was growth enhancing; 56% were rated

as adequate/custodial, meaning that they were neither growth enhancing nor growth harming; and 35% were rated as inadequate or
growth harming. Family day care and relative care are usually used
by parents of infants and toddlers because of the belief that the
homelike atmosphere is more conducive to children's development.
In theory, family day care and relative care can be good options.
However, the majority of family day care and relative care occurs
"underground" with providers being isolated from the child care
community and unknown to regulators. It has been estimated that
75% to 90% of family day care homes are unregulated. This
estimate is confirmed by the National Family Day Care Study noted
above, which found that only 12% of family day care homes are
regulated and only 1% of care by relatives is regulated (Galinsky,
Howes, Kontos, & Shinn, 1994).

In the most recent study on cost, quality, and child outcomes in
child care centers (Helburn et al., 1995), it was found that only
14% of centers could be regarded as providing good-quality care.
In the majority of centers in the study, it was found that the
environment is poor to mediocre, with almost half of all young
children being in centers that are less than minimal in quality.
Minimal quality was defined as follows: The children's basic health
and safety needs are not met; there is little, if any, evidence of
warmth and support provided by the adults to the children; and
few if any learning experiences or opportunities for learning are
provided.

The studies noted above on the quality of care also provided some
information on supply-and-demand issues. In the area of
availability of care for preschool children, there seems to be some
debate, with some arguing that a sufficient number of child care
slots exist to accommodate the need. Others point out, however,
that although the number of preschool child care slots has kept up
with demand, what is generally available is either of poor quality
or too expensive for most families, and when taking this into
account, it is evident that there is a lack of good-quality, affordable
child care for preschoolers. There are no disagreements on two
other aspects of the availability of care: one, that the demand for
care far exceeds supply for infant child care and school-age child
care and, two, that the need for child care services will continue to
increase into the next century not only because more mothers will

be working, but also because the job market is expected to tighten over the next decade causing competition for workers. With child care paying only minimal wages, it is likely that providers will leave the field and opt for higher-paying positions (Committee for Economic Development [CED], 1993).

Another major problem associated with child care is the lack of a coherent child care system. What we have in place currently is a patchwork of services, some delivered by individuals out of their homes, others operated by nonprofit and for-profit groups in a variety of settings (CED, 1993). Few of the services are of good quality, the majority are not, and, given the lack of a system, we are unable to make any improvements with any assurance that they will be implemented and sustained.

Policy Responses. Attempts to create a more coherent child care structure have resulted in calls for both lesser and greater government involvement in child care. Some groups advocate limiting the role of government to tax credits for parents (these currently exist, but their value is diminished for poor families who are not earning enough to realize benefits associated with tax credits). Others argue for increased government spending and involvement in such issues as the regulation of child care facilities. These and other views were represented in the hundreds of bills introduced in Congress in recent years, which culminated in the passage of the 1990 Child Care and Development Act, mentioned earlier in the chapter. In keeping with the trend toward the New Federalism evidenced over the past two decades, the law makes funding available to the states in the form of block grants, leaving room for interpretation and allowing allocation decisions to be made at the state level (Cohen, 1996). To some extent, this represents an opportunity because each state can respond more readily to its population's needs. However, in light of the nonuniform standards for child care that exist across the United States (Young, Marsland, & Zigler, in press) and the diversity of services within the existing nonsystem, this legislation does not represent any gain in terms of establishing a comprehensive, accessible, quality system of child care and family support in this country; it merely provides some additional funds.

The greatest concern is that passage of the Child Care and Development Act of 1990 is counterproductive because although

Congress has viewed it as the solution to the child care problem, its effect in terms of better meeting existing child care needs has been negligible, and the majority of states continue to have insufficient funds to address even basic needs for child care subsidies (Blank, 1994; Cohen, 1996). For example, the law targets 75% of the block grant funding to serve low-income families. Prior to enactment of the law, California was able to provide subsidies for the care of approximately 25% of the low-income children in need of care. With funding from the Child Care and Development Act, estimates indicate that these programs serve approximately 30% of low-income families. Although an increase, the funding still falls far short of meeting the needs of all low-income families.

Guiding Principles. It is clear that the 1990 Child Care and Development Act has not resulted in a comprehensive solution to the child care problem. Given the scope of the child care problem, we need a comprehensive system that is developed on the basis of what we know from child development research on the needs of children and the programs that can successfully meet these needs.

Toward this end, several guiding principles have been identified as necessary for developing an effective child care system (Zigler, 1987). First, the system must provide universal access to quality child care and include a sliding scale for parental fees as well as direct subsidies for low-income families through federal, state, and/or local funding. Second, child care must promote the optimal development of children and should focus on all developmental domains, including physical, social, emotional, and cognitive. This is emphasized because at times early interventions focus solely on cognitive development, neglecting to emphasize the development of the child as a whole. Third, child care must be predicated on a partnership between parents and providers. Successful programs, such as Head Start, have demonstrated that much of their success can be attributed to the active participation of parents in the services provided to their children (Zigler & Muenchow, 1992; Zigler & Valentine, 1979).

The fourth guiding principle underscores the crucial role providers have in the quality of care children receive, and calls for recognition and support of child care providers through training, the provision of benefits, and pay upgrades. Fifth, based on the need to appreciate the heterogeneity of children and parents and their differing needs for child care and support, any child care policy must ensure a flexible system that is adjustable to the needs of families and available to families on a voluntary basis.

Finally, we must build a stable, reliable, good-quality child care system that is integrated with the political and economic structure of society and is tied to a recognized and easily accessible societal institution such as the public school. The need for such a system is apparent given the lack of coherent structure in the current patchwork of child care services in the United States.

School of the 21st Century. These principles serve as the foundation for a school-based child care and family support program known as the School of the 21st Century (21C) (Zigler & Finn-Stevenson, 1989). 21C calls for implementing a child care system within the already existing educational system, where possible, making use of available school buildings. The components of 21C include all-day (matching the length of parents' workday), year-round child care for children ages 3, 4, and 5; before- and after-school and vacation care for school-age children up to age 12; parent education and support from birth to age 3, based on the Parents as Teachers home visitation program, which provides parents with knowledge on ways they can effectively interact with children; information and referral for other services children and their families may need; health and nutrition; and outreach to family day care providers. This latter component is included because family day care providers, who often care for infants and toddlers, are isolated from others in the child care community and do not receive training or other support. In 21C, the school serves as the hub for family day care providers in the neighborhood, providing them with training workshops and other services they may need.

The components of 21C ensure a comprehensive array of services for children and families and also make possible continuity of care and support for children to provide the foundation on which development and learning occur. The strength and ultimate potential of 21C stems from its comprehensive nature and integration with the education system. By eliminating the distinction between child care and education, 21C embraces and actualizes the notion that learning begins at birth and occurs in all settings, not just within the classroom. This guarantees the necessary consistency and continuity of care as well as enrichment opportunities for children to realize their developmental potential.

In 21C, the school is no longer seen as a building in which formal schooling is delivered during limited hours. Instead, the school becomes a place where formal schooling, child care, and family support occur together. Whereas ordinarily schools would operate from 8:00 in the morning to 3:00 in the afternoon, 9 months of the year, in 21C, the school building is open from 6:00 or 7:00 in the morning to 6:00 in the evening, 12 months a year to provide formal schooling and also core child care and family support services. Existing school and community programs, such as Head Start, other preschool or after-school services, and programs serving children with special needs, become a part of 21C, which enables coordination of services, activities, and resource sharing.

Using existing school buildings and the organizational structure of the school district is a cost-effective approach to building a child care system and means that good-quality, affordable child care can be made available to parents on a sliding scale fee system calibrated to family income. School districts do need, however, either to raise funds or reallocate money to cover a start-up period of about a year, and in many cases this has been done among schools implementing 21C. The program has been financed in a variety of ways. Generally, start-up funds to support renovations and purchase of materials and the operation of the program for the first year have been provided by community foundations and corporations or by enabling legislation (in Kentucky and Connecticut). After the first year, programs operate and even make a profit (which is put into the program to support various components and staff training) on the basis of parental fees for the child care services, which, as noted earlier, are based on a sliding scale schedule. In cases of low-income families, arrangements for public subsidies are made or, as some schools have done, a consortium of corporations in the area near the schools donate money to a scholarship fund that is used to offset tuition costs for needy families. Collaborating with Head Start programs, including special education children and using Chapter One funds, is among the other ways that schools have been able to expand the scope and reach of the program once it is implemented. Several schools have also become Medicaid case managers, and this has enabled them to realize a profit that is then put into the operation of the program (Lubker, 1995).

From a policy perspective, it is essential to approach 21C as an investment in human capital, not as a cost to be assessed in terms of present value. The long-term benefits that school districts and society stand to realize by investing in this program are detailed in several longitudinal studies on the effects of early childhood education efforts. These studies, detailed in a special issue of the *Future of Children* ("Long-Term Outcomes," 1995), reveal numerous benefits associated with early education, including improved grade retention rates, reduced use of special education and other special services, fewer graduates on welfare, increased rates of college attendance, and decreases in delinquency and social problems. In terms of costs and benefits, a conservative estimate indicates that for approximately every dollar invested in high-quality, developmentally appropriate preschool programs, a subsequent $7 savings will be realized (Barnett, 1992).

Although schools in a variety of urban, rural, and suburban communities have successfully implemented 21C, there are several issues associated with implementing the program. One concern is who operates the program. Given that professional educators, principals, and teachers are already overburdened and working tirelessly to enhance or just maintain the quality of schools, it is not appropriate to expect them to take on the responsibility of operating child care and family support services. Also, most school personnel do not have the training or expertise required in working with young children and their families. Instead, in 21C, services are headed by a person with a degree and training in early childhood education. The day-to-day care of children in the program is handled by staff trained in early childhood, child development, or a related field, with provisions made for ongoing staff development (Yale Bush Center in Child Development and Social Policy, 1992). Another implementation issue concerns space. At present, given increased enrollments, space in elementary schools is at a premium and schools have had to adjust by using modular units or renovating previously unused space. Space needs change as enrollments grow and decline over the years, and school districts have to adjust accordingly. In many communities, lower enrollments in elementary schools are predicted for the coming years as the "baby boomlet" subsides and also because the poor economy has resulted in fewer births. From a long-term perspective, however, it is important to plan for child care in the school. This had taken place for some years in the province of Ontario, Canada, where every school building built had to include space for child care.

Over 400 schools in 13 states have implemented 21C, providing an example of how, on the basis of the research and an understanding of the policy process, we can be instrumental in the development and implementation of needed programs and services. There is a need for other policies to address the needs of working parents (e.g., providing flexible work schedules and family leave so parents can take care of newborn infants or at times when children or other family members are ill). It is beyond the scope of this chapter to go into detail about these; suffice it to note, however, that researchers' involvement in these issues has been substantial (see, e.g., Zigler & Frank, 1988).

Divorce

Researchers have also been instrumental in contributing to the understanding and the development of policy directions and programs concerning children of divorce. Divorce has been cited as a contributing factor in the changes in family life as discussed in the background section of this chapter. Single-parent families, for example, are often the result of divorce. Also, for many women and children in particular, divorce contributes to a greatly reduced standard of living, often leading to poverty.

The number of children who experience the divorce of their parents rose dramatically between 1965 and 1979. Since 1979, the rate of divorce has declined and seems to have leveled off (Hernandez, 1988, 1995). Nevertheless, it is estimated that about 50% of children born in the past decade will experience the divorce of their parents and that most of these children will also experience the remarriage of one or both of their parents, and, after living for a period of time in a single-parent family, they will live in what has come to be known as a blended or reconstituted family (Hetherington, Hagan, & Anderson, 1989).

In their investigations of children's responses to the divorce and remarriage of their parents, researchers found that for some children, divorce may have some benefits in that the children do not have to continue to live in a dysfunctional family. However, most children experience changes in marital arrangements as stressful, and only some of them are able to cope with the changes and eventually adapt to their new family life (Hetherington et al., 1989). Many of the children suffer sustained developmental disruptions as a result of the changes in family life, and some appear to adapt well in the early stages of family reorganization but show delayed negative effects at a later time ("Children of Divorce," 1994; Wallerstein, 1988, 1991). Tschara, Johnson, Kline, and Wallerstein (1990) found that children had difficulty adjusting to the divorce if they were older, had prior psychological problems, and had parents with more marital conflict. Hetherington et al. (1989) found that the long-term effects of divorce and remarriage appear to be related to a number of factors, including the child's developmental status, sex, and temperament; the quality of the home environment; and availability of support systems both to the parents and to the child.

The number of stressors the child experiences is also a factor, because, as noted earlier, a single stressor typically does not carry with it appreciable psychiatric risk, but multiple stressors increase the risk for mental dysfunction (Rutter, 1980). In this regard, particular concern is noted for children whose custodial parent experiences extreme economic difficulties for an extended period of time and/or whose noncustodial parent fails to pay for child support. Children whose parents suffer emotional and psychological difficulties as a result of the divorce are also likely to experience multiple stressors. Researchers have found that when parents' distress is acute, the parents fail to attend to the needs of their children, they do not recognize the children's painful experience with the divorce, or they burden the children with their own adjustment difficulties (Kurdek & Blisk, 1983).

This knowledge about the effects of divorce on children has led to recent policy decisions in some states to make divorce more difficult to obtain (e.g., requiring a 1-year waiting period), with advocates of such policies noting that this is an effort to address the needs of children (Seppa, 1996). Such policy efforts are just now beginning, and researchers can contribute by engaging in research that would help illuminate whether children are better off experiencing the divorce of their parents and not staying in a dysfunctional family environment, or would they benefit in the long-term if their parents had to continue to remain married despite martial difficulties. This is not an easy question to settle, and the answer may vary depending on children's temperament as well as other factors and circumstances. Additionally, because some studies have shown that at times children may appear to be adjusting and only several years later present negative symptoms as a result of divorce, it is important to base policy decisions on findings from longitudinal research (Amato, 1994).

Among children of divorce, the most vulnerable are the children whose parents engage in legal battles over custody issues. The children are at substantial risk not only because of the adversarial environment in which they have to live, but also because custody battles can continue indefinitely. Judges attempt to make custody decisions on the basis of the best interests of the child. However, neither judges nor lawyers are prepared for the arduous task of determining the best interests of the child. Nor are they trained to interview the child, consider his or her developmental and emotional needs and concerns, or weigh the urgency of the child's condition and circumstances (Wallerstein, 1986; Wallerstein & Corbin, 1996). Recognizing the child as the hidden client in divorce proceedings, Goldstein, Freud, and Solnit (1973, 1979) have made an attempt to provide guidance to lawyers and judges by incorporating legal considerations within the framework of principles drawn from developmental psychology and psychiatry. They recommend that decisions regarding child custody be made quickly, that an effort be made to avoid prolonged proceedings, and that whatever decision is made have final effect that is not reversible. They further recommend that judges award full custody of the child to one "psychological parent." There is controversy surrounding this latter recommendation. Some psychiatrists emphasize the psychological value for some children of maintaining a close relationship with both parents, even those involved in a bitter dispute over custody issues (Guidibaldi, Cleminshaw, & Perry, 1983). Others maintain that as the developmental needs of children change with age, so should custody decisions (Kelly, 1994). However, although some of their recommendations are controversial, Goldstein et al. paved the way for other researchers to think about the use of knowledge and theoretical principles in establishing criteria for practical decisions that involve children.

Mediating the effects of divorce. Some researchers have advocated the use of mediation as a means of reducing the stressful effects of divorce on children. Some parents, for example, turn to trusted friends of family members or other professionals outside the judicial system (e.g., clergy) for advice on decisions pertaining to divorce (Bloom, Hodges, & Caldwell, 1982). Also, during the past decade, formal mediation for divorce in general and custody issues in particular has become increasingly available. In such an option, a mediator is assigned to assist parents in making decisions. Although some are concerned that mediation puts women at a disadvantage (Grillo, 1991), the need to protect children from prolonged divorce proceedings and legal battles over custody issues has led several states to enact laws mandating mediation as the first step in the process (Kelly, 1994). These laws will no doubt be refined over time as more knowledge from the research becomes available, but they are indicative of the uses of the research in the policy arena.

Although, as is evident in the discussion above, policymakers and legal professionals are seeking guidance from researchers in the matter of divorce and its effect on children, the accumulation of psychological knowledge has not kept up with rapid changes that have occurred in family law. Hetherington and Camara (1984) and Wallerstein (1986, 1988) make this point, indicating that knowledge about the effects of divorce on children and postdivorce parent-child relationships is still fragmentary, with several important questions remaining to be addressed. Behrman and Quinn (1994), in a review of studies on how policy and program changes can better serve the needs of children experiencing the divorce of their parents, also note the need for further research, but emphasize the importance of using current knowledge to educate parents, attorneys, and judges about the effect of divorce and marital conflict on children. Given what we know to date about the effects of divorce, other professionals who interact with children should also have access to the available knowledge base. Teachers, for example, need to be alerted to findings from the research on the effects of divorce on children and parents so they can be sensitive to any changes in children's behavior, counseling them on ways they can cope with the changes in their lives (Kurdek, 1981) and if necessary, providing them with support services.

Integrating Research and Policy

Family Support Service

The need for support services is noted not only in reference to children and parents who experience divorce but also in reference to other families. Families, like individuals, have a certain life course in which, at particular points, stresses and crises are a natural state of affairs. At those times, support programs can be invaluable in helping family members to use their strengths and rally to cope with the problem, thus warding off severe family dysfunction and mental health disorders (Riessman, 1986).

In response to the widespread need for such programs, a host of family support services has been developed and implemented in recent years. Although many of the programs were developed by the very people who need the support, others have been developed in collaboration with mental health professionals who have participated not only in the development and implementation of such programs (Weiss & Halpern, 1990), but also in attempts to evaluate them and ascertain which types of services are best suited for and have the most effect on children.

As a result of a cycle of experimentation and revision in the area of program development and evaluation, we have amassed a great deal of information on various family support services and on other types of programs as well ("Long-Term Outcomes," 1995; Price, Cowen, Lorion, & Ramos-McKay, 1988). This knowledge, derived from three decades of program research, "totally transforms the nation's capacity to improve outcomes for vulnerable children" (Schorr & Schorr, 1988, p. 3). It includes evidence on the effectiveness of a number of programs that reduce the burdens of risk factors in childhood, thereby reducing the probability of later damage (for a review of effective programs, see "Long-Term Outcomes," 1995; Price et al., 1988; Schorr & Schorr, 1988).

Besides the fact that information about effective programs exists, there is evidence to the effect that it is not necessary to change everything—the structure of opportunity, the neighborhood environment, and other aspects of the child's life—to make a crucial difference for children at risk (Hamburg, 1982). However, this knowledge is not being used to alter the life path of many of the children who are growing up under stressful conditions.

Problems in the Use of Research

The failure to use knowledge from the research stems from several problems. First, the information on effective programs is sometimes not shared with the public or with policymakers (White, 1988). Thus, programs, many of them at the demonstration stage, fail to be replicated on a larger scale. Even in cases where programs' potential benefits are known, there is skepticism that such programs, once they are replicated, will continue to be effective (Weiss & Halpern, 1990). Although this is a valid concern, Schorr and Schorr (1988) note that successful programs can be built on and expanded if we can attract and train enough skilled and committed personnel, if we devise a variety of replication strategies, and if we resist the lure of replication through dilution. This latter point is significant because, often, in an effort to serve as many children as possible, programs are diluted, thus diminishing their quality and potential benefits (Zigler & Berman, 1983).

Another problem standing in the way of using research in the policy arena is the uneasy relationship between researchers and policymakers. Describing the relationship, Maccoby, Kahn, and Everett (1983) note that policymakers often regard researchers as impractical and may be skeptical of policy recommendations coming from researchers who do not seem to understand the complexities of achieving a consensus among rival constituencies. Researchers, on the other hand, seem to regard policymakers as disingenuous and too willing to compromise even when the research evidence does not justify such action. Meltsner (1986) also observes that part of the tension and mistrust between policymakers and mental health researchers emanates from the assumption that knowledge from research is value free whereas policies are made in a value-laden context. However, this characterization of research and policy is misleading. Often, scientific research takes on the values of the investigators, as is evident in the questions asked, methodologies employed, and the interpretation and presentation of the findings.

In discussing the failure to translate research findings into large-scale programs and policies, Zervigon-Hakes (1995) notes that part of the problem stems from the fact that policymakers and researchers not only work in vastly different arenas, they have vastly different communication styles and different interests, and these differences stand in the way of creating collaborations.

The problems are further exacerbated by the fact that researchers are often perceived as unable to provide clear answers to policy questions or, looked at from another perspective, that policymakers are unable to ask questions in a way that would lead to valid and reliable research (Maccoby et al., 1983). In part, this problem stems from the unrealistic expectations policymakers have and their inability to appreciate the fact that single studies cannot, in and of themselves, provide definitive answers to questions. But researchers also contribute to the problem. White (1988) notes that often, researchers are unfamiliar with the policy process and/or are unable to "read" political issues. They hold to long, slow standards of proof and refutation that are, in the policy arena, "obstructive and nihilistic." Thompson (1993) makes a similar point, noting that often, policy issues do not lend themselves easily to research and that research findings are often limited in their applicability to policy because of sampling and measurement issues. Although it is imperative that researchers uphold their professional standards and credibility as scientists (Zigler & Finn-Stevenson, 1987), there are times when findings from the research, even if they are not entirely conclusive, can nonetheless provide a direction for policy. For example, the research on the effects of child care on children's development has been for a time controversial, yielding conflicting findings that serve to confuse the public and policymakers (Clarke-Stewart, 1989). Although research on the topic is continuing and would no doubt lead to clarifications as to which type of care affects children in what ways and at what particular age, researchers were able to convene and come to a consensus that indicated that as long as young children are in good-quality child care settings, they will not be adversely affected by their experiences in child care. This led to a policy recommendation for efforts to monitor the quality of care children receive and ensure that all children receive care that is conducive to optimal development (National Center for Clinical Infant Programs, 1988). It is apparent that there are circumstances—such as the reality of an increasing number of children in child care—when our awaiting definitive conclusions from the research is counterproductive, especially when action can be taken at the same time that research on a particular issue is continuing.

Strategies for Change

Understanding these and other problems that often impede the use of research in policy is important if mental health researchers are to have an effect in the policy arena. This point is made by Lindblom (1986), who identifies four general guidelines for researchers to follow to encourage the use of research in carving out policy directions: that researchers be concerned in a nonpartisan way with the values and interests of society in general and children in particular; that they take a practical approach and suggest policies that are feasible and have a chance of attracting widespread political and public support; that they respond to the needs of policymakers and provide them with recommendations for action on the basis of the knowledge from the research; and that they become cognizant of and responsive to the policy process.

It is also suggested that researchers make serious attempts to disseminate the findings from the research, not only to policymakers but to the general public through the mass media (Zervigon-Hakes, 1995). This suggestion is made in view of the fact that no society acts until it has a sense of the immediacy of the problem (Zigler & Finn, 1981). This is illustrated in the founding during the 1960s of the Great Society. During that time, social issues were covered in major newspapers and were in the forefront of national attention. There were daily stories on welfare mothers, reports on poverty, and expositions on hunger in the United States. Hence there was sympathy for the poor and public support for policies related to the War on Poverty (Zigler & Valentine, 1979).

Although for a time thereafter there was appreciably less interest in issues pertaining to children and families, there are some indications that this is changing. First, developmental psychologists, psychiatrists, and others in the mental health field are becoming aware of the need for enhancing public awareness on the needs of children (McCall, Gregory, & Murray, 1984). And, in a departure from their past practices, many mental health professionals are no longer satisfied with simply sharing information with one another. Rather, they disseminate their knowledge not only by presenting their findings directly to policymakers but also by taking steps to ensure that the information is covered in the popular media. Indeed, the dissemination of research in the context of the popular media has come to be accepted as an important aspect of the training received by some professionals in the field of mental health (Stevenson & Siegel, 1984).

Many professionals in disciplines related to child development are also receiving training in the integration of research and social policy, learning not only about the policy process but also about some of the ways to merge their knowledge with that of policymakers in the formation of programs and policies for children. The success of such efforts is evident in the numerous issues, such as child care, divorce, and the need for family support services, that only a few years ago were not discussed much but that now command national attention. The success of these efforts is further evident in the fact that an increasing number of policymakers are now acknowledging the importance of knowledge from the research in the formulation of policies and are actively seeking the collaboration of professionals in the field of mental health. If professionals from the research community and the policy arena continue to work together in this spirit of collaboration, we will be able to bring about much needed societal changes that will enhance child and family life.

The opportunity to make such changes is present in the *Healthy People 2010* initiative. Several recommendations are made in context of this effort, all of which are important. However, given our discussion in this chapter, additional objectives are warranted: that by 2010, all children would have access to good-quality child care and that provisions be made to increase the availability of support services to families. These objectives would enhance the *Healthy People 2010* initiative by focusing on the prevention of problems and may be included either as new objectives or as recommendations proposed for achieving existing objectives. In efforts to reduce the proportion of young people who use alcohol and drugs, for example (Objective 4.6), the availability of child care is noted as an important recommendation for action because the research has shown that young adolescents who are in supervised after-school programs are less likely than those who are not to abuse drugs and alcohol (Richardson, Dwyer, & McGuigan, 1989). Also, in efforts to reduce the prevalence of mental disorders among children and youth (Objective 6.3) most of the existing recommendations for action focus on interventions rather than prevention and would be enhanced if family support services were made available to families as may be needed from the birth of the child throughout the childhood and adolescent years. It is through such dual focus on prevention and intervention that we can achieve meaningful change that will be sustained over time.

References

Albee, G. W. (1986). Toward a just society: Lessons from observations on the primary prevention of psychopathology. *Journal of American Psychology, 41,* 891-898.

Allen, R. E., & Oliver, J. M. (1982). The effects of child maltreatment on language development. *Child Abuse & Neglect, 6,* 299-305.

Amato, P. R. (1994). Lifespan adjustment of children to their parents' divorce. *Future of Children, 4*(1), 142-164.

American Psychiatric Association. (1987). *Diagnostic and statistical manual of mental disorders* (3rd ed., rev.). Washington, DC: Author.

Barnett, W. S. (1992). Benefits of compensatory preschool education. *Journal of Human Resources, 27,* 279-312.

Behrman, R. E., & Quinn, L. S. (1994). Children and divorce: Overview and analysis. *Future of Children, 4*(1), 4-14.

Blank, H. (1994). *Protecting our children: State and federal policies for exempt child care settings.* National Association for the Education of Young Children. Washington, DC: Children's Defense Fund.

Bloom, B. L., Hodges, W. V., & Caldwell, R. A. (1982). A preventive program for the newly separated: Initial evaluation. *American Journal of Community Psychology, 10,* 251-264.

Bredekamp, S. (Ed.). (1987). *Developmentally appropriate practices in early childhood programs serving children from birth through age 8.* Washington, DC: National Association for the Education of Young Children.

Bronfenbrenner, U. (1979). *The ecology of human development: Experiments by nature design.* Cambridge, MA: Harvard University Press.

Brown, J. L., Gershoff, S. N., & Cook, J. T. (1992). The politics of hunger: When science and ideology clash. *International Journal of Health and Science, 22,* 44-60.

Bureau of Labor Statistics. (1992). *Current population survey, 1981, 1986, 1992.* Washington, DC: U.S. Department of Labor.

Burns, A., & Scott, C. (1994). *Mother headed families and why they have increased.* Mahwah, NJ: Lawrence Erlbaum.

Children of divorce. (1994). *Future of Children, 4*(1) [Special issue].

Children's Defense Fund. (1993). *State of America's children.* Washington, DC: Author.

Children's Defense Fund. (1994a). *Child care tradeoffs: States make painful choices.* Washington, DC: Author.

Children's Defense Fund. (1994b). *Protecting our children: State and federal policies for exempt child care settings.* Washington, DC: Author.

Clarke-Stewart, K. A. (1989). Infant day care: Maligned or malignant? *American Psychology, 44,* 266-273.

Cohen, A. J. (1996). A brief history of federal financing for child care in the U.S. *Future of Children, 6*(6), 26-40.

Coleman, J. S. (1987). Families and schools. *Educational Researcher, 16,* 32.

Committee for Economic Development. (1993). *Why child care matters.* New York: Author.

Friedman, D. (1987). *Family supportive policies: The corporate decision making process.* New York: Conference Board.

Galinsky, E., Howes, C., Kontos, S., & Shinn, M. B. (1994). *The study of children in family child care and relative care.* New York: Families and Work Institute.

Garmezy, M. (1985). Stress resistant children: The search for protective factors. In J. E. Stevenson (Ed.), *Recent research in developmental psychopathology* (pp. 213-233). Oxford: Pergamon.

Goldstein, J., Freud, A., & Solnit, A. (1973). *Beyond the best interests of the child.* New York: Free Press.

Goldstein, J., Freud, A., & Solnit, A. (1979). *Before the best interests of the child.* New York: Free Press.

Gore, S. (1980). Stress-buffering functions of social supports: An appraisal and clarification of research models. In B. S. Dohrenwend & B. P. Dohrenwend (Eds.), *Stressful life events: Their nature and effects.* New York: John Wiley.

Gormley, W. T., Jr. (1995). *Everybody's children.* Washington, DC: Brookings Institution.

Greenberger, E., & Bronfenbrenner, U. (1989, August). *Maternal employment and the perception of young children.* Paper presented at the 97th annual convention of the American Psychological Association, New Orleans.

Grillo, T. (1991). The mediation alternative: Process changes for women. *Yale Law Journal, 100,* 1545-1610.

Guidibaldi, J., Cleminshaw, H. K., & Perry, J. D. (1983). The effects of divorce on child development. *School Psychology Review, 13,* 300-323.

Hamburg, D. (1982). An outlook on stress research and health. In G. Elliot & C. Eisdorfer (Eds.), *Stress and human health.* New York: Springer.

Hayes, C. D., Palmer, J. L., & Zaslow, M. (Eds.). (1990). *Who cares for America's children?* Washington, DC: National Academy Press.

Helburn, S., Culkin, M., Morris, J., Mocan, N., Howes, C., Phillipsen, L., Bryant, D., Clifford, R., Cryer, D., Peisner-Feinberg, E., Burchinal, M., Kagan, S. L., & Rustici, J. (1995). *Cost, quality, and child outcomes in child care centers.* Final report. Denver: University of Colorado.

Hernandez, D. J. (1988). Demographic trends and the living arrangements of children. In E. M. Hetherington & I. D. Arsteh (Eds.), *Impact of divorce, single-parenting, and step-parenting on children* (pp. 3-22). Hillsdale, NJ: Lawrence Erlbaum.

Hernandez, D. J. (1995). Changing demographics: Past and future demands for services. *Future of Children, 5*(3), 145-160.

Hetherington, E. M., & Camara, K. A. (1984). Families in transition: The process of dissolution and reconstitution. In R. D. Parke (Ed.), *Review of child development research: Vol. 7. The family* (pp. 93-116). Chicago: University of Chicago Press.

Hetherington, E. M., Hagan, M. S., & Anderson, E. R. (1989). Marital transition: A child's perspective. *American Psychology, 44,* 303-312.

Hofferth, S. L., & Wissoker, D. A. (1992). Price, quality, and income in child care choice. *Journal of Human Resources, 27,* 70-111.

Hoffman, L. W. (1986). Work, family and the child. In M. S. Pallak & R. O. Perloff (Eds.), *Psychology and work: Productivity, change and employment.* Washington, DC: American Psychological Association.

Hoffman, L. W. (1989). Effects of maternal employment in the two-parent family. *American Psychology, 44,* 283-292.

Huston, A. C., McLoyd, V. C., & Garcia-Coll, C. (1994). Children in poverty: Issues in contemporary research. *Child Development, 65,* 275-282.

Institute of Medicine. (1989). *Research on children and adolescents with mental, behavioral and developmental disorders.* Washington, DC: National Academy Press.

Joint Commission on Mental Health of Children. (1969). *Crisis in child mental health: Challenge for the 1970s.* New York: Harper & Row.

Kashani, J. H., Beck, N. C., & Hoepper, E. W. (1987). Psychiatric disorders in a community sample of adolescents. *American Journal of Psychiatry, 144,* 584-589.

Kazdin, A. E. (1993). Psychotherapy for children and adolescents: Current progress and future research directions. *American Psychology, 48,* 644-657.

Kelly, J. (1994). The determination of child custody. *Future of Children, 4*(1), 121-142.

Klerman, L. (1991). *Alive and well? Health care for children in America.* New York: National Center for Children in Poverty.

Knitzer, J. (1993). Children's mental health policy: Challenging the future. *Journal of Emotional and Behavioral Disorders, 1*(1), 8-16.

Kurdek, L. A. (1981). An integrative perspective on children's divorce adjustment. *American Psychology, 36,* 856-866.

Kurdek, L. A., & Blisk, D. (1983). Dimensions and correlates of mothers' divorce experiences. *Journal of Divorce, 6,* 1-24.

Lindblom, C. E. (1986). Who needs what social research for policy making? *Knowledge: Creation, Diffusion, Utilization, 7,* 345-366.

Long-term outcomes of early childhood programs. (1995). *Future of Children, 5*(3) [Special issue].

Lubker, M. (1995). *Schools' involvement in Medicaid.* Newsletter of the School of the 21st Century and Family Resource Centers. New Haven, CT: Yale Bush Center in Child Development and Social Policy.

Maccoby, E. E., Kahn, A. L., & Everett, B. A. (1983). The role of psychology research in the formation of policies affecting children. *American Psychologist, 38,* 80-84.

Margolis, L., & Farran, D. (1985). Consequences of unemployment. *The Networker, 4,* 1-3. (Available from the Bush Center in Child Development and Social Policy, Yale University, New Haven, CT)

McCall, R. B., Gregory, T. G., & Murray, J. P. (1984). Community developmental research results to the general public through television. *Developmental Psychology, 20,* 45-54.

McLeod, J. D., & Shanahan, M. J. (1993). Poverty, parenting and children's mental health. *American Sociological Review, 58,* 351-366.

Meltsner, A. L. (1986). The seven deadly sins of policy analysis. *Knowledge: Creation, Diffusion, Utilization, 7,* 367-382.

Miringoff, M. (1993). *The index of social health*. New York: United Nations Children's Fund.

Moen, P., & Dempster, M. C. (1987). Employed parents: Role strain, work time and preferences for working less. *Journal of Marriage and Family, 49,* 579-590.

National Center for Children in Poverty. (1993). *Five million children: An update.* New York: Author.

National Center for Children in Poverty. (1995). States making investments toward the well-being of children. *News & Issues, 5,* 1. (Published by National Center for Children in Poverty, New York)

National Center for Clinical Infant Programs. (1988). *Who will mind the babies?* Washington, DC: Author.

National Commission on Children. (1990). *Beyond rhetoric: A new agenda for children and families.* Washington, DC: U.S. Government Printing Office.

Nelson, J. R., Jr. (1982). The politics of federal day care regulation. In E. Zigler & E. Gordon (Eds.), *Day care: Scientific and social policy issues* (pp. 267-306). Boston: Auburn House.

Office of Technology Assessment. (1986). *Children and mental health: Problems and services* (Background Paper No. OTA-BP-H33). Washington, DC: U.S. Government Printing Office.

Phillips, D. (1987). *Quality child care: What does the research tell us?* Washington, DC: National Association for the Education of Young Children.

Phillips, D. (1995, August). *The future of children.* Presented at the annual meeting of the American Sociological Association, Washington, DC.

President's Commission on Mental Health. (1978). *Task panel reports submitted to the President's Commission on Mental Health* (Vols. 1-4). Washington, DC: U.S. Government Printing Office.

Price, R. H., Cowen, E. L., Lorion, R. P., & Ramos-McKay, J. (Eds.). (1988). *Fourteen ounces of prevention: A casebook for practitioners.* Washington, DC: American Psychological Association.

Rice, D. P., Kelman, S., & Dunmeyer, S. (1990). *The economic costs of alcohol and drug abuse and mental illness: 1985* (Report to the Office of Financing and Coverage Policy, Alcohol, Drug Abuse and Mental Health Administration, U.S. Department of Health and Human Services). San Francisco: University of California, Institutes for Health & Aging.

Richardson, J., Dwyer, K., & McGuigan, K. (1989). Drug and alcohol use among eighth grade children who look after themselves after school. *Pediatrics, 84,* 556-566.

Riessman, F. (1986). Support groups as preventive intervention. In M. Kessler & S. E. Goldstone (Eds.), *A decade of progress in primary prevention.* Hanover, NH: University Press of New England.

Roupp, R., Travers, J., Glantz, F., & Coelen, L. (1979). *Children at the center: Final report of the national day care study* (Vol. 1). Cambridge, MA: Abt.

Rutter, M. (1976). Institute of psychiatry, department of child and adolescent psychiatry. *Psychological Medicine, 6,* 505-516.

Rutter, M. (1980). *Changing youth in a changing society.* Cambridge, MA: Harvard University Press.

Rutter, M. (1983). *Developmental neuropsychiatry.* New York: Guilford.

Rutter, M. (1987). Parental mental disorder as a psychiatric risk factor. In R. Hales & A. Frances (Eds.), *Annual review* (Vol. 6, pp. 647-663). Washington, DC: American Psychiatric Press.

Salkind, N. J. (1983) The effectiveness of early intervention. In E. M. Goets & K. E. Allen (Eds.), *Early childhood education: Special environmental, policy, and legal considerations* (pp. 39-55). Gaithersburg, MD: Aspen.

Sameroff, A. J., Seifer, R., & Zax, M. (1987). Early indicators of developmental risk: The Rochester longitudinal study. *Schizophrenia Bulletin, 13,* 383-394.

Schorr, L. B., & Schorr, D. (1988). *Within our reach: Breaking the cycle of disadvantage.* New York: Doubleday.

Select Panel for the Promotion of Child Health. (1981). *Better health for our children: A national strategy.* Washington, DC: U.S. Government Printing Office.

Seppa, N. (1996, June). Should states keep families together? *APA Monitor,* p. 4.

Stevenson, H. W., & Siegel, A. E. (Eds.). (1984). *Child development research and social policy.* Chicago: University of Chicago Press.

Takanishi, R., DeLeon, P., & Pallak, M. S. (1983). Psychology and public policy affecting children, youth, and families. *American Psychologist, 38,* 67-69.

Tennant, C. (1988). Parental loss in childhood. *Archives of General Psychiatry, 45,* 1045-1050.

Thompson, R. (1993). Developmental research and legal policy: Toward a two-way street. In D. Cicchetti & S. Toth (Eds.), *Child abuse, child development and social policy.* Norwood, NJ: Ablex.

Thompson, R. A., & Wilcox, B. L. (1995). Child maltreatment research: Federal support and policy issues. *American Psychologist, 50,* 789-793.

Tschara, J. M., Johnson, J. R., Kline, M., & Wallerstein, J. S. (1990). Conflict, loss, change and parent-child relationships: Predicting children's adjustment during divorce. *Journal of Divorce, 13,* 1-22.

Tuma, J. M. (1989). Mental health services for children. *American Psychologist, 44,* 188-199.

U.S. Bureau of the Census. (1988). *Money, income, and poverty status of families and persons in the United States* (Current Population Reports). Washington, DC: Author.

U.S. Department of Health and Human Services, Public Health Service. (1991). *Healthy people 2000: National health promotion and disease prevention objectives* (DHHS Publication No. PHS 91-50212). Washington, DC: U.S. Government Printing Office.

U.S. Department of Health and Human Services, Public Health Service. (1995). *Healthy people 2000: Midcourse review and 1995 revisions.* Washington, DC: U.S. Government Printing Office.

Wallerstein, J. (1986). Child of divorce: An overview. *Behavioral Science and Law, 4,* 105-118.

Wallerstein, J., & Corbin, S. (1996). The child and the vicissitudes of divorce. In M. Lewis (Ed.), *Child and adolescent psychiatry: A comprehensive textbook* (pp. 1118-1126). Baltimore: Williams & Wilkins.

Wallerstein, J. S. (1988). *Surviving the breakup.* New York: Basic Books.

Wallerstein, J. S. (1991). Tailoring the intervention to the child in the separating and divorced family. *Family and Conciliation Courts Review, 29,* 448-459.

Weiss, H., & Halpern, R. (1990). *Community-based family support and education programs: Something old or something new.* New York: National Center for Children in Poverty.

White, S. (1988, September). Review of *Within Our Reach. Young Children,* pp. 66-70.

Whitebook, M., Howes, C., & Phillips, D. (1990). *Who cares? Child care teachers and the quality care in America: Final report of the national child care staffing study.* Oakland, CA: Child Care Employee Project.

Women's Bureau. (1994). *1993 handbook on women workers: Trends and issues.* Washington, DC: U.S. Department of Labor.

Yale Bush Center in Child Development and Social Policy. (1992). *The School of the 21st Century: Guidelines for implementation.* New Haven, CT: Yale University, Bush Center in Child Development and Social Policy.

Young, A., Marsland, K., & Zigler, E. (in press). *State regulation governing child care.*

Zeitlin, J. (1989). *Work and family responsibilities: Achieving a balance.* New York: Ford Foundation.

Zervigon-Hakes, A. M. (1995). Translating research findings into large-scale public programs and policy. *Future of Children, 5,* 175-191.

Zigler, E. (1987). A solution to the nation's child care crisis: The School of the 21st Century. In *Parents as Teachers National Center: Investing in the beginning.* St. Louis, MO: Parents as Teachers National Center.

Zigler, E. (1989). The School of the 21st Century. *American Journal of Ortho-psychiatry, 36,* 31-32, 55-59.

Zigler, E., & Berman, W. (1983). Discerning the future of early childhood intervention. *American Psychology, 38,* 894-906.

Zigler, E., & Finn, M. (1981). From problem to solution: Changing public policy as it affects children and families. *Young Children, 36,* 31-32, 55-59.

Zigler, E., & Finn-Stevenson, M. (1987). Applied developmental psychology. In M. Lamb & M. Bornstein (Eds.), *Developmental psychology: An advanced textbook.* Hillsdale, NJ: Lawrence Erlbaum.

Zigler, E., & Finn-Stevenson, M. (1989). Child care in America: From problem to solution. *Educational Policy, 3,* 313-329.

Zigler, E., & Finn-Stevenson, M. (1996). Funding child care and public education. *Future of Children, 6*(6), 104-121.

Zigler, E., & Frank, M. (Eds.). (1988). *The parental leave crisis: Toward a national policy.* New Haven, CT: Yale University Press.

Zigler, E., & Muenchow, S. (1992). *Head Start: The inside story of America's most successful educational experiment.* New York: Basic Books.

Zigler, E., & Styfco, S. (Eds.). (1993). *Head Start and beyond: A national plan for extended childhood intervention.* New Haven, CT: Yale University Press.

Zigler, E., & Valentine, J. (Eds.). (1979). *Project Head Start: A legacy of the War on Poverty.* New York: Free Press.

Zill, N., Sigal, H., & Brim, O. G., Jr. (1983). Development of childhood social indicators. In E. Zigler, S. L. Kagan, & E. Klugman (Eds.), *Children, families, and government: Perspectives on American social policy.* New York: Cambridge University Press.

Defining and Implementing School Readiness: Challenges for Families, Early Care and Education, and Schools

SHARON L. KAGAN

MICHELLE J. NEUMAN

There is widespread popular sentiment that readying young children for school is important not only to their school success but to their long-term life success. Such sentiment is not unfounded; confirming what has been recognized by parents and child development experts for years, new brain research indicates that the first years of life have important long-lasting effects on children's brain functioning and their overall development (Carnegie Task Force on Meeting the Needs of Young Children, 1994). This research, along with decades of work that has preceded it, points to the critical need for attending to children's early years—to providing them with a healthy start that readies them for school and later life.

Beyond broad agreement about the importance of readying children for school, the readiness waters are murky. First, there is little consensus on precisely what constitutes readiness. Is readiness simply the recitation of simple facts, numbers, shapes, and colors, or is it more fundamental? Does and should readiness include how children approach learning? Does and should it include children's health and mental health? How, indeed, do we define readiness?

Beyond such definitional ambiguity, there is a lack of clarity regarding how the nation should go about implementing readiness and who should be responsible for doing so. Are parents responsible for their children's readiness? Should communities offer universal early care and education[1] services to children under age 5, as they do educational services to children over 5? Should parents be expected to pay for these services or are they a public responsibility? Are parents entitled to parenting education and family support services or should they remain services restricted to the few?

The purpose of this chapter is to explore these issues—to first examine what is really meant by readiness and then to discuss how readiness should be implemented, considering the serious issues associated with such implementation. Building on this discussion, we offer policy recommendations to be considered for inclusion in *Healthy People 2010*. We suggest that the two major themes of this chapter—defining and implementing readiness—are not unrelated; how we define readiness may affect who is responsible for its implementation, and conversely, who implements readiness may dramatically influence how it is defined. Our premise is that a narrow definition of readiness and a narrow construction of who is responsible for its implementation will yield youngsters and a society unprepared to meet each others' needs. Therefore, we suggest that readiness must be defined broadly, and relatedly, there must be broad and shared responsibility for its implementation. We urge the acceptance of the National Education Goals Panel (NEGP) definition of readiness and advocate that readiness be the responsibility of families and an array of institutions including early care and education, family support, schools, and communities.

Defining Readiness: What Does It Really Mean?

Historical Definitions of Readiness

Debated for decades, definitions of readiness vary both over time and within given periods of time. Historically, two major constructs—readiness for learning and readiness for school—have competed with each other and undergird much of the readiness confusion. Leading theorists in child development and learning have defined *readiness for learning* as the average age at which individuals reach a level of development capable of learning specific material. When elaborating on this definition, theorists offer individual interpretations of the definition. For example, Gagne (1970) suggests that readiness for learning involves attentional set, motivation, and developmental status. Piaget (1970) focuses on the importance of the learner's internal forces—such as how children integrate new stimuli with previously acquired information. Bruner (1960) and colleagues attribute greater significance to external, environmental forces. But all share the belief that readiness for learning is intimately tied to developmental processes that evolve in fairly predictable ways. Indeed, children are truly born ready to learn.

Though conceptually confounded with readiness for learning, *readiness for school* is an entirely different construct. It is linked to children's knowledge at a moment in time of specific cognitive and linguistic skills, such as the ability to identify colors by name, or being able to copy a square. The more rigid construct of school readiness historically has most often been equated with reading readiness. It is also manifest in other subject areas that demand a fixed level of physical, intellectual, and social development sufficient to enable children to fulfill school requirements and to assimilate curriculum content.

These two constructs—readiness for learning and readiness for school—have given birth to a third, *maturational readiness,* which has evolved from the tension between the two. In line with the basic tenet of school readiness, maturational readiness expects children to attain a certain specified standard before entering school, yet like readiness to learn, it acknowledges individual variation. It recognizes that not all children will attain a common standard at the same time. Consequently, many maturationists advocate that children be retained from entering formal schooling until they are determined to be maturationally or developmentally ready.

A fourth construct, advanced by Vygotsky (1978), claims that children grow into the intellectual life around them and that their development is stimulated by learning. Consequently, rather than considering readiness as a gate, keeping the "unready" out of school, this construct opens the gates and says all should come because learning takes place within the context of social interactions. Vygotskians, therefore, support the notion that schools must be ready for children, for all children, regardless of what cognitive factoids children do or do not possess.

A More Recent Definition

However accurate, these approaches have failed to yield a consensus on what constitutes child readiness. The lack of such consensus became publicly apparent in the early 1990s when the NEGP declared as the first national educational goal that by the year 2000, all children should start school ready to learn. Initial response to this goal was swift and critical: Early childhood educators claimed that children begin life ready to learn; evaluation specialists said that tools were not available to measure the goal; others noted that the very constructs that defined readiness were not delineated.

To address these concerns, the NEGP appointed a Technical Planning Group to forge a consensus regarding the definition of children's early learning and development. Building on past work, five dimensions were identified: physical health and motor development, social and emotional development, approaches toward learning, language usage, and general knowledge. To amplify these dimensions and thereby more precisely define readiness, 30 papers by nationally recognized scholars were commissioned, and based on their work and that of others, a synthesis document was prepared. The synthesis document was widely reviewed by over 500 researchers, practitioners, parents, and politicians before it was finalized (Kagan, Moore, & Bredekamp, 1995). It should be noted that none of the dimensions or their amplification presented in the synthesis was new; rather, the document represented a codification of what was already known regarding children's early learning and development.

More specifically, the first dimension addresses the physical well-being and motor development of children, conditions that are central to their entire learning experience. Physical well-being—physical development—includes children's overall rates of growth, levels of physical fitness, body physiology, and physical abilities such as gross and fine motor skills and sensorimotor skills. It also includes the context of development—the perinatal context, caregiving environment, and use of health care.

The second dimension relates to children's social development—the ability to form and sustain social relationships with both peers and adults—and emotional development—how children express their own feelings and how they manifest sensitivity and empathy to the feelings of others. Patterns of emotion, for example, joy, fear, grief, or delight, result from children's interactions and help to shape a young child's self-concept. Emotional development also affects how children express their own feelings and how they manifest sensitivity and empathy to the feelings of others. Social development is the ability to form and sustain social relationships with peers and adults and encompasses variables such as cooperation, companionship, and support for others.

Approaches toward learning—the third dimension—is the least understood and least researched dimension. It includes both children's predispositions and learning styles. Predispositions such as gender, temperament, and cultural patterns and values are genetically and culturally embedded early on and influence the way a child both thinks about and acts on learning opportunities. Learning styles are the way that a child approaches the process of learning, for example, through openness, curiosity, initiative, imagination, or invention.

The fourth dimension focuses on language development, how a child acquires linguistic forms and procedures as well as rules and customs for expression and interpretation. Both verbal language and emerging literacy, two important components of language development for young children, are strongly dependent on children's experiences within their homes and communities. Verbal language comprises listening, speaking, and vocabulary use among other skills. Emerging literacy includes both extracting meaning from printed symbols as well as decoding words. It is important to note that previous definitions of language development have failed to account for how English proficiency is acquired by children whose primary language is not English. The NEGP document notes that when educators assess youngsters' cognitive and linguistic abilities, they must be aware of cultural and linguistic factors that influence the way children express themselves.

Finally, the fifth dimension—cognition and general knowledge—is the one most frequently associated with early development and learning. Although the public generally limits cognition and general knowledge dimension to social-conventional knowledge—such as the names for colors and numbers—in fact, this dimension is far more complex and involves all types of knowledge. For example, it includes physical knowledge, which is the knowledge of objects in external reality, and logico-mathematical knowledge, which refers to the relationships created in the mind among objects, events, or people. Through the interaction of these three kinds of knowledge, children develop cognitive competencies, including problem solving, mathematical knowledge, social knowledge, and imagination. Often, children's cognitive competencies are a reflection of cultural preferences and patterns.

Caveats Associated With Defining Readiness

Although this document has been widely accepted, several major caveats characterize it and would—in all likelihood—characterize most efforts to define readiness. First, they are inextricably linked. The five dimensions—the very idea of readiness—must be considered as a totality to capture the complex interconnectedness of early development and learning. Second, the amount of information and the state of knowledge on each of the dimensions is not even. Consequently, some of the dimensions of readiness are more clearly delineated than others. Third, individual child performance is multidimensional, episodic, and highly variable across the dimensions. As a result, it is impossible to establish a threshold for readiness, above which children are deemed developmentally ready and below which they are deemed unready for school. Instead, the dimensions need to be considered as an attempt to amplify the range of variables associated with early development and learning. Fourth, conventional definitions of early development and learning have not attended to individual, cultural, and contextual variation. Rather, they have tended to focus on genetic and/or developmental variation, with the result that cultural and contextual differences have often been misinterpreted as deficiencies. Moreover, approaches to assessment that have been predicated on developmental variation in the absence of cultural and contextual variation have de facto ignored cultural competence and used majority-culture norms to measure competence. In contrast, the NEGP report attempted to recognize that individual, cultural, and contextual variables are critical to children's understanding of the world, how they process information, interpret experiences, and present themselves.

Finally, whether children attain healthy development on all of these dimensions is highly influenced by available family and community services and supports. Indeed, the report—as any definition of readiness should—emphasizes the importance of families and communities in shaping children's early experiences and encounters with their environments. The important role of communities in supporting children and in supporting parents in their own roles as nurturers and providers must be considered central to understanding readiness. In other words, readiness was conceptualized as not simply inherent to the child, but inherent to the community and society. As a result, the report called for increasing the commitment to children's well-being as a social imperative—one that is essential to the future well-being of the nation. Moreover, it noted that the healthy development of young children can only be achieved with the cooperation and support of societal institutions including government, corporate America, the media, schools, and families.

Adopting much of the thinking that characterized the NEGP work, this chapter—like the NEGP document—does not use the word *readiness* to refer to a specific set of skills or abilities demonstrated by children at a given point in time. Rather, we use readiness to suggest an overall condition of children, families, support institutions, and communities that promotes the healthy development and learning of young children. Readiness is not a finite product or state to be used to gauge or label the status of an individual child; rather, readiness herein connotes the overall state of the nation's commitment to its young children. As such, we now turn to discuss how various institutional players can and must adopt a renewed commitment to young children. We term this *implementing readiness*.

Implementing Readiness:
The Role of Families and Family Support Programs

Without families who are ready to support and nurture their young children, youngsters' early learning and development will be thwarted. Families are not simply the cornerstone of life for the young child; they are the instruments through which children come to see, understand, and interpret their worlds. Families are the primary and most responsible agents who craft children's early development and learning; they are the very foundation on which readiness is built. Acknowledging the importance of families to children's lives, a specific objective of the first education goal is that every parent will be a child's first teacher and devote time each day to helping his or her preschool child learn (Kagan et al., 1995). More generally, the objective suggests that parents and families must engage in behaviors that contribute to children's development. Recognizing that such parenting is not innate, but demands skills and resources, the objective calls for access to training and support that parents need to fulfill this responsibility. We turn to a discussion of the behaviors and attitudes that contribute to healthy development and then discuss the new family support movement as a means of fostering such behaviors.

Family Behaviors and Attitudes That Contribute to Children's Early Development and Learning

Research confirms the importance of families to children's development and school success (Moore, 1990; Powell, 1990, 1995). Compelling longitudinal research indicates that maternal attitudes and child-rearing attitudes and practices in the first years of life are linked to a child's subsequent performance in school. In a Stanford University study, measures of maternal attitudes and behavior correlated with child readiness at age 5 or 6 and later school achievement at age 12. The maternal measures—which included expectations of achievement, affective tone and style, maternal teaching and communication styles, strategies for controlling child behavior, and attributions of child success and failure in school—were a much stronger predictor of child outcomes than socioeconomic status, and the correlation between maternal variables and school achievement was not a function of maternal IQ (Hess, Holloway, Dickson, & Price, 1984). There is also evidence that the quality of the home environment—the level of parental support of early cognitive and social-emotional development— during the first years of life correlates with school achievement (Bradley & Caldwell, 1984). Parents who are supportive of their preschool-age children are likely to be supportive of their school-age children, although the family's influence in school achievement for older children may subside as the influences of school and peers take on a larger role (Powell, 1995).

Parental attitudes and behavior are intertwined with their daily interactions with their children. Therefore, it is difficult to isolate the most important parental influences on children's early development and learning (Powell, 1995). In fact, there does not seem to be one single parental attitude or action that predicts school readiness or achievement more than others. Rather, research points to a group of parental beliefs and practices that mesh to positively influence children's early development and learning (Powell, 1995):

- Parents with a constructivist perspective on development (who view development as a complex process that involves the child as an active contributor to his or her own development) promote children's cognitive outcomes.

- Parents who have an accurate understanding of their child's intellectual abilities create an environment that enhances their child's intellectual performance.

- The most effective parental teaching strategies are those that stimulate the child's own thinking and promote active verbal engagement in task, provided that this is appropriate to the child's developmental level.

- Attentive, warm, and nonrestrictive maternal behaviors during infancy and preschool years foster intellectual development.

- Direct control tactics in teaching and disciplinary situations are negatively related to school-related abilities, possibly because children learn that the capability to solve problems belongs primarily to the adult.

- Parents may create a positive environment for their children to acquire reading skills by providing access to reading and writing materials and limiting the amount of television they watch. The quantity and quality of parental reading to the child contributes to children's early literacy.

Although desirable, how prevalent are these behaviors among parents and families today? In reality, the pressures on families today are overwhelming as parents must balance their work and child-rearing responsibilities. Indeed, with over 60% of mothers in the workforce, almost half of those with children under 1 year of age, it is not surprising that two thirds of parents with children under 18 feel that they do not have enough time to spend with their children (Families and Work Institute, 1994). The limited time that parents and children have together makes how that time is spent all the more important.

Frequently used indexes of parenting include how often parents read to and actively engage in activities with their children. According to the National Center for Education Statistics, family members read to 78% of all preschoolers three or more times a week in 1993, up from 71% in 1991. About 41% of preschoolers are told stories several times per week and about 39% of preschoolers visit the library once per month. More than a third of 3- to 6-year-olds learn songs or music regularly from their parents, and one third engage in arts and crafts with their parents on a regular basis (Wright, Hausken, & West, 1994). Other studies suggest that parents spend very little instructional time with their young children. Survey data from the early 1980s found that 3- to 5-year-old children spent only 7 minutes per day reading or being read to, whereas they spent almost 2 hours watching television during the week and slightly more on weekends (Timmer, Eccles, & O'Brien, 1985).

Are there differences in the ways in which different parents spend time and engage in activities with their children? Research indicates that parents with more formal education spend more time reading to their children and watch less television than those with less education (Eccles, O'Brien, & Timmer, 1985-1986; Timmer et al., 1985; Wright et al., 1994). Some variability within socioeconomic groups regarding the amount of stimulating experiences children encounter in their home environments (Heath, 1983; Teale, 1986) has been found, with low-income families engaging their children in storybook reading less frequently than middle- and upper-income counterparts (Teale, 1986).

Employment may relate to how much time parents spend with their children. Although mothers who work outside the home spend less total time with their children, several studies suggest that employed mothers are more highly interactive with their young children than homemakers (Zaslow, Pedersen, Suwalsky, Cain, & Fivel, 1985). Working mothers spend an average of 11 minutes a day reading, conversing, or playing with their children during the week, and 30 minutes a day on weekends. Homemakers spend 30 minutes each day during the week, and 36 minutes a day on weekends. The time fathers spend with their children does not seem to change according to whether or not their spouse is in the workforce (Eccles et al., 1985-1986; Timmer et al., 1985).

Although these data suggest that there are very low levels of instructional exchanges between parents and young children, there are opportunities to enhance parents' participation in their children's early education. Parents want to spend their precious time with their children in a manner that supports their early learning. In fact, there is evidence that parents are committed to and interested in promoting their children's growth and development (Powell, 1990), but lack the guidance or the resources to do so.

Engaging Parents and Families:
A Case for Family Support

What do families need to strengthen their roles as their children's first teachers? Families need information and support. Today, a growing number of volumes on parenting and preparing children for school line bookstore shelves and close to a hundred parenting magazines are thriving. Parents are going on-line to get advice on child-rearing issues over the Internet, and more than 2 million parents have called one of the many helplines in the United States (Shore, 1994). Despite the use of reading material, media, and other information sources, parents still rely on friends and relatives, as well as on formal and informal interactions with professionals, to gather information on parenting. Indeed, helping professionals have been found to be more useful sources of parenting information than mass media sources (Crase, Carlson, & Kontos, 1981; Hughes & Durio, 1983; Keopke & Williams, 1989; Mullis & Mullis, 1983). Parenting education programs—home visiting programs and child-rearing classes—have become part of a burgeoning set of services.

Such programs form the basis for an emerging movement deemed "family support programs." These family support efforts provide emotional, informational, and instrumental supports to families as they confront the challenging task of raising their children. Family support began in the late 1970s as a grassroots movement, largely characterized by scattered programs where staff provided informal support services to parents with young children. Diverse and highly idiosyncratic, the programs existed independently of one another, although they shared a desire to serve entire families and to do so in a way that was nonjudgmental, highly inclusive of all family members, and preventive in orientation. During this early era, discrete programs proliferated, with few opportunities for linkage among them.

Scattered programs slowly became aware of one another and decided to come together to share their work, philosophies, and concerns. During this period, in the early to mid-1980s, meetings were held, organizations were formed, and the ideas that framed the individual programs were codified into a working set of principles: decentralized decision making, according power to the consumer, preventing problems before they occur, family inclusiveness, and voluntary participation. Once codified, these principles guided the development of many new programs and formed the basis for the emergence of family support to the public agenda.

As family support emerged as a set of principles, it became apparent that its ideas were not unique to these programs. Similar ideas were being discussed as part of reform efforts that were taking hold in other domains—business, education, consumer protection, and preventive and mental health care. In fact, the ideas that undergirded family support became popular and began to transcend "the programs originally designed to contain them" (Kagan & Weissbourd, 1994, p. 475). Family support became an approach not limited to discrete family support programs but one that could be adapted and infused into mainstream social institutions, including public schools, health care, and social services. And isolated institutions began to adopt a family support approach.

As family support burgeoned from programs to principles to an approach, its ideas have caught on. More and more, family support is finding its way into diverse facets of the American agenda. Family support has been manifest in legislation; it has been infused into corporate policies, striving to make business and industry more family supportive; and it has been embraced by many conventional social services bureaucracies. Already a movement, presently family support appears to be on the cusp of creating a new normative system of family support. Such a normative system suggests that family support will no longer be considered haphazard or unique; it will become what is normal, what prevails. Family support would become so enmeshed in the social fabric of this nation that it would not be regarded as a treatment or intervention, but as a condition of life (Garbarino & Kostelny, 1994). Today, it is estimated that some 2,500 family support programs exist, with federal funding supporting some of them. Moreover, family support principles characterize many more programs, institutions, and corporations.

As progress is made, the challenges to becoming a normative system reveal themselves. First and foremost among current issues in family support is quality. To date, there has been limited attention to defining quality for family support programs for several reasons. For the past decade, as noted earlier, efforts have focused on developing basic principles and communicating them to the field and to the public. The pragmatic need to plan and sustain programs superseded academic efforts to define quality. There have been only limited opportunities for leaders in the field to come together for this purpose. The field has also been in a stage of experimentation and exploration regarding what family support means; it has not been ready to define quality. Yet the need for specifying quality in family support is crucial. Without a definition and standards of quality for programs, it is difficult to encourage and guide new programs, train workers for the field, frame policy to safeguard quality, and evaluate quality (Kagan, 1994).

Recently, however, the Family Resource Coalition's Best Practice Project has convened a national constituency of practitioners, academicians, and leaders in the field to define what constitutes excellence in family support practice. The volume, *Guidelines for Family Support Practice* (Family Resource Coalition, 1996) discusses guidelines for implementing family support principles, giving examples of best practices from the field. The question is not whether good practice exists—it certainly does. Rather, the challenge is to capitalize on what we know and to make this information accessible as the movement grows and family support programs spread across the nation (Kagan, 1994).

A second and related issue in family support is professionalization. Some are concerned that if family support—always a grassroots movement—becomes overly professionalized, it will lose the very vitality, responsiveness, and inclusiveness that distinguishes family support from conventional social services. Another school of thought suggests that without professionalization, the movement will not mature to its potential or garner recognition and autonomy for its workers. Irrespective of which stance is advocated, how such professionalization would unfold is being considered. According to conventional approaches to professionalization, to become a profession family support would need to define a body of knowledge, discern the content of training, and determine standards for credentialing its workers (Kagan & Weissbourd, 1994). Not necessarily under the rubric of professionalization, many of these efforts are currently under way. The clear challenge is for these efforts to continue without losing the field's unique commitment to inclusiveness and diversity.

Clearly, family support as an active movement has outpaced family support as a purely analytic endeavor; nowhere is this more apparent than in the data on program effectiveness. Indeed, it has been noted specifically that family support program expansion has outpaced research on its implementation and effectiveness (Powell, 1994). Fueled in part by the need for programs, there are several important methodological considerations that have impeded the rapid evolution of evaluative data. In part, this is due to the lack of availability of valid and reliable measures. But this is not the sole or primary reason for the slow evaluation pace. Indeed, research methodology is not highly advanced because family support programs are very difficult to evaluate. Programs, and therefore sample sizes, are often very small, and because each program differs, research designs must be tailored to the particular program. Random assignment is often impossible due to ethical, political, and logistical reasons; quasi-experimental designs with lower reliability and validity are used instead. Staff are rightly concerned that most evaluation tools do not capture all the effects of programs on families, especially family functioning. Similarly, economic assessment is still in early stages of development.

Evaluating family support programs remains an urgent, but complicated, task. Yet there are some promising evaluation efforts (see Powell, 1994). For example, some involve participants and program staff in the evaluation process. Others describe program implementation and identify the contributions of program and population characteristics to program outcomes. There has been growing interest in context; research questions have been refined to include data that can be used for improving program design. In addition, the national evaluation of family support programs has used the theories of change approach, which suggests that there is an implicit theory that every person brings to the table about what is to be changed in programs or in communities. The approach asks practitioners and parents to identify their short- and long-range goals (usually in terms of specific outcomes), activities that they feel lead to these outcomes, and how this change is expected to occur. The benefit of a theories of change approach is that it enables the clear specification of activities and desired outcomes. In making change processes quite explicit, the approach serves as a guide for practitioners and researchers as they coconstruct the evaluation design. Despite these challenges that family support must confront in the coming years, the family support movement represents an important asset to the nation as it considers readying children for their futures. Few other efforts so honor families while providing them with the support and resources to carry out their parenting responsibilities effectively.

Implementing Readiness: The Role of Early Care and Education

Early care and education services also play an essential role in enabling children to succeed in school. Such settings can expose children to opportunities for social, cognitive, emotional, and physical development. Despite this possibility and despite the reality that 98% of all children actually have some form of out-of-home services before first grade, American early care and education is as fraught with problems as it is with possibilities. Several are discussed below, with their implications for implementing readiness.

The Quality Imperative and the Quality Problem

Quality early care and education prepares children for later educational achievement. Recent studies have linked quality early care and education to the healthy cognitive, social, and emotional development of all young children (Cost, Quality, and Child Outcomes Study Team, 1995) and in particular to low-income children's later social and cognitive functioning (Barnett, 1995; Gomby, Larner, Stevenson, Lewit, & Behrman, 1995; Phillips, 1995; Schweinhart, Barnes, & Weikart, 1993; Yoshikawa, 1995). Children who develop reasoning and problem-solving skills within a quality early care and education environment are likely to be more cooperative and considerate of others and to have more self-esteem. Many of these positive effects may linger and contribute to children's increased cognitive abilities, positive classroom learning behavior, long-term school success, and even improved likelihood of long-term social and economic self-sufficiency (Gomby et al., 1995; Poersch, Adams, & Sandfort, 1994; Schweinhart et al., 1993). Children attending lower-quality programs, in contrast, are more likely to encounter difficulties with language and social development and less likely to have mastered age-appropriate behaviors or expected levels of development (Whitebook, Howes, & Phillips, 1989).

In spite of this child development research, quality early care and education is scant. The recent Cost, Quality, and Child Outcomes four-state study found that 86% of child care centers provided mediocre- to poor-quality care (Cost, Quality, and Child Outcomes Study Team, 1995). The United States also faces a quality crisis in family child care. Another recent study found that 16% of regulated family child care homes and up to 50% of unregulated homes offered substandard care (Galinsky, Howes, Kontos, & Shinn, 1994).

The quality crisis in early care and education has many roots. Historically, the care and education of young children has been considered the primary responsibility of the family and, therefore, outside the realm of government. Public and private institutions only intervened when families failed or were deemed deficient. This deficit approach continues today. Treated as necessary evils of a humane society, the American public funds many social services—including early care and education—with reluctance. It is therefore not surprising that such targeted programs carry with them great stigma and low funding levels. In contrast, financial support and government intervention in early care and education for nonpoor families has only taken place during periods of crisis, such as during World War II or the Great Depression. With the end of the crisis, public support and financial backing for universal early care and education has quickly waned. Unlike support for the public school system, early care and education for all children has never held a prominent place on the U.S. social agenda.

Social ambivalence toward motherhood has also contributed to the low levels of commitment to a quality early care and education system. Instead of viewing early care and education as an important opportunity for children's learning, the United States has resisted policies and programs that appear to intervene in any way with family life and motherhood. Indeed, many Americans continue to believe that out-of-home care is harmful, despite evidence to the contrary (Gomby et al., 1995; Hayes, Palmer, & Zaslow, 1990; National Institute of Child Health and Human Development, 1996; Phillips & Howes, 1987). Additionally, Americans dismiss the care of young children as mindless, custodial work, devaluing the contributions of stay-at-home mothers. Although the public continues to uphold national policies that lead to nonparental care for more and more young children, it stops short of calling for policies to protect its youngest citizens from harm and promote their development while in out-of-home care. Such attitudinal ambivalence has manifested itself in ambivalence in early care and education policy, leaving support for early care and education open to recurrent debate and inconsistent investment of resources.

The Access Imperative and the Access Problem

If the United States expects all children to start school ready to learn, universal access to quality early care and education services must be a national priority. Although more than 13 million children from birth to age 5 in the United States attend early care and education programs on a regular basis (U.S. Department of Education, National Center for Education Statistics, 1995), consistent quality services are far from universal. Unlike education, which is an entitlement for all children, early care and education enrollment is not equally distributed throughout the population. Low-income children are much less likely to attend early care and education programs than their higher-income peers (U.S. General Accounting Office, 1993). Only 50% of children living in households with incomes of $10,000 or less regularly attend early care and education, compared to more than 75% of children in households with incomes in excess of $75,000 (U.S. Department of Education, National Center for Education Statistics, 1995).

Looking at preschool enrollment in 1990, only 35% of poor and near-poor 3- and 4-year-olds participated in preschools compared to 45% of the nonpoor population. The highest participation rates—60%—were among children with annual family incomes above $63,370 for a family of four (U.S. General Accounting Office, 1993). Minority children—Hispanic preschoolers in particular—are less likely than other children to have early childhood program experience before beginning school (West, Hausken, &

Collins, 1993). The U.S. General Accounting Office found that children from immigrant families or linguistically isolated households, families where parents did not work, families where parents had not completed high school, and single-parent families had substantially lower rates of preschool participation than other children. Furthermore, poor or near-poor children in these groups—those most in need of quality early care and education services to support their development and learning—had the lowest rates of preschool participation (U.S. General Accounting Office, 1993).

Even within Head Start, the nation's primary federal program to prepare poor children to start school ready to learn, access is limited. Head Start reaches a fraction of those eligible, and those served by Head Start are not representative of poor families in general (Hofferth, 1995). More broadly, there is growing concern that Head Start, because it is predominantly composed of part-day programs, may be inaccessible to single parents who are struggling to combine child rearing and work (Hofferth, 1995).

Access to early care and education services appears to be particularly low for working-poor and blue-collar families who neither qualify for subsidies nor can afford child care fees (Phillips, Voran, Kisker, Howes, & Whitebook, 1994; Whitebook et al., 1989). Findings from these studies suggest that race and income determine whether children will begin school with quality early care and education experiences to ready them for school success.

Indeed, when disadvantaged children do have access to early care and education, they often do not receive quality services. The General Accounting Office found that more than half—59%—of the disadvantaged children who do attend preschool are in programs that may not provide the full range of child development, health, and parent services that are needed to optimize school readiness (U.S. General Accounting Office, 1995a). The children who would benefit the most from quality early care and education programs are the least likely to be attending them.

The Infrastructure Problem

Accessible quality early care and education programs cannot be achieved in isolation; they must be part of a quality system. To date, the early care and education field has focused on promoting direct services, the programs that touch the lives of children and families day to day. However, a system depends on essential functions that act behind the scenes to support direct services—the infrastructure. Scholars have identified five key elements to the essential functions of the infrastructure: parent information and engagement; professional development; facility licensing, enforcement, and accreditation; funding and financing; and government and planning. As with any system of services, quality early care and education will function effectively only when all the components work together.

In each component of the infrastructure, scattered reform efforts are now under way, and some progress has been made. However, what resembles an infrastructure is fragmented and reform efforts are too few and far between to support consistent quality programs across the country. The lack of commitment to the development of an infrastructure is made even more complicated by the lack of coordination in direct service programs themselves. Programs emerge episodically and inconsistently, emanating from different legislative mandates, funding streams, regulatory systems, and administrative agencies. Some programs fall under the jurisdiction of state departments of education, others are overseen by departments of health, and still others by departments of welfare or social services (Kagan, Goffin, Golub, & Pritchard, 1995). A recent study documented 90 different federal programs sitting in 11 federal agencies and 20 offices (U.S. General Accounting Office, 1995b). Equally inconsistent, state-supported programs vary from state to state and even within states. Given attitudinal ambivalence toward early care and education generally and the confusion of an uncoordinated set of programs specifically, it is not surprising that little attention has been given to the development of an early care and education infrastructure.

The Financial Problem

For all children to have access to quality early care and education programs, the system must be adequately funded. Children of all incomes, races, and needs do better in higher-quality programs than in lower-quality programs, and these programs cost somewhat more (Cost, Quality, and Child Outcomes Study Team, 1995). Furthermore, the components of the infrastructure to support a quality system discussed earlier also depend on adequate funding. Thus, current underinvestment in early care and education prevents a quality early care and education system from developing and prevents children across the United States from obtaining needed services.

Inadequate public funding burdens parents with the majority of the costs of early care and education and contributes to inequitable service delivery. Roughly 80% of all early care and education costs are absorbed by families, with the remaining 20% distributed among the government (via program and consumer subsidies), foundations, and corporations. Families with lower incomes bear a larger burden of the early care and education expense—and receive lower-quality services in return. A national study found that employed mothers with incomes under $15,000 spent about 25% of their income on early care and education (averaging $63 per week), whereas those with an annual family income of $50,000 or more spent 6% of their income on early care and education programs for their young children (averaging $85 per week) (Hofferth, Brayfield, Deich, & Holcomb, 1991). Those families who cannot afford the full cost of early care and education must rely on the small stream of public subsidies to enroll their children in programs. However, in five of six states surveyed in a 1994 study, parents were on waiting lists for subsidies to purchase early care and education, but these subsidies were not forthcoming because of limited funding (U.S. General Accounting Office, 1994). Limited subsidies constrain parents' early care and education choices. Without financial assistance, lower-income parents are often forced to settle with lower-quality care for their children.

Low public investment in early care and education also jeopardizes children by forcing programs to operate with inadequate funds to provide quality. Whereas the average of $5,800 that governments spend per child on a year of public school pays for just 30 hours of education a week for about 40 weeks a year, the combined parent and government spending of $3,000 to $5,000 per child for a year of full-time early care and education pays for 35 to 50 hours of early care and education per week for 50 to 52 weeks per year (Casper, 1995; Cost, Quality, and Child Outcomes Study Team, 1995; Hofferth et al., 1991; Sugarman, 1995). Early care and education workers subsidize the underfunded system with their low wages. Consequently, the field struggles to retain and nurture a well-qualified workforce as staff turnover remains high. Given the relatively large number of hours paid for by the relatively small investment in early care and education compared to school, it should not be surprising that the quality of early care and education is so low. As with families, early care and education needs support to fulfill its responsibility for readying children for school success.

Implementing Readiness: The Role of Schools

Children begin school with a range of experiences and backgrounds. Teachers face the challenge of meeting the needs of children who are both demographically and developmentally diverse. A recent study found that of 4-year-olds, 9 out of 10 could button their own clothes and hold a pencil properly, and 7 out of 10 could identify primary colors by name. However, only 6 out of 10 could count to 20 and recognize the letters of the alphabet (Zill, Collins, & Hausken, 1995). The sociodemographic risk factors that children bring with them to kindergarten have been found to correlate with accomplishments and difficulties across developmental domains. Specifically, researchers have identified five family risk factors that negatively affect a child's development (Zill et al., 1995): mothers with less than a high school education; families below the poverty line; mothers who are non-English-language dominant; mothers who were unmarried at the time of the child's birth; and single-parent families. In general, children with more risk factors are more likely to experience more developmental difficulties and fewer accomplishments, even after controlling for other child and family characteristics. This is a serious finding given that half of all preschoolers are affected by at least one risk factor, and 15% by three or more. Furthermore, these risk factors are associated with children's learning difficulties after they enter school. As a recent study notes, "While there has always been variation in children entering kindergarten, the commitment to meeting the educational and developmental needs of *all* children in an increasingly diverse society presents greater challenges to teachers and schools" (Zill et al., 1995, p. viii). In the classroom, teachers face the delicate balance of promoting the development of children with early literacy and numeracy while encouraging basic skills in children without them.

Accommodating the differing needs of young students is not an easy charge. It requires teachers with warmth, sensitivity, and patience as well as with adequate training and resources. Kindergartens have taken various approaches to promote early school success and reduce the risk of school failure. The first (and less favored) approach expects children to be ready for schools by structuring homogeneous kindergartens for a heterogeneous population. The second approach—flexible programs to meet the needs of demographically diverse students—gives schools the responsibility of being ready for children.

Entrance Age and Extra-Year Programs

Favoring a maturationist view that older children may be more developmentally ready to learn and succeed in school, schools and parents have called for raising the entrance age to kindergarten (see Powell, 1995). In addition, some parents—especially middle-class and wealthy parents—choose to keep their children out of school an extra year and enroll them at age 6 rather than the traditional age 5 (Goal One Ready Schools Resource Group, 1995). These parents fear pushing their children beyond their developmental level (Graue, 1993a) and hope that an extra year of social, cognitive, and physical maturation will prime them for kindergarten success (Goal One Ready Schools Resource Group, 1995). Children of lower-income parents who may not be able to afford quality early care and education programs for an additional year may be disadvantaged by such redshirting. On the other hand, holding children out of kindergarten may not even be effective. Research shows that within kindergarten classrooms, younger children do receive slightly lower scores on standardized tests through at least first grade (Sheehan, Cryan, Wiechel, & Bandy-Hedden, 1991; Shepard & Smith, 1986). However, by third grade differences in test performance between older and younger children disappear (Shepard & Smith, 1986).

Programs that give children the "gift of time" gained popularity in the 1980s (Powell, 1995). Developmental or junior kindergartens aim to give children considered developmentally immature 2 years of formal schooling before entering first grade. The first year resembles a preschool program, and the second is similar to traditional kindergarten. Transitional first grade enrolls children who have completed kindergarten but are deemed unready for first grade. Children may also be retained for an additional year of regular kindergarten. Although these extra-year programs try to reduce the risk of school failure, studies have found this approach to be ineffective in the long term (Graue, 1993b; Gredler, 1992; Karweit & Wasik, 1994; Meisels, 1992; Shepard, 1989).

Not only do these approaches have limited long-term success, but they place the burden on children to be ready for school. Separating "unready" children from their peers may hurt their self-esteem by making them feel different or that they are being punished (Bredekamp & Shepard, 1988). More important, if schools were committed to accommodating the variation among children's development and competencies, there would be no reason to hold back children (Goal One Ready Schools Resource Group, 1995). Indeed, all schools need to ready themselves for all children, regardless of children's apparent developmental readiness.

Transitions and Developmentally Appropriate Schools

The transition to formal schooling is a huge change for children and their families. All families can benefit from support during this period as their children leave the comfort of home or an early care and education setting for schools. Children learn and develop better if they experience continuity between the time periods and spheres of their lives. Children who do not make successful transitions may be less successful in school, have difficulties making friends, and may be vulnerable to mental health and adjustment problems (Goal One Ready Schools Resource Group, 1995). Facilitating transitions so that children and families adjust to the new learning environment is a crucial part of sharing the responsibility for preparing children for school success. It requires interaction among homes, schools, early care and education programs, and communities. Unfortunately, research suggests that this support is not widespread.

Instead of placing the burden on the child to demonstrate readiness, schools can accept that children will arrive in their classroom with varying levels of development. Schools can ready themselves for children by adopting developmentally appropriate practices—including flexible program structures and curricula—that accommodate children's age and individual differences. For example, some schools have experimented with multiage grouping that enables teachers to account for the range of competencies among students and within an individual child. Multiage grouping allows children to learn from each other and reduces same-age peer comparisons that can make children feel inadequate (Katz, Evangelou, & Hartman, 1990). Holistic, integrated instruction, not didactic teaching such as worksheets and drill and practice, optimizes children's early school experiences. Developmentally appropriate curriculum emphasizes the whole child. Active learning flows from the child's interest. Children participate in concrete activities that are relevant to their young lives, and subject matter is integrated throughout children's work (Boyer, 1991; Bredekamp, 1987; Goal One Ready Schools Resource Group, 1995; National Association of State Boards of Education, 1991).

Children make easier transitions to formal schooling through opportunities to visit and familiarize themselves with the new classroom. However, nationally representative samples of schools and school districts in the National Transition Study found that less than half of schools had formal programs for school visitation by parents (Love, Logue, Trudeau, & Thayer, 1992). Schools can establish continuity between families and institutions by supporting parents as their children's first teachers. Teachers and schools must recognize that language, values, behavioral codes, and expectations may differ between children's homes or early care and education programs and the school, making it difficult for children to adjust without efforts to make them feel comfortable and supported. Attention to and respect for this diversity—during parent-teacher meetings and in teacher-child classroom interactions—are an essential part of developmentally appropriate practice.

Unfortunately, research suggests that developmentally appropriate or "ready" schools are not widespread. One statewide study found that only 20% of randomly selected kindergartens met the criterion of developmental appropriateness (Bryant, Clifford, & Peisner, 1991). The implementation of developmentally appropriate practices may be inhibited by different attitudes and beliefs held by teachers and parents. In determining whether a child is ready for kindergarten, parents emphasize social and emotional maturity (Eisenhart & Graue, 1990). However, compared to kindergarten teachers, parents stress academic skills and favor classroom practices that are more academically oriented (Knudsen-

Lindauer & Harris, 1989). A U.S. Department of Education study found that parents were six to eight times more likely than teachers to rate counting to 20 and knowing the alphabet and three times more likely to rate the ability to use pencil and paintbrushes as very important or essential for kindergarten readiness (West et al., 1993).

Parents and teachers need to come together to discuss their goals and beliefs about readiness. Because both teachers and parents play a large role in preparing children for school success, their disparate goals may have far-reaching effects on children's development and learning. As Knudsen-Lindauer and Harris (1989) suggest, the closer parents' and teachers' attitudes and expectations are, the easier it is for them to work together to facilitate children's successful transitions to kindergarten and promote their school success.

Fortunately, teachers are enthusiastic about involving parents to improve children's early school success. A recent survey found that 64% of more than 7,000 kindergarten teachers surveyed indicated that parent education is the most important goal to pursue in addressing school readiness (Boyer, 1991). Parents can and should be treated as partners in their children's education and should be allowed to take strong decision-making roles in schools.

This section has focused on a vertical transition—that which occurs as children move up from one grade or class to the next. However, children also experience horizontal transitions, those which occur during a given day as children move from one caretaking/educational setting to another (Kagan, 1991; Zigler & Kagan, 1982). For some children, this may entail moving from home to care by a grandparent to half-day Head Start to child care back to the grandparent and then home. As discussed earlier, young children are increasingly in nonfamilial care settings—sometimes many different care situations per day. Kindergarten programs that are developmentally appropriate build on what children have learned in preschools and through other early childhood experiences. Communication between preschool and kindergarten teachers can help ensure compatible program philosophies. However, nationally representative samples of schools and school districts found that in only 10% of schools did regular communication occur between kindergarten teachers and previous caregivers or teachers about the entering kindergarten children. Only 12% of schools had curricula that build on preschool programs (Love et al., 1992).

Children with disabilities are faced with another kind of horizontal transition—the transition from special services to mainstream classrooms. Just as there is a need to link child care and school settings, there is often the need to link within school settings around the needs of particular children. Finally, schools need to establish linkages with neighborhoods, communities, and community institutions. These relationships should be infused in school structure and curricula. Teachers need to be able to draw on resources beyond the classroom for help and support. Tutors, health professionals, and technology specialists should be available for children and families. Working with social service and health agencies, making referrals and following up on them, schools can enhance the lives of children and their families. Schools should maintain contact with community-based institutions—those that offer before-school, after-school, or weekend programs for young children and their families. In addition, by collaborating with cultural institutions such as libraries and museums, schools can create a community of learners (Goal One Ready Schools Resource Group, 1995).

Readying children to succeed in school commands serious attention by families, schools, and communities to all of these transitions. In a climate of block grants and diminishing resources, collaboration, communication, and service integration among the different parties and institutions that touch the lives of children and families is a social imperative.

Assessment

Schools that are ready for young children understand the need for and the dilemmas surrounding assessment. It is true that readiness assessment can help gauge how well families, institutions, and communities are preparing children for success in school. Collecting data around readiness can garner attention and focus support around early childhood issues. Assessment can drive policy and allow the field to create better, more appropriate instruments. It can lead to better observations of child behavior and give the nation information on how well it is fulfilling its commitment to children.

However, young children are notoriously difficult to assess. Traditional paper-and-pencil tests are inappropriate for very young children, who are restless test takers with very short attention spans. Furthermore, young children's growth is rapid and episodic;

test results only report children's performance at one given point in time and therefore are not useful for generalizations about further growth and development. Meisels (1988, 1989) has noted that few valid and reliable assessment instruments have been developed, and other scholars have been rightly concerned about how the results of tests will be used (National Association for the Education of Young Children, 1988). A California study of standardized testing to sort children in and out of programs and classify them for retention or promotion found that boys were retained more often than girls, and children with English as a second language were more likely to be retained than those whose home language was English (Agee & California State Department of Education, 1988). Such methods segregate children—often based on the results of a single test—and challenge commitments to educational equity.

The NEGP has proposed the development of an early childhood assessment system that would achieve some of the goals of assessment without compromising the well-being of young children at the earliest stage of their education. The proposed system would be grounded in several principles to ensure that it would not jeopardize, label, or stigmatize individual children. First, the assessment system would respect the diversity among children and families—linguistically, culturally, and racially. Second, it would shift from collecting information on any given child to collecting social indicator data—data on children and communities. Third, the system would not resemble traditional tests but would assess using teacher input, parent input, and children's work samples, for example, block constructions, scribble stories, dictation. As a result of this assessment system, teachers would be better observers; parents would be involved in the assessment process; and national, solid empirically based data would be available to policymakers. Finally, such a system would shift the readiness burden from children to communities and schools.

Policy Recommendations

As our discussion indicates, readying children for school success is a complex and challenging task that must be shared by many stakeholders. No longer the burden of individual children, the major individuals and institutions that touch the lives of our youngest citizens—families, early care and education, schools— must come together to define and implement readiness.

Healthy People 2000 recognized the importance of the early years to children's school and later success. One of its services and protection objectives called for access to quality early care and education for all disadvantaged children and children with disabilities to prepare them for school and increase their prospects for school performance, problem behaviors, and mental and physical health (U.S. Department of Health and Human Services, Public Health Service, 1991). Yet early care and education is just one critical component to prepare children for school success. Although important, this objective alone is not sufficient to implement readiness for *all* children. *Healthy People 2010* has an opportunity to focus more attention on the critical needs of young children by setting more, specific objectives that support readiness. The following recommendations build on the information presented earlier and offer concrete policy steps for the future. We urge the *Healthy People 2010* report to consider including these recommendations in the laudable effort to promote the health and well-being of our children, our families, our institutions, and our society.

1. Consistent with the Healthy People 2000 preventive orientation, give more attention to children and the importance of the early years before school.

Americans must recognize their social obligation to support policy and practice that promote young children's early development and learning. More research on children's early brain development is needed; the findings from studies must be circulated widely—in layperson's language—to parents, early childhood educators, and policymakers. Working with the media and others, we should make these players aware of what they can do to support children's healthy growth and development, including their early literacy and numeracy. With increased public attention to the link between children's early experiences and their later functioning, families, early care and education, and schools will be more likely to recognize and accept their responsibility to ready children for school success.

*2. Conceptualize readiness as children's readiness, family
readiness, school readiness, and community readiness.*

Defining readiness has plagued the early childhood field for
years. Now, with the NEGP's conception of children's early
development and learning, the field finally has a widely accepted
definition. More research is needed on each of the five dimensions,
and funding should be made available to support this. In addition,
efforts should be made to ensure that the five dimensions are
understood as influenced by families, schools, and communities. It
is no longer appropriate to place the burden for children's readiness
on children alone. It is a responsibility that must be dispersed and
shared more widely.

*3. Generate adequate assessment systems for children, schools,
and communities.*

Serious attention to defining readiness opens the door for more
substantive work on assessment. Clearly, steps have been taken
toward inventive assessments strategies—including portfolio
development, the work sampling system—that can be used diagnos-
tically and can be used to improve pedagogy and instruction. Far
more work is needed to assess children for accountability purposes
in ways that consider young children's learning and assessment
styles. Furthermore, work needs to be done to conjure appropriate
mechanisms to hold the nation accountable for what it is doing to
promote school readiness. We need to establish mechanisms for
evaluating schools' readiness for children and communities' readiness for supporting young children.

4. Consider children and families holistically.

Early care and education, family support, and health services
need to be more closely aligned in terms of goals/principles and
service delivery. The early care and education and family support
movements are linked conceptually; both adhere to similar principles. Both movements acknowledge that the responsibility for
education transcends formal schooling. As a result, quality
programs promote the education and development of young
children before they begin school. In addition, both early care and

education and family support uphold universal and equitable service delivery as essential to promoting early development and learning for all children.

However, although these conceptual commonalities exist between early care and education and family support, few practical links connect the two movements. In part, this results from the fact that the two movements have reached different stages of development. Although early care and education services in the United States remain fragmented and highly idiosyncratic, there is still a more advanced infrastructure and more secure funding streams for early care and education than for family support. Family support needs to create an accepted definition of quality, a professionalized workforce, and advanced evaluation methodology. Most important, the two movements must forge operational links with one another to assure a holistic orientation to the development of young children.

In addition to linking family support and early care and education, far more work needs to be done to infuse health and health services into the development of ready children and ready communities. Given the increasingly vulnerable health status of America's children and the proven correlations between health and development, universal access to comprehensive screening and appropriate health services must be part of a national focus on readiness. In short, children's services can no longer be envisioned as categorical efforts that work to "fix" health, education, or family services. Rather, adopting a preventive and holistic orientation, one that regards readiness as a collective national effort, is required if we are to have a nation composed of healthy children and healthy families.

Finally, a quality early care and education infrastructure is needed to support quality programs that promote children's health and development. Comprehensive programs devoted to meeting children's needs across domains would acknowledge the strengths of individual children and their cultural and developmental differences. Attention would focus on easing children's transitions as they move from caregiver to caregiver and from early care and education to formal schooling. A quality infrastructure would include a system for licensing facilities and individuals who work with young children so that they are protected from harm. Governance structures at the state and local levels would hold the system accountable. Parents would have access to the information they need to be effective consumers of early care and education services. Employers and programs would support parents to be engaged as partners in their children's early care and education experiences. Finally, the system would be adequately funded with the financial burden shared among government, parents, employers, and the public at large.

Taken together, these recommendations are not simple; they represent a tall order. Yet for America to stand tall, it can no longer beg the issue of the importance of the early years. The time for action is now and *Healthy People 2010* represents one promising path for action.

Note

1. The term *early care and education* is used by the field to connote all nonparental care for young children, including those services that take place in centers and family child care homes. Early care and education includes nonprofit and for-profit child care, Head Start and other comprehensive development programs, Title I and other school-based prekindergarten programs, and part-day nursery schools. Home-based programs include family child care.

References

Agee, J. L., & California State Department of Education. (1988). *Here they come: Ready or not! A report of the School Readiness Task Force.* Sacramento: California State Department of Education.

Barnett, W. S. (1995). Long-term effects of early childhood programs on cognitive and school outcomes. *Future of Children, 5*(3), 25-50. [Special issue: Long-Term Outcomes of Early Childhood Programs]

Boyer, E. (1991). *Ready to learn: A mandate for the nation.* Princeton, NJ: Carnegie Foundation for the Advancement of Teaching.

Bradley, R. H., & Caldwell, B. M. (1984). The relation of infants' home environments to achievement test performance in first grade: A follow-up study. *Child Development, 55,* 803-809.

Bredekamp, S. (Ed.). (1987). *Developmentally appropriate practice in early childhood programs serving children from birth through age 8.* Washington, DC: National Association for the Education of Young Children.

Bredekamp, S., & Shepard, L. A. (1988). How to best protect children from inappropriate school expectations, practices, and policies. *Young Children, 44,* 14-24.

Bruner, J. (1960). *The process of education*. Cambridge, MA: Harvard University Press.

Bryant, D. M., Clifford, R. M., & Peisner, E. S. (1991). Best practices for beginners: Developmentally appropriateness in kindergarten. *American Educational Research Journal, 28,* 783-803.

Carnegie Task Force on Meeting the Needs of Young Children. (1994). *Starting points: Meeting the needs of our youngest children: The report of the Carnegie Task Force on Meeting the Needs of Young Children.* New York: Carnegie Corporation of New York.

Casper, L. M. (1995). What does it cost to mind our preschoolers? In *Current Population Reports: Household Economic Studies* (Report No. P70-52). Washington, DC: U.S. Department of Commerce.

Cost, Quality, and Child Outcomes Study Team. (1995). *Cost, quality, and child outcomes in child care centers.* Denver: University of Colorado at Denver, Department of Economics.

Crase, S. J., Carlson, C., & Kontos, S. (1981). Parent education needs and sources as perceived by parents. *Home Economics Research Journal, 9,* 221-231.

Eccles, J. L., O'Brien, K., & Timmer, S. G. (1985-1986). How families use time. *ISR Newsletter, 3-4.* (University of Michigan Institute for Social Research)

Eisenhart, M. S., & Graue, M. E. (1990). Socially constructed readiness for school. *International Journal for Qualitative Studies in Education, 3,* 253-269.

Families and Work Institute. (1994). *Employers, families, and education: Facilitating family involvement in learning.* New York: Author.

Family Resource Coalition. (1996). *Guidelines for family support practice.* Chicago: Author.

Gagne, R. M. (1970). *The conditions of learning* (2nd ed.). New York: Holt, Rinehart and Winston.

Galinsky, E., Howes, C., Kontos, S., & Shinn, M. (1994). *The study of children in family child care and relative care.* New York: Families and Work Institute.

Garbarino, J., & Kostelny, K. (1994). Family support and community development. In S. L. Kagan & B. Weissbourd (Eds.), *Putting families first: America's family support movement and the challenge of change* (pp. 297-320). San Francisco: Jossey-Bass.

Goal One Ready Schools Resource Group. (1995). *Ready schools for young children.* Washington, DC: National Education Goals Panel.

Gomby, D. S., Larner, M. B., Stevenson, C. S., Lewit, E. M., & Behrman, R. E. (1995). Long-term outcomes of early childhood programs: Analysis and recommendations. *Future of Children, 5*(3), 6-24. [Special issue: Long-Term Outcomes of Early Childhood Programs]

Graue, M. E. (1993a). Expectations and ideas coming to school. *Early Childhood Research Quarterly, 8,* 53-75.

Graue, M. E. (1993b). *Ready for what? Constructing meanings of readiness for kindergarten.* Albany: State University of New York Press.

Gredler, G. R. (1992). *School readiness: Assessment and educational issues.* Brandon, VT: Clinical Psychology.

Hayes, C. D., Palmer, J. L., & Zaslow, M. J. (Eds.). (1990). *Who cares for America's children?* Washington, DC: National Research Council, Panel on Child Care Policy, National Academy Press.

Heath, S. H. (1983). *Ways with words: Language, life, and work in communities and classrooms.* New York: Cambridge University Press.

Hess, R. D., Holloway, S. D., Dickson, W. P., & Price, G. G. (1984). Maternal variables as predictors of children's school readiness and later achievement in vocabulary and mathematics in sixth grade. *Child Development, 55,* 1902-1912.

Hofferth, S. L. (1995). Caring for children at the poverty line. *Children and Youth Services Review, 17*(1-2), 1-31.

Hofferth, S. L., Brayfield, A., Deich, S., & Holcomb, P. (1991). *National child care survey, 1990.* Washington, DC: Urban Institute.

Hughes, R., & Durio, H. F. (1983). Patterns of child care information seeking by families. *Family Relations, 32,* 203-212.

Kagan, S. L. (1991, September). *The strategic importance of linkages and the transition between early childhood programs and early elementary school.* Keynote presentation, National Policy Forum on Early Childhood Education, Chevy Chase, MD.

Kagan, S. L. (1994). Defining and achieving quality in family support. In S. L. Kagan & B. Weissbourd (Eds.), *Putting families first: America's family support movement and the challenge of change* (pp. 375-400). San Francisco: Jossey-Bass.

Kagan, S. L., Goffin, S., Golub, S., & Pritchard, E. (1995). *Toward systemic reform: Service integration for young children and their families.* Falls Church, VA: National Center for Service Integration.

Kagan, S. L., Moore, E., & Bredekamp, S. (Eds.). (1995). *Reconsidering children's early development and learning: Toward shared beliefs and vocabulary.* Washington, DC: National Education Goals Panel.

Kagan, S. L., & Weissbourd, B. (1994). Toward a new normative system of family support. In S. L. Kagan & B. Weissbourd (Eds.), *Putting families first: America's family support movement and the challenge of change* (pp. 473-490). San Francisco: Jossey-Bass.

Karweit, N. L., & Wasik, B. A. (1994). Extra-year kindergarten programs and transitional first grades. In R. E. Slavin, N. L. Karweit, & B. A. Wasik (Eds.), *Preventing early school failure: Research, policy, and practice* (pp. 102-121). Boston: Allyn & Bacon.

Katz, L., Evangelou, D., & Hartman, J. A. (1990). *The case for mixed age grouping in early education.* Washington, DC: National Association for the Education of Young Children.

Keopke, J., & Williams, C. (1989). Child-rearing information: Resources parents use. *Family Relations, 38,* 462-465.

Knudsen-Lindauer, S. L., & Harris, K. (1989). Priorities for kindergarten curricula: Views of parents and teachers. *Journal of Research in Childhood Education, 4,* 51-61.

Love, J. M., Logue, M. E., Trudeau, J. V., & Thayer, K. (1992). *Transitions to kindergarten in American schools. Final report of the National Transition Study.* Portsmouth, NH: RMC Research.

Meisels, S. J. (1988). Developmental screening in early childhood: The interaction of research and social policy. *Annual Review of Public Health, 9,* 527-550.

Meisels, S. J. (1989, April). High-stakes testing in kindergarten. *Educational Leadership,* pp. 16-22.

Meisels, S. J. (1992). Doing harm by doing good: Iatrogenic effects of early childhood enrollment and promotion practices. *Early Childhood Research Quarterly, 7,* 155-174.

Moore, E. (1990). *Increasing parental involvement as a means of improving our nation's schools.* Washington, DC: U.S. Department of Education, Office of Planning, Budget, and Evaluation.

Mullis, A. K., & Mullis, R. L. (1983). Making parent education relevant. *Family Perspectives, 17,* 167-173.

National Association for the Education of Young Children. (1988). Position statement on standardized testing of young children 3 through 8 years of age. *Young Children, 43,* 42-47.

National Association of State Boards of Education. (1991). *Caring communities: Supporting young children and families.* Report of the National Task Force on School Readiness. Alexandria, VA: Author.

National Institute of Child Health and Human Development. (1996). *Infant child care and attachment security: Results of the NICHD study of early child care.* Washington, DC: U.S. Department of Health and Human Services.

Phillips, D. A. (Ed.). (1995). *Child care for low-income families: Summary of two workshops.* Washington, DC: National Academy Press.

Phillips, D. A., & Howes, C. (1987). Indicators of quality in child care: Review of research. In D. Phillips (Ed.), *Quality in child care: What does the research tell us?* (pp. 1-19). Washington, DC: National Association for the Education of Young Children.

Phillips, D. A., Voran, M., Kisker, E., Howes, C., & Whitebook, M. (1994). Child care for children in poverty: Opportunity or inequality? *Child Development, 65,* 440-456.

Piaget, J. (1970). *Science of education and the psychology of the child.* New York: Orion.

Poersch, N., Adams, G., & Sandfort, J. (1994). *Child care and development: Key facts.* Washington, DC: Children's Defense Fund.

Powell, D. R. (1990). *Parents as the child's first teacher: Opportunities and constraints.* Washington, DC: U.S. Department of Education, Office of Planning, Budget, and Evaluation.

Powell, D. R. (1994). Evaluating family support programs: Are we making progress? In S. L. Kagan & B. Weissbourd (Eds.), *Putting families first: America's family support movement and the challenge of change* (pp. 441-470). San Francisco: Jossey-Bass.

Powell, D. R. (1995). *Enabling young children to succeed in school.* Washington, DC: American Educational Research Association.

Schweinhart, L. J., Barnes, H. V., & Weikart, D. P., with Barnett, W. S., & Epstein, A. S. (1993). *Significant benefits: The High/Scope Perry Preschool Study through age 27.* Ypsilanti, MI: High/Scope.

Sheehan, R., Cryan, J. R., Wiechel, J., & Bandy-Hedden, I. (1991). Factors contributing to success in elementary schools: Research findings for early childhood educators. *Journal of Research in Childhood Education, 6,* 1-10.

Shepard, L. A. (1989). A review of research on kindergarten retention. In L. A. Shepard & M. L. Smith (Eds.), *Flunking grades: Research and policies on retention* (pp. 64-78). Philadelphia: Falmer.

Shepard, L. A., & Smith, M. L. (1986). Synthesis of research on school readiness and kindergarten retention. *Educational Leadership, 44,* 78-86.

Shore, R. (1994). *Family support and parent education: Opportunities for scaling up.* Report of a meeting convened by Carnegie Corporation of New York, November 16-17, 1994.

Sugarman, J. (1995). *Comparison of expenditures for public school education and early childhood programs.* Washington, DC: Center on Effective Services for Children.

Teale, W. H. (1986). Home background and young children's literacy development. In W. H. Teale & F. P. Stafford (Eds.), *Time, goods, and well-being* (pp. 353-382). Ann Arbor: University of Michigan, Institute for Social Research.

Timmer, S. G., Eccles, J., & O'Brien, K. (1985). How children use time. In F. T. Juster & F. P. Stafford (Eds.), *Time, goods, and well-being* (pp. 353-382). Ann Arbor: University of Michigan, Institute for Social Research.

U.S. Department of Education, National Center for Education Statistics. (1995). *1995 national household education survey.* Washington, DC: Author.

U.S. Department of Health and Human Services, Public Health Service. (1991). *Healthy people 2000: National health promotion and disease prevention objectives* (DHHS Publication No. PHS 91-50212). Washington, DC: U.S. Government Printing Office.

U.S. General Accounting Office. (1993). *Poor preschool-aged children: Numbers increase but most not in preschool* (Report No. 93-111). Washington, DC: Author.

U.S. General Accounting Office. (1994). *Child care: Working poor and welfare recipients face service gaps* (Report No. 94-87). Washington, DC: Author.

U.S. General Accounting Office. (1995a). *Early childhood centers: Services to prepare children for school often limited* (Report No. 95-21). Washington, DC: Author.

U.S. General Accounting Office. (1995b). *Early childhood programs: Multiple programs and overlapping target groups* (Report No. 95-4FS). Washington, DC: Author.

Vygotsky, L. S. (1978). *Mind in society: The development of higher psychological processes.* Cambridge, MA: Harvard University Press.

West, J., Hausken, E. G., & Collins, M. (1993). *Readiness for kindergarten: Parent and teacher beliefs* (Report No. NCES 93-257). Washington, DC: U.S. Department of Education, Office of Educational Research and Improvement, National Center for Education Statistics.

Whitebook, M., Howes, C., & Phillips, D. (1989). *Who cares? Child care teachers and the quality of care in America: Final report of the National Child Care Staffing Study.* Oakland, CA: Child Care Employee Project.

Wright, J., Hausken, E. G., & West, J. (1994). *Family-child engagement in literacy activities: Changes in participation between 1991 and 1993* (Report No. NCES 95-689). Washington, DC: U.S. Department of Education, Office of Educational Research and Improvement, National Center for Education Statistics.

Yoshikawa, H. (1995). Long-term effects of early childhood programs on social outcomes and delinquency. *Future of Children, 5*(3), 51-75. [Special issue: Long-Term Outcomes of Early Childhood Programs]

Zaslow, M. J., Pedersen, F. A., Suwalsky, J. T. D., Cain, R. L., & Fivel, M. (1985). The early resumption of employment by mothers: Implications for parent-infant interaction. *Journal of Applied Developmental Psychology, 6,* 1-16.

Zigler, E., & Kagan, S. L. (1982). Child development knowledge and educational practice: Using what we know. In A. Lieberman & M. McLaughlin (Eds.), *Policy making in education. Eighty-first yearbook of the National Society for the Study of Education.* Chicago: University of Chicago Press.

Zill, N., Collins, M., & Hausken, E. G. (1995). *Approaching kindergarten: A look at preschoolers in the United States.* National Household Education Survey (No. NCES 95-280). Washington, DC: U.S. Department of Education, Office of Educational Research and Improvement, National Center for Educational Statistics.

Schools and the Enhancement of Children's Wellness: Some Opportunities and Some Limiting Factors

EMORY L. COWEN

This chapter starts with a preamble that lightly sketches its ultimate direction. Its main corpus describes the thinking and experiences behind that sense of direction, and it develops further the vision to which they lead.

School psychology, school social work, and school mental health are generic, field-designating terms used to describe the work that school-based professionals do in seeking to ameliorate or contain children's school adjustment problems. These activities are shaped by a regnant world-view of what school professional roles are about and the educational and training experiences that subserve that view. Should a field's guiding objectives be recast, associated professional training must also change; that is, new roles and activities that vivify the shift must be articulated.

The school helping professions first came into being a century ago. At that time their prime goals were to identify (diagnose) blatant problems children were experiencing and deal with them as best they could. Although that guiding mandate has remained largely constant over the years, the technology used to carry it out has become far more sophisticated.

Understandably, school mental health has always mirrored the objectives and practices of the broader mental health field of which it is part. It still does. One noteworthy recent trend in these fields is a growing interest in before-the-fact prevention (Cowen, 1994, 1996; Durlak & Wells, 1997; Mrazek & Haggerty, 1994). When prevention is the goal, malleable young children become ideal targets and schools ideal settings for such work (Cowen et al., 1996; Durlak, 1995).

The point to highlight, however, is that different views of school mental health's basic goals (e.g., repair vs. wellness enhancement) produce different scenarios for allocating professional time and implicate qualitatively different roles and activities. To the extent that building wellness from the start is viewed as a legitimate, high-priority goal, professional activities in schools must move beyond diagnosing and repairing things that have already gone wrong, indeed even beyond ontogenetically early secondary prevention, toward innovative, proactive contributions that schools are in an especially good position to make as part of a broader societal quest to enhance wellness. Children are important people and schools have important (but not exclusive) roles to play both in their early formation and in continuing steps dedicated to enhancing their wellness.

Implicit in the preceding statement is the conviction that the underlying goals and objectives (e.g., enhancing wellness vs. preventing further failure in the already failing, vs. early repair of incipient dysfunction), *not* simply location (i.e., schools vs. other places), must crucially shape professional roles and activities in *all* settings, including schools. To think of fields such as school psychology and school social work without embeddedness in a guiding context of such objectives is to put the cart before the horse. Hence a core premise of this chapter is that we stand to profit from a conception of school mental health services built around thoughtful answers to the question: "What useful roles can schools play as part of a concerted social effort targeted to the enhancement of children's wellness?" Answers to that question can help to crystallize recommendations for *Healthy People 2010*.

A brief, way-station answer to be fleshed out in the body of the chapter, is: "many important roles," including, no doubt, some that entail practical, repair-oriented steps. The latter, however, should comprise but one element in a broader matrix of wellness enhancement efforts—an element that will need to unfold in concert with other steps within a framework of reallocated priorities. New roles that are likely to become more salient as wellness enhancement objectives achieve greater visibility include engineering health-promoting school and class environments, building proactive health-facilitating curricula, and developing fluid outreach systems to families and community settings in the service of enhancing children's early wellness.

Four Decades of Formation:
The PMHP Experience

Over the past 40 years, the bulk of my professional efforts have been invested in developing, implementing, evaluating, and disseminating school-based prevention programs for young children. The sections that follow describe the school mental health issues our work has addressed and the program models we have developed and applied in this context. Finally, learnings from these experiences are used to formulate guidelines and suggestions for (school) mental health programming in the early 21st century.

Much of what we have done and learned in the school mental health arena in the past four decades is built around a master entity called the Primary Mental Health Project (PMHP), a program for early detection and prevention of young children's school adjustment problems. PMHP's early development (i.e., its first 15 years) was described in a book by Cowen et al. (1975); its subsequent growth and evolution are described in a new volume (Cowen et al., 1996). The existence of those two volumes obviates the need for detailed accounts of PMHP's rationale, course of emergence, and accomplishments. Here we provide only a bare-bones summary of that information, enough, it is hoped, to establish a foundation for several conclusions and recommendations for the future.

PMHP began in 1957 as a small pilot-experimental project, fueled both by observations about children in schools and concerns about the predominant thrust and insufficiencies of existing mental health approaches. The hows and whys of PMHP's emergence cannot be understood independent of those concerns. As prestigious review bodies of the time (Joint Commission on Mental Illness and Health, 1961) pointed out, the mental health fields were then beset by vexing problems, including (a) shortages of professional personpower; (b) uneven distribution of resources that sharply limited access of underserved groups such as poor people and children to the system's scarce and costly services; and, perhaps deadliest of all, (c) the fact that the system's limited resources were targeted primarily to people with already rooted, often refractory, problems—precisely those with the poorest prognoses. Under the latter conditions, even the most effectively delivered restorative services have limited potential.

These vexing problems formed the backdrop that shaped PMHP's early development (Cowen et al., 1996). In contrast with the conceptualizations and practices that guided the then-dominant mental health delivery system, the initial PMHP and its later programmatic extensions were carved out in the image of three masters: *prevention,* rather than repair, as the overarching goal; *young children,* rather than adults, as prime targets; and *schools,* because they offered systematic access to young children, as the prime locus.

At its core, PMHP is built on four structural pillars: (a) a focus on primary graders before problems root and fan out; (b) systematic use of screening and early detection procedures to identify at-risk young children as soon as possible; (c) using carefully selected, trained, supervised nonprofessional child associates as the program's prime, direct help-agents with these early identified children; and (d) modifying professional roles to feature systematic early screening to identify children at risk; selection, training, and supervision of child associates; and consultative roles with teachers and other school personnel. The basic goals of this revamped delivery system are to bring prompt preventively oriented help to young children when it can do the most good, and to extend the reach of effective early services to children in need.

PMHP works as follows: Brief, objective screening measures that we have developed are used to profile children's school-related problems and competencies (see, e.g., Hightower et al., 1987; Hightower et al., 1986). Information derived from those measures, along with feedback from teachers and parents, is reviewed at an initial assignment conference early in the school year. If significant indicators of ineffective functioning (e.g., acting-out, shy-anxious, or learning problems) are identified, children are referred to PMHP and intervention goals are established. After parent permission has been received, child associates begin to see referred children regularly—most individually, but some in small groups. Associates are selected for their human qualities (e.g., warmth, caring for children) rather than prior education and training. They receive some training before they start, further on-the-job training and supervision, and later specialty training to broaden their skills. Half-time associates, working under professional supervision, can see roughly 12-15 children a week.

A typical school-based PMHP team includes project professionals, child associates, primary grade teachers, and a school administrator. After the initial assignment conference, team members continue to exchange pertinent information and coordinate goals on the child's behalf. Midyear progress conferences are held to review each child's current situation and, when needed, to realign goals and approaches. End-of-year conferences evaluate children's overall progress in PMHP and, if needed, formulate plans for further helping steps. Program consultants provide support, stimulation, and inputs regarding especially challenging children and troublesome issues.

PMHP is built on meaningful interfaces between service and research. Many of its studies are addressed to concrete program issues and many of its research findings are fed back to strengthen program services. Several program developments that extend PMHP's reach, or strengthen its applicability to particular children, have evolved over the years as a product of this service-research marriage. Those include mini-programs for (a) seeing children in small groups; (b) bridging between schools and families (i.e., "parent" associates); (c) using limit-setting approaches with acting-out children; (d) crisis intervention; and (e) planned short-term intervention. These "add-on" programs come about in much the same way structurally. First, the need for a program is identified and a pilot program to meet that need is developed and explored. Promising pilot models are evaluated more extensively and, when found to be effective, they are incorporated into PMHP's mainstream through program-relevant training for child associates. In the aggregate, these new options have added considerably to PMHP's flexibility and reach (Cowen et al., 1996).

Research has been central to PMHP since Day 1. Research studies have explored diverse program-related matters, including (a) child and family variables associated with children's school adjustment; (b) attributes of effective child associates; (c) the nature of the associate-child interaction process in PMHP; (d) children with whom the program is more, versus less, effective; and (e) the efficacy of new program offshoots. Cowen et al.'s (1996) review of PMHP's research noted that outcome studies have been the most extensive aspect of this work. Spanning nearly 40 years, such studies have evaluated PMHP's efficacy in a broad range of settings and with diverse populations. Several of these studies have been truly massive, including one documenting program efficacy based on 47,000 children seen through PMHP in some 200 California school districts, over a 5-year period (Cowen et al., 1996).

Among the key conclusions from these many program evaluation studies are the following: (a) Overall, PMHP effectively strengthens the behavioral adaptation and school performance of young, at-risk children; (b) initial short-term program gains endure over time; (c) because the approach works well with children reflecting diverse sociocultural backgrounds, it is a good way to reach underserved populations; and (d) PMHP is cost-effective compared to other forms of intervention with children.

In its first two decades, PMHP laid the basic program model in place, fine-tuned and extended it, and developed a sound empirical base documenting its efficacy. After those early credentializing steps were completed (Cowen et al., 1975), more effort was invested in two other types of activities, that is, program dissemination and new primary prevention programming. Again, because the recent PMHP volume (Cowen et al., 1996) details both these developments, they are described only briefly here.

A next natural question, following documentation of PMHP's efficacy, was how this hard-come-by knowledge could best be applied to extend program benefits to many more children in need around the country. This challenge stimulated a set of dissemination activities that PMHP has pursued for two decades. These include (a) conducting national workshops to elevate consciousness about the program, (b) doing consultative visits to implementing districts and providing short-term internships for their personnel in PMHP demonstration schools, (c) establishing regional PMHP demonstration centers each based on its own successful program, and (d) working with state offices to promote within-state program dissemination.

The last of these steps led to the passage of specific PMHP enabling legislation, with supporting budget, in four states (New York, California, Washington, and Connecticut), and to extensive but less formal program development in other states (and countries). As a result of these dissemination activities, PMHP programs are now operating in more than 700 school districts in this country and elsewhere (e.g., Australia, Canada, Israel). These programs serve sociodemographically diverse children and range from stress-ridden, inner-city settings (Meller, Laboy, Rothwax, Fritton, & Mangual, 1994) to new consortia of 4-6 underresourced rural school districts that share program services (Farie, Cowen, & Smith, 1986). As such, they illustrate an appealing feature of the PMHP model, that is, its potential adaptability across diverse settings and circumstances, including programs for historically neglected populations.

Collectively, this family of PMHP programs now brings early, effective, preventively oriented help to many thousands of young schoolchildren at risk annually. This development has helped to modify how school mental health services are conceptualized and delivered and, in that sense, has contributed to the elusive goal of bringing about constructive social change.

PMHP's early development demonstrated that the program model made good sense both as a concept and empirically in relation to traditional, after-the-fact, repair-oriented school mental health approaches. Although we saw this as a significant forward stride in effective, ontogenetically early secondary prevention, two realities raised cautions in our minds: (a) Because PMHP was directed primarily to children in whom warning signs had already been detected, it remained a somewhat reactive program, rather than one that served all children in health-enhancing ways; and (b) even though PMHP was effective overall, some children were not helped by it.

As these awarenesses grew, a more basic challenge began to crystallize: "What could schools do to optimize the wellness and school adaptation of *all* children from the start, beyond targeting programs to the identifiable fraction at risk?" That question highlights one key goal of primary prevention, a generic name for a family of programs that seeks to enhance wellness as well as to avert psychological difficulties (Cowen, 1994, 1996; Durlak, 1995; Durlak & Wells, 1997). Thus, we have also sought, in the past 20 years, to develop primary prevention program models that broaden PMHP's scope by reaching children more proactively. The approaches we have explored reflect three strategies: (a) teaching children adjustment-enhancing skills and competencies, (b) modifying class environments and practices to improve educational and behavioral outcomes, and (c) developing programs that teach adaptive coping skills to children at risk by virtue of exposure to significant life stress.

Four such developments are described briefly here—two class-based, for all children, and two non-class based, targeted to youngsters with specific risk histories. One set, that is, competence training programs (Gesten, Flores de Apodaca, Rains, Weissberg, & Cowen, 1979; Gesten et al., 1982; Spivack, Platt, & Shure, 1976; Spivack & Shure, 1974), seeks to train in interpersonal, or social, problem solving skills (e.g., recognizing feelings in self and others, generating alternative solutions to interpersonal problems, evaluating the consequences of solutions, and taking the role of the other) and self-control or adaptive assertiveness skills (Rotheram, Armstrong, & Booraem, 1982) known to relate to good adjustment. The goal of such skill training is to enhance children's adjustment and school adaptation.

Another of our primary prevention steps was to develop programs built around planful change in class environments. One such approach, called the "jigsaw" classroom (Aronson, Blaney, Stephan, Sikes, & Snapp, 1978), rests on the assumption that perceived class attributes such as order and organization, affiliation, and involvement promote positive student outcomes (Moos, 1979). Jigsaw classrooms use structures and practices designed to enhance such perceptions. Specifically within PMHP, Wright and Cowen (1985) developed a jigsaw program based on mixed gender and ability-level groups of five children in fifth-grade social studies classes. Each group member had to learn one segment of a larger curriculum unit and teach it to groupmates. This approach was found to be effective in terms of both academic and interpersonal outcomes. A related, later PMHP-developed program called Study-Buddy (Hightower, Avery, & Levinson, 1988) pairs students, who work together in dyads three to five times a week over the school year, to promote reciprocal peer learning and cooperative peer relationships (Cowen et al., 1996).

Two other of our primary prevention programs are targeted to children at risk. The first, the Children of Divorce Intervention Program (CODIP), was the product of two convergent strands: (a) sharply rising divorce rates and referral rates of children of divorce to PMHP; and (b) observational and empirical data documenting the negative effects of divorce on children's adjustment and school performance. To date, six versions of CODIP have been developed for urban and suburban, kindergarten to eighth-grade children. Although these programs share common objectives, their technology varies as a function of the age and sociodemographic attributes of the target populations. As minimal common denominators, however, all CODIP programs provide support; teach appropriate ways to identify and express feelings; clarify divorce-related misconceptions; teach problem solving, communication, and anger control skills; and enhance children's perceptions of self and family. Research findings document CODIP's adjustment-enhancing effects for diverse groups (Pedro-Carroll & Alpert-Gillis, in press; Pedro-Carroll, Alpert-Gillis, & Cowen, 1992; Pedro-Carroll & Cowen, 1985; Pedro-Carroll, Cowen, Hightower, & Guare, 1986).

A final primary prevention probe, called the Rochester Child Resilience Project (RCRP), is still evolving. Targeted to young profoundly stressed urban children, the RCRP has identified child variables (e.g., perceived self-worth, social problem solving skills, empathy, realistic control attributions), through testing, and developmental and family milieu variables (e.g., easy early temperament; a warm, caring child-parent relationship; father involvement in child care; and sound, authoritative discipline practices), through in-depth interviews with parents, that correctly classified 85% of these highly stressed youngsters as having stress-resilient or stress-affected adjustment outcomes (Cowen et al., 1992; Hoyt-Meyers et al., 1995; Wyman et al., in press; Wyman, Cowen, Work, & Parker, 1991; Wyman et al., 1992). These findings offer a base on which to develop preventive interventions for children at risk for unfortunate personal and academic outcomes because of chronic exposure to major life stress. We have begun to develop a program model for preventive intervention with such youngsters (Cowen, Wyman, Work, & Iker, 1994).

Although program manuals have been developed for each of these new primary prevention projects, as a group they are less extensively explored, or evaluated, than PMHP. Even so, their emergence has modified PMHP's focus and resource allocations. Whereas, initially, 100% of our efforts were invested in the basic PMHP model, about 50% of our resources are now allocated to "vintage" PMHP, and 25% each to program dissemination and new primary prevention program initiatives. More important, the field at large has undertaken increasingly serious exploration of well-ness-oriented, primary prevention program options that go far beyond our own limited probes. The latter wholesome development is considered later in the chapter.

The PMHP Experience: Accomplishments and Limitations

The preceding section described PMHP. Backing off from those trees to glimpse a larger forest, the last half of the chapter overviews accomplishments and limitations of the PMHP development and uses that analysis as a base for considering (a) the future place of ontogenetically early secondary prevention programs in schools; and (b) needed types of complementary programs.

The PMHP development has been exciting and socially contributory. Its special blend of components offers a cohesive package that provides early, effective, preventively oriented services to many more children than traditional school mental services can reach. Focusing such services on primary graders holds potential for reducing the flow of later, more serious school- and life-adjustment problems. Moreover, because PMHP has been shown to be effective with diverse groups, it can be targeted specifically to underserved populations in which the need for services is strong. Schools find PMHP to "make sense," that is, it well addresses many vexing, everyday problems they experience. Consumer satisfaction with the program, its extensive documentation, and its flexible application potential are all big pluses for dissemination. Also, the productive marriage between service and research in PMHP has made it an ever-evolving, ever-improving program that continues to reach more children effectively.

The preceding accomplishments are substantial. They suggest that the PMHP model that has evolved offers a balanced set of early preventive options that merit consideration as one key element in a multifaceted plan for future school mental health services. Although such a component is needed, it will not fully address all the child learning and adjustment problems that many schools are called on to engage daily. The demurrer in the last sentence leads to a consideration of things PMHP has *not* done so well, and educated guesses about *why* not. Such an analysis is motivated neither by modesty nor self-derogation; rather, it is a needed, reality-based step in developing recipes for future school mental health services.

PMHP's most obvious limitation is that it does not work well for *some* children. Although it is hard to attach exact numbers to the term "work well," a recent, 5-year program outcome study involving 47,000 children from several hundred California school districts suggests that 65% of PMHP-seen children do very well, 20% show modest gains, and the remaining 15% gain little or not at all (Cowen et al., 1996). Those numbers describe only how children looked when the intervention ended and say nothing about the durability of those early outcomes. But even within a short-term framework, they make it clear that PMHP does not always work.

There are several reasons why PMHP is not effective for all children. First, even though its innovative child associate approach is sensible and effective overall, not all associates are equally effective, and not all associate-child pairings are made in heaven. In practice, some fraction of those pairings range from poor to marginal. This is less an intrinsic flaw in the program model and more a failing in the mechanics of its execution.

Other less than satisfactory PMHP outcomes come from misapplications of the approach. PMHP was never intended to be all things for all children. It was designed as an early preventive intervention, not as a restorative program for children with deeply rooted, pervasive problems (e.g., profound conduct disorder; major childhood depression). Nevertheless, in some settings, children with long-standing, serious problems *do* enter the program for any of several reasons. The latter include (a) pressures from teachers to do something about "difficult" children (e.g., chronic acter-outers), even if it is just to get them out of the classroom for brief respites; (b) professionals sometimes endow PMHP with an (unwarranted) infallibility and agree to see children whose problems are serious enough to overtax the best of what it can offer; and (c) in some communities that lack mental health facilities, because PMHP is the "only show in town," children are either seen within its auspices or not at all. Because PMHP is not an approach of choice in the preceding situations, it may at best be minimally effective with children who fall into those categories. These situations, too, less reflect a shortcoming in the program model and more an overextension in its application.

With regard to limitations of applicability that we have identified, PMHP has sought, from the start, to develop correctives to extend the program's reach and improve its batting average. Some of those efforts have been very effective, others less so. Examples of successful extensions include offshoot programs for small group intervention (Terrell, McWilliams, & Cowen, 1972), work with acting-out children (Cowen, Orgel, Gesten, & Wilson, 1979), and planned short-term interventions (Winer-Elkin, Weissberg, & Cowen, 1988) that have enhanced PMHP's reach and versatility.

Early experience with PMHP also made it clear that however effective this early secondary prevention model was with the children it reached, it was still reactive, reaching only some children showing early risk signs, and was less than 100% successful. This realization fueled exploration of primary prevention approaches designed to enhance the wellness of all children, in the belief that such proactive steps are much needed and will become an increasingly important aspect of future mental health programming in schools.

The steps we have thus far taken in this direction are more exploratory and paradigmatic than comprehensive and definitive. Collectively, they comprise only a tiny fraction of a rising tide, involving many groups and approaches seeking to develop mass-oriented, proactive program models that differ qualitatively from past restorative approaches. Several recent sources provide rationales for these largely school-based primary prevention programs and cite promising examples (Consortium on the School-Based Promotion of Social Competence, 1994; Cowen, 1994, 1996; Durlak, 1995; Elias & Tobias, 1995; Lorion, 1990; Price, Cowen, Lorion, & Ramos-McKay, 1988). Discussion of this development here is limited to several outstanding illustrations of the approach, primarily to concretize what has thus far been said abstractly. Weissberg and Greenberg's (1997) recent scholarly, thought-provoking review of this area offers a much richer consideration of the topic and describes a number of effective wellness-oriented programs (primarily school-based) for children and youth ages 0-18. Their review is "must-reading" for those with interest in the current status, and promise, of a competence enhancement approach.

The development of interpersonal problem solving training programs for children (Spivack et al., 1976; Spivack & Shure, 1974) is an early competence-building approach that has had substantial enduring value. This work rests on a generative knowledge base showing that maladapted groups are deficient in such social problem solving (SPS) skills as generating alternative solutions and evaluating their consequences. Hence curricula were developed to train young children in these skills. The heuristic value of this work stemmed both from early findings and, importantly, from the fact that it modeled an appealing new health-building paradigm. SPS training, in which we too were involved (Gesten et al., 1979; Gesten et al., 1982; Weissberg, Gesten, Carnrike, et al., 1981; Weissberg, Gesten, Liebenstein, Schmid, & Hutton, 1980; Weissberg, Gesten, Rapkin, et al., 1981), has continued over the years both in the form of freestanding programs and condensed modules that are elements in expanded social competence training programs (Durlak, 1995; Elias & Clabby, 1992; Elias & Tobias, 1995).

As several limiting realities of the initial SPS approach became clear, work in this area went through some metamorphoses (Consortium on the School-Based Promotion of Social Competence, 1994; Weissberg & Elias, 1993). One such reality was that encapsulated (one-shot) SPS programs were found to have restricted initial value and limited staying power (Durlak, 1983). Also, evolving generative knowledge bases identified relationships between other (non-SPS) families of variables (e.g., impulse control, empathy, communication and stress management skills) and positive adjustment outcomes. These realities led to the development of second-generation social competence training programs, in which SPS training was but one element in more sophisticated, comprehensive curricula that (a) extended over multiple years, (b) introduced new competencies at developmentally appropriate times, (c) included boosters for skills previously taught at simpler levels, and (d) created class and school mechanisms to promote real-life application of program learnings after the formal program ended.

There now exist multiple examples of effective social competence training programs of this type. These programs have yielded such positive outcomes as enhanced self-control; problem-solving, decision-making, and conflict resolution skills; and lowered anxiety and susceptibility to alcohol and substance use (see, e.g., Caplan et al., 1992; Cowen, 1994; Elias, Gara, Schuyler, Branden-Muller, & Sayette, 1991). Their success in terms of both proximal and longer-term, bellwether outcomes has stimulated exploration of third-generation social competence training programs that are continuous from kindergarten to 12th grade, introducing new components as children's interests and cognitive capabilities mature (Consortium on the School-Based Promotion of Social Competence, 1994; Weissberg & Elias, 1993; Weissberg & Greenberg, 1997). These programs seek to promote a full spectrum of core social competencies known to undergird wholesome adjustment in children.

The Child Development Project (CDP) is a different, systemic approach to enhancing children's wellness. CDP seeks to modify the total school environment in wellness-enhancing ways (Battistich, Solomon, Watson, Solomon, & Schaps, 1989; Developmental Studies Center, 1994; Solomon, Watson, Delucchi, Schaps, & Battistich, 1988). With coordinated inputs from schools, families, and children, CDP strives, at its core, to create a "caring school environment," from kindergarten through sixth grade, in ways that build on children's prime motivational needs for autonomy, belongingness, and competence (Deci & Ryan, 1985). To promote autonomy support, CDP uses a schoolwide discipline approach in which children are responsible for setting and upholding class rules. This is intended both to empower them and to foster democratic values. Children's sense of belongingness is promoted by using cooperative learning formats at all grade levels and a buddy program that pairs older and younger children. Reading and instructional materials are selected to help children better understand themselves and others and to promote prosocial values. CDP rests on the assumption that children will engage better in, and profit more from, the school experience if it is intrinsically interesting and if they have genuine shaping inputs in what they do.

Empirical findings support that assumption. Classroom observations showed that the program was implemented as intended. Thus, program classes at all grade levels exceeded comparison classes in terms of judged warmth and supportiveness, mutual help activities and cooperative work formats, emphasis on interpersonal understanding and personal values, opportunities for student autonomy, and discipline formats that promoted responsible behavior.

In terms of program outcomes, CDP children were found to be more cooperative and considerate than controls, better able to express their views and resolve conflicts, and more willing to include peers in group decision-making steps. They exceeded controls in self-esteem, empathy, and, importantly, perceived sense of community. They had more friends, felt better accepted by peers and more competent socially, had less anxiety, and evidenced a better understanding of others. Their academic performance was at least as good as comparison children's—better in some areas (e.g., reading comprehension).

Follow-up, 3 years later, when participants were seventh and eighth graders in new schools, showed that early program gains were maintained and that there were important new benefits such as lower rates of alcohol and marijuana use and fewer delinquent or violent behaviors (Battistich, Schaps, Watson, & Solomon, 1995). Schools highest in fidelity of program implementation had the best outcomes. Significant program gains were also found in schools with high proportions of poverty-level students. A variable that favored positive program outcomes, and overrode the typical negative effects of poverty, was student perception of the school as a caring community (Battistich, Solomon, Kim, Watson, & Schaps, 1995). CDP's initial demonstrations of significant program benefit are now being replicated around the country.

Both second-generation social competence training and CDP's social system modification programs are promising approaches that (a) are integrated naturally into a school's way of operating, (b) reach all children in a school building, (c) extend over multiple school years, and (d) share the prime goal of enhancing children's wellness. Such population-oriented wellness programs, relatively new to the school scene, rest on ways of thinking, targetings, and practices that differ qualitatively from the past repair-dominated approaches in school mental health. It is hoped that this new thrust will be a significant aspect of future school mental health programming, with concomitant modifications in the training of school mental health professionals.

Although the wellness enhancement programs described seem timely and promising, even the best and most comprehensive of them may be too little and too late for increasing numbers of children whose formation and early life experiences so markedly shape the outlook and problems they bring to school, that the school's mission may, de facto, be defeated before it starts. These are the children who grow up in the shadow of profound, chronic stressors (e.g., neighborhood crime and violence; family chaos and disorganization; exposure to substance abuse, poverty, and squalid living conditions) that exact staggering tolls. Increasingly, educators see these youngsters as prime candidates for school failure and its many unfortunate associated life sequelae if poor starts are not reversed by third grade. Given the severity of their problems and life situations, there is little reason to expect that 20 meetings with a compassionate, caring adult, or even the best executed wellness enhancement program for that matter, should turn a bleak situation of such magnitude and chronicity around. Innovative new approaches that call for new roles and activities by schools are needed to meet this vexing and potentially destructive challenge (Carnegie Foundation Report, 1996).

Wellness Enhancement: Levels of Address

The unexplained term *wellness enhancement* is broad and projective. Like the concept of prevention, it can be viewed in ways that range, at one extreme, from trying to help the already very sick to be less sick, to promoting wellness in all people at the other. Wellness objectives can be pursued in many different ways and at different points along such a hypothetical continuum. This can be illustrated using three arbitrarily selected points.

The first level, reflecting school mental health's origins, and prime, current modus operandi, consists of efforts to diagnose and repair things that have already gone wrong. This costly, labor-intensive approach reaches only a small fraction of those in need, that is, children with the most serious, entrenched problems that resist change and have the poorest prognoses. Although such repair activities will undoubtedly remain focal in future school mental health services (whether through inertia, in response to immediate pressures, or for reasons of compassion), their payoff value, as suggested earlier, is limited. It is hoped such services will absorb only a fraction of school mental health's limited total resources, in ways that do not restrict the development and application of other promising approaches.

A second level of services, that is, systematic early detection and early secondary prevention, is well reflected in PMHP's model. Advantages of this strategy over reactive approaches targeted to already florid problems are that it reaches many more children at risk sooner, before such problems root and fan out, and can thus offer meaningful correctives earlier. Accordingly, programs such as PMHP that combine systematic early detection and prompt, effective intervention for identified children at risk should figure prominently in a balanced portfolio of future school mental health services.

Primary prevention activities represent a third set of roles for school mental health professionals that differ from the two prior ones both in intent and substance. Their prime objective is to promote wellness in all children proactively, rather than struggling reactively to minimize existing problems. This promising set of still-evolving roles is not yet either widely perceived or meaningfully incorporated into the preparation of school mental health professionals. The primary prevention or wellness enhancement programs that are currently best known to professionals are those that (a) train children in skills and competencies that promote wellness outcomes; and (b) modify class and school environments and practices with that same goal in mind. Yields from this work to date suggest that a significant shift in the school mental health activities in these directions can help many young children adapt more effectively to school, and to life.

Although the types of primary prevention programs described are surely promising "in general" (Durlak & Wells, 1997; Mrazek & Haggerty, 1994), they may be insufficient for many children in modern society whose lives before school are characterized by chronic exposure to profound stressors that exact major tolls. Such stressors can be so overwhelming and pervasive for a family that the child's educational experience pales into insignificance next to them.

This reality, viewed from a broader wellness enhancement perspective, calls for earlier, more basic steps in children's formation than the most that schools can offer after the fact. The phrase "more basic steps" is meant to include (a) social change to enhance living conditions, opportunities, and hope for many people in modern society; and (b) preceding school programs with family and community outreach programs that seek to enhance the wellness and school preparedness of children at serious risk from the very start.

Mounting evidence of considerable importance suggests that such comprehensive early wellness enhancing steps for children and families can contribute importantly to the prevention of later costly and damaging personal and social outcomes, for example, delinquency (Tolan & Guerra, 1994; Yoshikawa, 1994, 1995; Zigler, Taussig, & Black, 1992). In this arena, it appears that sound building in the first place is much to be preferred to the best of all possible repairs. Parent education programs before the child is born (Olds, 1988); active outreaching programs for parents after the child is born (Broussard, 1989; Greenspan, 1981); and effective, comprehensive early childhood programs such as Head Start (Schweinhart, Barnes, & Weikart, 1993; Zigler, 1994; Zigler & Styfco, 1994) exemplify the types of important steps that are needed to establish wholesome early bases in the quest for wellness. Schools, particularly urban schools, must have greater future involvements in planning, conducting, and supporting programs that precede the school experience and seek to optimize the benefits that children derive from schooling.

Society's concerns about the many children who begin school unprepared, and who thus do not profit from school, has grown steadily. The unfortunate effects of such adverse starts are increasingly evident. Many escalate into major academic and behavioral problems, at great cost to the affected children, schools, and society. Schools that have been witness to these problems for many years can readily attest to their magnitude.

A point implicit in this discussion is that there are strong continuities between the nature of the child's formation and early experiences, and what happens in school (i.e., what the child can derive from the school experience). In this arena, schools cannot be islands unto themselves. Unless the chronic, overwhelming problems that many children experience before they enter school, and concurrently with their schooling, can be short-circuited and healthier starts promoted, school failure will remain a high likelihood for them.

The preceding reality has stimulated consideration of new types of school-community partnerships designed to enhance children's early adjustment and increase their preparedness for school. In this context, Dryfoos (1994) developed a sweeping proposal for "full-service schools" in communities with high proportions of multiple-risk children. These settings would provide high-quality education for children as well as other essential services (e.g., health and social services) to families. The ultimate goal behind providing coordinated and readily accessible services in a single setting (i.e., "one-stop shopping") is to facilitate the adaptation of families and thereby establish a path toward meaningful and effective educational experiences for the child.

Others (Wang, Haertel, & Walberg, 1995) have focused on this same theme. A recent special issue of *Professional Psychology* summarized current thinking and recommendations in this area (Paavola et al., 1996; Talley & Short, 1996). In this forum, Paavola et al. (1996) formulated the underlying issue as follows: "The unmet needs of children and families have continued to grow. These conditions are particularly serious for impoverished minority populations. Support has grown for a paradigm shift for service delivery strategies, toward the use of coordinated and collaborative services . . . particularly with respect to the role of schools" (pp. 34, 39). The general approach proposed in those sources includes both school-based and school-linked services, and entails new foci and activities, including some outside the school's walls, for school mental health professionals. A note of caution, however: Neither a full-service school model nor the proposed new type of school-community partnership structures is per se sure to work. Because function is at least as important as structure, the utility of such partnerships may depend on the extent to which they focus on wellness enhancement and school preparedness, not just remediating florid problems. The Carnegie Foundation Report (1996) takes a similar position in calling for a "practical, prevention-oriented approach" that includes (a) universal access to high-quality early care and education for all 3- and 4-year-olds; (b) expansion of parent support and education programs; and, most basically, (c) a prime focus on early prevention rather than later remediation. These worthy objectives highlight wellness goals and implicate new school-community linkages and new professional roles.

On Goals and Roles

One nicety of a book titled *Healthy Children 2010* is that it encourages recommendations about future directions. On the basis of the thinking and programmatic experiences described in this chapter, several issues touched on, but not fully developed, in the preamble can be revisited. One concerns future roles and activities for school mental health professionals.

Earlier, we sketched out three different (not mutually exclusive) levels of school mental health functions along a hypothetical wellness enhancement continuum. That analysis offers a framework, depicted skeletally in Figure 4.1, for considering both how school mental health roles have evolved, and perceived needs for future role changes. When this field first came into being, and for many years thereafter, its roles reflected only Level 1 (containment and repair) activities. Although such activities still comprise the dominant core of school mental health services, recurrent problems not solved by such an approach stimulated explorations of ontogenetically early secondary prevention and wellness-oriented primary prevention programs. Sound prototypic models for the latter approaches are now available and in growing use. As these models are fine-tuned, and clinical-observational and empirical evidence of their efficacy cumulates, such approaches will grow in number and diversity, and professional roles needed to bring them off effectively will be more fully articulated. Indeed, enough is already known about the efficacy and promise of several of these emergent approaches to warrant recommendations by *Healthy People 2010* for needed new school professional roles and changes in training to facilitate the effective conduct of those roles.

One obvious justification for moving in these directions is that the new roles offer intrinsically appealing, heuristic options. A second, less obvious but nonetheless important, one is the growing realization that enhancing children's wellness per se may be the best and most pragmatic route to preventing problems (Cowen, 1994)—a route that schools can help significantly to pave. Pursuing these evolving options calls both for primary prevention roles in the schools and new school-community partnerships designed to enhance children's early wellness and increase their school preparedness, well before the official moment of school entry.

The variables in Figure 4.1 are oversimplified and arbitrarily selected. Levels of function are less pure and less discrete than their representation, and role evolutions over time have been more complex and continuous than what is suggested by the three arbitrarily depicted cross-cuts in time. Finally, the absolute percentages of investment entered for each type of function, at each

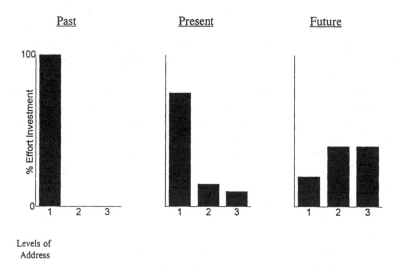

Figure 4.1. Evolution of School Mental Health Roles
NOTE: Level 1 = containment/restoration; Level 2 = early detection and ontogenetically early secondary prevention; Level 3 = primary prevention/wellness enhancement.

time-point (surely for the future), reflect lots of guesswork. Indeed, for that very reason, another useful objective for *Healthy People 2010* would be to gather information about actual, current deployments of school professionals' time across activity categories to establish a baseline for informed recommendations about needed role changes. The intent of Figure 4.1 is simply to portray broad trends, both actual and needed, in the evolution of school mental health roles.

Overview, Summary, and Next Steps

Important changes are taking place in the concepts and practices that guide the mental health fields, particularly school mental health. One is a broadening of its past dominant mandate (i.e., to repair problems), to include before-the-fact prevention—indeed, more basically the enhancement of wellness. Explorations of this broadening purview have led both to the development of sound, useful programs for systematic early detection and prevention of school adjustment problems, and increasingly effective steps toward developing wellness enhancement programs for all children. The latter include second-generation social competence training programs and creating proactive, wellness-targeted school environments.

Although both these developments merit strong representation in future school mental health portfolios, they are not likely to be sufficient to address the vexing school adjustment problems that stem, for some children, from profoundly difficult early life situations. For such youngsters, and they are not few in number, school mental health activities restricted by the Procrustean beds of location (i.e., in school) and addressable issues (i.e., doing the best that can be done for a child with already pervasive problems) are likely to remain limited in value. Rather, the pervasiveness and devastating effects of the problems described suggest a strong need for structures and programs designed to enhance children's wellness and readiness from the start. Such a shift in orientation necessarily implicates new types of community outreaches and interfaces for schools, new alliances with other agencies, and direct involvements in programs that will help children to profit from school. For many children, societal wellness enhancement strategies must begin at birth or before, and continue actively in the early childhood period to optimize formation of solid foundations and the skills and attitudes needed for meaningful gain to accrue from the school experience.

Schools will continue to play a vital role in children's formation and in the maintenance and the enhancement of their wellness. To deliver effectively on that promise, however, calls for programs and activities that differ qualitatively from what has traditionally comprised the defining corpus of school mental health. For notions of prevention and wellness enhancement to take hold in the next century, substantially greater proportions of the total school mental health effort must be invested in proactive activities that strive to enhance wellness outcomes. Such a changing focus will require cognate modifications in the preparation and training of school, and other, mental health professionals. To the extent that high priority is accorded to the goal of enhancing children's wellness, the objectives suggested in the two preceding sentences offer a mini-framework within which *Healthy People 2010* can formulate needed future recommendations.

References

Aronson, E., Blaney, N., Stephan, C., Sikes, J., & Snapp, M. (1978). *The jigsaw classroom.* Beverly Hills, CA: Sage.

Battistich, V., Schaps, E., Watson, M., & Solomon, D. (1995). Prevention effects of the Child Development Project: Early findings from an ongoing multisite demonstration trial. *Journal of Adolescent Research, 11,* 12-35.

Battistich, V., Solomon, D., Kim, D., Watson, M., & Schaps, E. (1995). Schools as communities, poverty levels of student populations, and students' attitudes, motives and performance: A multilevel analysis. *American Educational Research Journal, 32,* 627-658.

Battistich, V., Solomon, D. S., Watson, M., Solomon, J., & Schaps, E. (1989). Effects of an elementary school program to enhance prosocial behavior and children's cognitive social problem solving skills and strategies. *Journal of Applied Developmental Psychology, 10,* 147-169.

Broussard, E. B. (1989). The Infant-Family Resource Program: Facilitating optimal development. In R. E. Hess & J. DeLeon (Eds.), *The National Mental Health Association: 80 years of involvement in the field of prevention* (pp. 179-224). New York: Haworth.

Caplan, M. Z., Weissberg, R. P., Grober, J. S., Sivo, P. J., Grady, K., & Jacoby, C. (1992). Social competence promotion with inner-city and suburban young adolescents: Effects on social adjustment and alcohol use. *Journal of Consulting and Clinical Psychology, 60,* 56-63.

Carnegie Foundation Report. (1996). *Carnegie Task Force on Learning in the Primary Grades.* New York: Carnegie Foundation.

Consortium on the School-Based Promotion of Social Competence. (1994). The school-based promotion of social competence: Theory, research, practice, and policy. In R. J. Haggerty, L. R. Sherrod, N. Garmezy, & M. Rutter (Eds.), *Stress, risk, and resilience in children and adolescents: Processes, mechanisms, and interventions* (pp. 268-316). New York: Cambridge University Press.

Cowen, E. L. (1994). The enhancement of psychological wellness: Challenges and opportunities. *American Journal of Community Psychology, 22,* 149-179.

Cowen, E. L. (1996). The ontogenesis of primary prevention: Lengthy strides and stubbed toes. *American Journal of Community Psychology, 24,* 235-249.

Cowen, E. L., Hightower, A. D., Pedro-Carroll, J. L., Work, W. C., Wyman, P. A., & Haffey, W. G. (1996). *School-based prevention for children at risk: The Primary Mental Health Project.* Washington, DC: American Psychological Association.

Cowen, E. L., Orgel, A. R., Gesten, E. L., & Wilson, A. B. (1979). The evaluation of an intervention program for young schoolchildren with acting-out problems. *Journal of Abnormal Child Psychology, 7,* 381-396.

Cowen, E. L., Trost, M. A., Lorion, R. P., Dorr, D., Izzo, L. D., & Isaacson, R. V. (1975). *New ways in school mental health: Early detection and prevention of school maladaptation.* New York: Human Sciences Press.

Cowen, E. L., Work, W. C., Wyman, P. A., Parker, G. R., Wannon, M., & Gribble, P. A. (1992). Test comparisons among stress-affected, stress-resilient and non-classified 4th-6th grade urban children. *Journal of Community Psychology, 20,* 200-214.

Cowen, E. L., Wyman, P. A., Work, W. C., & Iker, M. R. (1994). A preventive intervention for enhancing resilience among young highly stressed urban children. *Journal of Primary Prevention, 15,* 247-260.

Deci, E. L., & Ryan, R. (1985). *Intrinsic motivation and self-determination in human behavior.* New York: Plenum.

Developmental Studies Center. (1994). *The Child Development Project: Summary of findings in two initial districts and the first phase of an expansion to six additional districts nationally.* Oakland, CA: Author.

Dryfoos, J. G. (1994). *Full service schools: A revolution in health and social services for children, youth and families.* San Francisco: Jossey-Bass.

Durlak, J. A. (1983). Social problem-solving as a primary prevention strategy. In R. D. Felner, L. A. Jason, J. N. Moritsugu, & S. S. Farber (Eds.), *Preventive psychology: Theory, research and practice* (pp. 31-48). Elmsford, NY: Pergamon.

Durlak, J. A. (1995). *School-based prevention programs for children and adolescents.* Thousand Oaks, CA: Sage.

Durlak, J. A., & Wells, A. M. (1997). Primary prevention programs for children and adolescents. *American Journal of Community Psychology, 24.*

Elias, M. J., & Clabby, J. F. (1992). *Building social problem-solving skills: Guidelines from a school-based program.* San Francisco: Jossey-Bass.

Elias, M. J., Gara, M. A., Schuyler, T. F., Branden-Muller, L. R., & Sayette, M. A. (1991). The promotion of social competence: Longitudinal study of a school-based program. *American Journal of Orthopsychiatry, 61,* 409-417.

Elias, M. J., & Tobias, S. E. (1995). *Social problem solving: Interventions in the schools.* New York: Guilford.

Farie, A. M., Cowen, E. L., & Smith, M. (1986). The development and implementation of a rural consortium program to provide early, preventive school mental health services. *Community Mental Health Journal, 22,* 94-103.

Gesten, E. L., Flores de Apodaca, R., Rains, M. H., Weissberg, R. P., & Cowen, E. L. (1979). Promoting peer-related social competence in schools. In M. W. Kent & J. E. Rolf (Eds.), *The primary prevention of psychopathology: Social competence in children* (pp. 220-247). Hanover, NH: University Press of New England.

Gesten, E. L., Rains, M. H., Rapkin, B. D., Weissberg, R. P., Flores de Apodaca, R., Cowen, E. L., & Bowen, R. (1982). Training children in social problem-solving competencies: A first and second look. *American Journal of Community Psychology, 10,* 95-115.

Greenspan, S. I. (1981). *Psychopathology and adaptation in infancy and early childhood: Principles of clinical diagnosis and preventive intervention.* Clinical Infant Report No. 1. New York: International Universities Press.

Hightower, A. D., Avery, R. R., & Levinson, H. R. (1988, April). *An evaluation of the Study Buddy Program: A preventive intervention for 4th and 5th grades.* Paper presented at the meeting of the National Association of School Psychologists, Chicago.

Hightower, A. D., Cowen, E. L., Spinell, A. P., Lotyczewski, B. S., Guare, J. C., Rohrbeck, C. A., & Brown, L. P. (1987). The Child Rating Scale: The development and psychometric refinement of a socioemotional self-rating scale for young school children. *School Psychology Review, 16,* 239-255.

Hightower, A. D., Work, W. C., Cowen, E. L., Lotyczewski, B. S., Spinell, A. P., Guare, J. C., & Rohrbeck, C. A. (1986). The Teacher-Child Rating Scale: A brief objective measure of elementary children's school problem behaviors and competencies. *School Psychology Review, 15,* 393-409.

Hoyt-Meyers, L. A., Cowen, E. L., Work, W. C., Wyman, P. A., Magnus, K., Fagen, D. B., & Lotyczewski, B. S. (1995). Test correlates of resilient outcomes among highly stressed 2nd-3rd grade urban children. *Journal of Community Psychology, 23,* 326-338.

Joint Commission on Mental Illness and Health. (1961). *Action for mental health.* New York: Basic Books.

Lorion, R. P. (Ed.). (1990). *Protecting the children: Strategies for optimizing emotional and behavioral development.* New York: Haworth.

Meller, P. J., Laboy, W., Rothwax, Y., Fritton, J., & Mangual, J. (1994). *Community School District #4: Primary Mental Health Project, 1990-1994.* New York: Community School District #4.

Moos, R. H. (1979). *Evaluating educational environments.* San Francisco: Jossey-Bass.

Mrazek, P. J., & Haggerty, R. J. (Eds.). (1994). *Reducing risks for mental disorders: Frontiers for preventive intervention research.* Washington, DC: National Academy Press.

Olds, D. L. (1988). The prenatal/early infancy project. In R. H. Price, E. L. Cowen, R. P. Lorion, & J. Ramos-McKay (Eds.), *Fourteen ounces of prevention: A casebook for practitioners* (pp. 9-23). Washington, DC: American Psychological Association.

Paavola, J. C., Carey, K., Cobb, C., Ilback, R. J., Joseph, H. M., Routh, D. K., & Torruella, A. (1996). Interdisciplinary school practice: Implications of the service integration model for psychologists. *Professional Psychology, 27,* 34-40.

Pedro-Carroll, J. L., & Alpert-Gillis, L. J. (in press). Preventive interventions for children of divorce: A developmental model for 5 and 6 year old children. *Journal of Primary Prevention, 18.*

Pedro-Carroll, J. L., Alpert-Gillis, L. J., & Cowen, E. L. (1992). An evaluation of the efficacy of a preventive intervention for 4th-6th grade urban children of divorce. *Journal of Primary Prevention, 13,* 115-130.

Pedro-Carroll, J. L., & Cowen, E. L. (1985). The children of divorce intervention program: An investigation of the efficacy of a school-based prevention program. *Journal of Consulting and Clinical Psychology, 53,* 603-611.

Pedro-Carroll, J. L., Cowen, E. L., Hightower, A. D., & Guare, J. C. (1986). Preventive intervention with latency-aged children of divorce: A replication study. *American Journal of Community Psychology, 14,* 277-290.

Price, R. H., Cowen, E. L., Lorion, R. P., & Ramos-McKay, J. (Eds.). (1988). *Fourteen ounces of prevention: A casebook for practitioners.* Washington, DC: American Psychological Association.

Rotheram, M. J., Armstrong, M., & Booraem, C. (1982). Assertiveness training in fourth- and fifth-grade children. *American Journal of Community Psychology, 10,* 567-582.

Schweinhart, L. J., Barnes, H. V., & Weikart, D. P., with Barnett, W. S., & Epstein, A. S. (1993). *Significant benefits: The High/Scope Perry Preschool study through age 27.* Ypsilanti, MI: High/Scope.

Solomon, D., Watson, M. S., Delucchi, K. L., Schaps, E., & Battistich, V. (1988). Enhancing children's prosocial behavior in the classroom. *American Educational Research Journal, 25,* 527-554.

Spivack, G., Platt, J. J., & Shure, M. B. (1976). *The problem-solving approach to adjustment.* San Francisco: Jossey-Bass.

Spivack, G., & Shure, M. B. (1974). *Social adjustment of young children: A cognitive approach to solving real life problems.* San Francisco: Jossey-Bass.

Talley, R. C., & Short, R. J. (1996). Social reforms and the future of school practice: Implications for American psychology. *Professional Psychology, 27,* 5-13.

Terrell, D. L., McWilliams, S. A., & Cowen, E. L. (1972). Description and evaluation of group-work training for nonprofessional aides in a school mental health program. *Psychology in the Schools, 9,* 70-75.

Tolan, P. H., & Guerra, N. G. (1994). Prevention of delinquency: Current status and issues. *Applied and Preventive Psychology, 3,* 251-273.

Wang, M. C., Haertel, G. D., & Walberg, H. J. (1995). The effectiveness of collaborative school-linked services. In L. C. Rigsby, M. C. Reynolds, & M. C. Wang (Eds.), *School/community connections: Issues for research and practice* (pp. 283-309). New York: Jossey-Bass.

Weissberg, R. P., & Elias, M. J. (1993). Enhancing young children's social competence and health behavior: An important challenge for educators, scientists, policy makers and funders. *Applied and Preventive Psychology, 2,* 179-190.

Weissberg, R. P., Gesten, E. L., Carnrike, C. L., Toro, P. A., Rapkin, B. D., Davidson, E., & Cowen, E. L. (1981). Social problem-solving skills training: A competence building intervention with 2nd-4th grade children. *American Journal of Community Psychology, 9,* 411-424.

Weissberg, R. P., Gesten, E. L., Liebenstein, N. L., Schmid, K. D., & Hutton, H. (1980). *The Rochester Social Problem-Solving (SPS) Program: A training manual for teachers of 2nd-4th grade children.* Rochester, NY: Primary Mental Health Project.

Weissberg, R. P., Gesten, E. L., Rapkin, B. D., Cowen, E. L., Davidson, E., Flores de Apodaca, R., & McKim, B. J. (1981). Evaluation of a social problem-solving training program for suburban and inner-city third-grade children. *Journal of Consulting and Clinical Psychology, 49,* 251-261.

Weissberg, R. P., & Greenberg, M. T. (1997). School and community competence-enhancement and prevention programs. In W. Damon (Series Ed.), I. E. Siegel, & K. Renninger (Vol. Eds.), *Handbook of child psychology: Vol. 5. Child psychology in practice* (5th ed.). New York: John Wiley.

Winer-Elkin, J. I., Weissberg, R. P., & Cowen, E. L. (1988). Evaluation of a planned short-term intervention for school children with focal adjustment problems. *Journal of Clinical Child Psychology, 17,* 106-115.

Wright, S., & Cowen, E. L. (1985). The effects of peer teaching on student perceptions of class environment, adjustment and academic performance. *American Journal of Community Psychology, 13,* 413-427.

Wyman, P. A., Cowen, E. L., Work, W. C., Hoyt-Meyers, L. A., Magnus, K., & Fagen, D. (in press). Developmental and caregiving factors differentiating parents of young stress-affected and stress-resilient urban children: A replication and extension. *Development and Psychopathology, 9.*

Wyman, P. A., Cowen, E. L., Work, W. C., & Parker, G. R. (1991). Developmental and family milieu interview correlates of resilience in urban children who have experienced major life-stress. *American Journal of Community Psychology, 19,* 405-426.

Wyman, P. A., Cowen, E. L., Work, W. C., Raoof, A., Gribble, P. A., Parker, G. R., & Wannon, M. (1992). Interviews with children who experienced major life stress: Family and child attributes that predict resilient outcomes. *Journal of the American Academy of Child and Adolescent Psychiatry, 31,* 904-910.

Yoshikawa, H. (1994). Prevention as cumulative protection: Effects of early family support and education on chronic delinquency and its risks. *Psychological Bulletin, 115,* 28-54.

Yoshikawa, H. (1995). Long-term effects of early childhood programs on social outcomes and delinquency. *Future of Children, 5,* 51-75.

Zigler, E. (1994). Reshaping early childhood intervention to be a more effective weapon against poverty. *American Journal of Community Psychology, 22,* 37-48.

Zigler, E., & Styfco, S. J. (1994). Head Start: Criticisms in a constructive context. *American Psychologist, 49,* 127-132.

Zigler, E., Taussig, C., & Black, K. (1992). A promising preventative for juvenile delinquency. *American Psychologist, 47,* 997-1006.

• CHAPTER 5 •

Mental Health Services for Children and Adolescents

MARY JANE ROTHERAM-BORUS

Policymakers have motivated the nation to address children's mental health needs by setting a series of goals for communities (Fleming, 1996; U.S. Department of Health and Human Services, Public Health Service [DHHS], 1991, 1995). These goals have included reducing the prevalence of psychiatric disorder, increasing the delivery of mental health services, and targeting specific problems, such as reducing the prevalence of suicidal behaviors, physical fighting, weapons possession, and the high school drop-out rate. Many of these goals will not be met by the year 2000; in fact, the mid-decade review acknowledges that some adolescent mental health problems are becoming worse (e.g., the increasing rate of suicide attempts) (DHHS, 1995; Fleming, 1996). This chapter will review the progress on meeting the nation's existing mental health goals for adolescents and identify issues that will have to be considered in setting new goals. To assist

AUTHOR'S NOTE: This chapter was prepared with support from the National Institute of Mental Health Grant No. 5U01-MH54278 to the author. Thanks are made to Roger Weissberg, Ph.D., Leonard Bickman, Ph.D., Coleen Cantwell, B.A., Sutherland Miller, Ph.D., Nancy Herrera, Ph.D., Madeline Zwart, B.A., Mary Rogers, Kris Langabeer, B.S., Eric Agdeppa, B.S., and Jason Saculles, B.A., for help in the preparation of this chapter. Address correspondence to Dr. Mary Jane Rotheram-Borus, Department of Psychiatry, UCLA, 10920 Wilshire, Suite 1103, Los Angeles, CA, 90024. Phone: (310) 794-8278; fax: (310) 794-8297; E-mail: mjrotheram@npimain.medsch.ucla.edu.

in the process, it will be necessary to identify a theoretical model guiding emerging policy issues that will influence our ability to achieve substantial changes in children's mental health problems (e.g., the increase of managed care, categorical funding) and to provide recommendations to understand factors that are likely to shape how communities can set new, realistic, and achievable goals for the year 2010.

Significance and Scope of the Problem

Need for Services

A substantial number of children need mental health services; therefore, 10 years ago we set a national goal to reduce the need for mental health services to 10% of children (DHHS, 1991; revised to 17% in 1995, DHHS, 1995). When the goal was set, there were no national data documenting the need for services. The presence of a psychiatric disorder is one traditional index of need. In 1989, it was estimated that 7.5 million children (12% of the child population) were in need of mental health services based on the presence of a mental disorder (U.S. Congress, Office of Technology Assessment, 1986).

In contrast to this estimate, substantially higher rates of psychiatric disorder consistently emerge in nonclinical samples of children assessed by different investigators using various assessment methods (Anderson, Williams, McGee, & Silva, 1989; Bird et al., 1988; Brandenburg & Friedman, 1990; Costello et al., 1988; Offord et al., 1987; Velez, Johnson, & Cohen, 1989). Between 17.6% and 22% of children in nonclinical settings are reported to have one or more psychiatric diagnoses, a rate similar to that obtained in the recent Methodology for Epidemiology in Children and Adolescents (MECA) trial (21%) (Lahey et al., 1994). About twice this percentage are anticipated to be subsyndromal for disorder (Angst & Hochstrasser, 1994; Judd, Rapaport, Paulus, & Brown, 1994), that is, at higher risk for developing mental health problems in the future and more likely to have a cluster of risk factors (Institute of Medicine, 1994). Children with more than one disorder are particularly likely to follow a negative developmental course, with increasing mental health problems with age (Coie et al., 1993; Lewinsohn, Rohde, & Seeley, 1995). As the overall rate of psychopathology is similar across these studies, so also are the rates of specific diagnoses, such as attention deficit hyperactivity disorder (ADHD) (4.2%), oppositional disorder (6.3%), conduct disorder (3.7%), and the combined externalizing behavior disorders (10.4%). Anxiety and depressive disorders rates are also similar across studies, 13.6% and 6.2%, respectively. These data support the assertion that mental illness is the number one cause of disabilities for those aged 10-18 years (National Institute of Child Health and Human Development, 1990). However, the data suggest that the goal of a 17% rate of psychiatric disorder in children will not be met by the year 2000 for specific subgroups (low income, ethnic minority children) and must be reexamined for feasibility and relevance for the year 2010.

One area that leads to reexamination of the goals is the dramatic gender and age differences found in the rates of psychopathology. Overall, young males have higher rates of disorder than young females and are more likely to have a disruptive behavior diagnosis (Bird et al., 1988). Males and females report similar rates of disorder in adolescence; however, the type of disorder varies. Affective disorders are far more common among adolescent females than males (Berman & Schwartz, 1990; Costello, 1989; Lewinsohn et al., 1995). There are a few studies of ethnic differences (including the MECA data set), but the data gathered are highly variable. Ethnic differences in scores of a single dimension of adjustment (e.g., depression) have been assessed (Reynolds & Graves, 1989); however, a national study of ethnic differences in need for mental health services is only currently being conducted (Utilization, Needs, Outcomes, and Costs for Child and Adolescent Psychopathology, or UNOCCAP), and the results will take several years to emerge. Socioeconomic status and community factors appear to influence rates significantly (Swanson, Holzer, & Ganju, 1993), with poverty increasing risk for a mental disorder.

To set a national goal, the definition of need for mental health, particularly among youth in disadvantaged socioeconomic groups and ethnicities, must be examined. In addition to psychiatric disorder, the functional impairment and adaptive functioning of children must be assessed to determine need for services (Halfon, English, Allen, & DeWoody, 1994). Children who are experiencing symptoms may or may not demonstrate functional impairments in daily life (Berman & Jobes, 1995; Berman & Schwartz, 1990). Given past research, about 40% of adolescents and children are believed to have a mental health disorder currently or in the past, or be subsyndromal for disorder (D. P. Cantwell, personal communication, June 18, 1994). These youth can be considered at high risk for multiple negative outcomes: dropping out of school, having contact with the criminal justice system, pregnancy and teenage motherhood, substance abuse, HIV infection, and unemployment. If 40% of the nation's children are at risk, a review of fundamental structural factors that shape mental health and our definitions of national goals may need to be readjusted.

Unmet Need for Services

Given the number of youth at risk, the number of children whose needs are being addressed by community service systems is low. When setting goals for the year 2000, the nation recognized that only one in eight young people who needed services actually received those services. Currently, while 20% to 40% of youth have a need for mental health services (based on MECA data) about 3% to 33% of youth receive such care (U.S. Congress, Office of Technology Assessment, 1986), between 3.5% and 6% of young people (Manderscheid et al., 1993). As increasing fiscal pressures are placed on community service providers, the percentage of youth who receive services appears to be decreasing, not increasing.

One major caveat exists in our evaluation of our ability to assess the mental health services provided to children. Children with mental health problems are more likely to present in special education, foster care, primary health care, the juvenile justice system, and substance abuse treatment than in the mental health system. Between 8% and 12% of schoolchildren are in special education classes, and almost half of those in special education are likely to have mental health problems (Knoff & Batsche, 1990; Sailor, Gerry, & Wilson, 1991; Urban Strategies Council, 1992). Children with mental disorders are more likely than their peers to seek care in primary health care settings (Costello et al., 1988; Horwitz, Leaf, Leventhal, Forsyth, & Speechley, 1992; Miranda, Hohmann, Attkisson, & Larson, 1994), although most receive help only from their doctor, rather than being referred for mental health care (Horwitz et al., 1992). For example, children with untreated mental health problems are likely to use double the resources in primary health care compared to children without mental health problems (Borus et al., 1985). This trend is likely to increase with the introduction of managed care, reliance on family practitioners, and reductions in spending. For example, child welfare programs (including foster and kinship care, group home, and residential care) serve between 30% and 65% of the children seen in mental health settings (Halfon, 1992; Halfon et al., 1994; Halfon & Klee, 1987; Hochstadt, Jaudes, Zimo, & Schachter, 1987; Schorr, Both, & Copple, 1991; Takayama, Bergman, & Connell, 1994; Weinstein & LaFleur, 1990), often delivering inappropriate, incomplete, and poorly coordinated care (Frank, 1980; Klee & Halfon, 1987). In addition, children of different ethnic groups receive care at very different rates (e.g., 1 of 13 African Americans vs. 1 of 401 Asian Americans) (McGlynn, Norquist, Wells, Sullivan, & Libernian, 1983). Juvenile justice also serves a large portion of children in need of mental health services (e.g., 37%) (Urban Strategies Council, 1992), with the criteria very unclear about who receives mental health care versus probation (Cohen et al., 1990; Elliott, Huizinga, & Menard, 1989; Paulson, Coombs, & Landsverk, 1990). Ethnicity appears to be a primary criteria for triaging youth to one setting or another. In particular, African Americans are far more likely to receive services in the juvenile justice sector when demonstrating the same number of mental health symptoms as Anglo peers being served in the mental health system (Wordes, Bynum, & Corley, 1994). Because most children with mental health problems are comorbid for multiple disorders, many disturbed youth are found in substance abuse programs (Berman & Schwartz, 1990; Brunswick & Menzel, 1988; Friedman, Utada, Glickman, & Morrissey, 1987; Hughes et al., 1990; Mannuzza, Klein, Bonagura, Konig, & Shenker, 1988; Windle, 1990). Finally, adolescent children at risk for mental health problems are far more likely to be identified by social service systems; the kinds of problems these youth can create (theft, teenage parenthood, car accidents, suicide) are of greater concern to society than the types of problems that younger children can create.

Many children served in other sectors are at risk for mental health problems, and these children are often using multiple services, although the pattern of use has not been well documented (Urban Strategies Council, 1992). Clearly, it is critical to understand the movement of children at risk for mental health problems among the various social service systems and how counties assign responsibility for the care of these children. There will clearly be ethnic-, gender-, and age-specific developmental pathways for youth without mental health problems in the same communities.

Thus, setting national goals for the delivery of services must stop using a sector approach to understanding the delivery of mental health services to children. By setting a goal that targets delivery in only one sector (e.g., more children will receive mental health care in the mental health sector), we fail to recognize the complexity of the problem and of the potential solutions. For example, clearly the easiest route to the delivery of mental health care for children and adolescents will be in the school or primary health care sectors. These sectors must consider their responsibility for achieving the positive, long-term mental health adjustment of children by developing integrated, comprehensive goals that will monitor integrated, comprehensive programs for youth. Considering the issues of pathways to services, it is necessary to examine the entire community service network. Adequate mental health services for children can only be realized when the efforts of multiple service sectors are recognized as interrelated.

Factors Influencing Goals in the Year 2010

Theoretical Model

National goals can only be met at the local level, especially when the goals necessitate the interface of individual children's problems and local-level service provision by therapists in their agency or office.

Thus, multiple factors at multiple levels (e.g., state, county, community, institutional, family, and individual) will influence the nation's ability to meet its health goals. For example, community factors dramatically influence the need and unmet need for mental health services in children (Kelly, 1979; Rutter, Maughan, Mortimore, Ouston, & Smith, 1979). High levels of poverty, overcrowding, crime, and poor housing are associated with high rates of conduct disorder (Hawkins, Catalano, & Miller, 1992; Rutter &

Giller, 1983). D. P. Cantwell (personal communication, June 18, 1994) estimates a 10-point difference in the mean level of the Children's Global Assessment Scale (CGAS) in children in two adjacent counties in southern California, based on community stressors. Structural, social, and health indicators of the community will be associated with children's need for mental health care. Building on paradigms that have been used to analyze access (Aday & Anderson, 1981) and quality of care (Donabedian, 1980; Mc-Glynn et al., 1983), and economic (Manning, Wells, Duan, Newhouse, & Ware, 1986) and clinical outcomes (Hoagwood, Hibbs, Brent, & Jensen, 1995) in previous mental health services research, an interdisciplinary team of researchers from the University of California, Los Angeles (Rotheram-Borus, Leibowitz, et al., 1994) and a consortium of universities have developed a model (see Figures 5.1 and 5.2) that can be used to examine structural factors at the community and service sector levels that, together with family factors, influence the process and outcomes associated with responding to children's mental health needs. Parallel frameworks have been used to investigate cultural processes (Gallimore, Goldenberg, & Weisner, 1993; Weisner, 1984; Weisner, Gallimore, & Jordan, 1988), developmental processes (Rogoff, 1995; Rogoff, Baker-Sennett, Lacasa, & Goldsmith, 1995), and educational (Artiles & Trent, 1994) and family settings for the developmentally disabled (Gallimore, Tharp, & Rueda, 1989). Figure 5.1 outlines the primary structural factors that influence the delivery and outcomes of care for communities and individuals. In this figure, the system of care refers to structural and family factors affecting need, access, the process of care, and outcomes. Each of these factors must be assessed from multiple perspectives and at multiple levels. In Figure 5.2, access refers to the ability to gain entry to mental health care; utilization refers to the amount of care received (Gillespie & Marten, 1978). Communities vary widely in the degree of integration of their mental health services for disturbed children. For example, in one county in California, all children entering the juvenile justice system are screened for mental health problems; about one third are in need of services, which are paid for by the juvenile justice system. This structural difference in the organization of care is likely to influence access to care and utilization.

In addition to structural features of the organizational setting predicting pathology and associated need for mental health services,

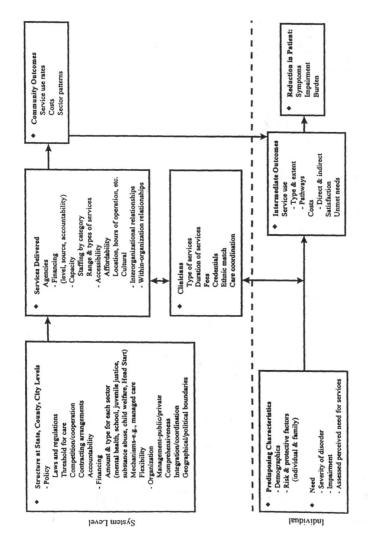

Figure 5.1. Model of a System of Care for Mental Health Services

131

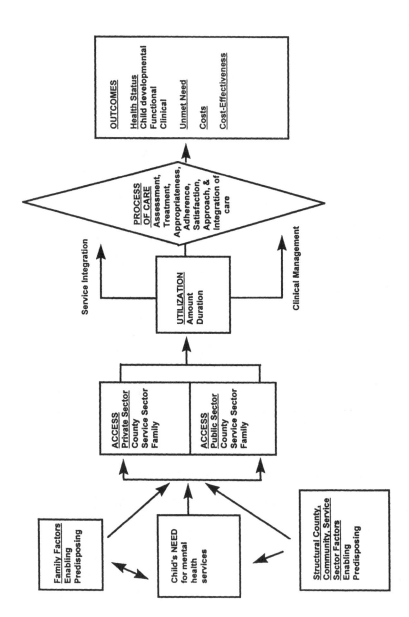

Figure 5.2. Theoretical Model Outlining Sets of Factors Influencing Children's Needs, Access, Utilization, and Outcomes

so do social disadvantage, marital discord, overcrowding or large family size, paternal criminality, maternal mental disorder, family behavioral management practices, and admission into child welfare services (Biederman et al., 1993; Bird, Gould, Yager, Staghezza, & Canino, 1989; Dishion & Loeber, 1985; Hetherington, 1989; Klee & Halfon, 1987; Rutter et al., 1979; Williams, Anderson, McGee, & Silva, 1990). While able to increase children's risk for mental health problems, families can also be protective. Having a small family, with children well spaced; supportive parental (Rutter, 1985) and sibling relationships; and adequate rule setting (Werner, 1986) protects children from disorder. Future national goals must target increases in family protective factors (e.g., alcohol-limited environments for families) and decreases in family-related risk factors (e.g., high rates of out-of-home placements) associated with the need for mental health services (Bird et al., 1989; Blank, Melaville, & Asayesh, 1992; Goldenberg & Gallimore, 1991). Similar to the manner in which we narrowly set a goal for mental health problems to be served by the mental health sector, we must recognize that children's adjustment will be related to environmental issues such as parents' employment and availability of low-cost child care. In addition, parents of different ethnic origins are likely to construct the meaning of their children's mental health symptoms quite differently and have very different thresholds for seeking mental health care for their children. While we need research that generates basic descriptions of the family's influences on the emergence and maintenance of its children's mental health problems (Coie et al., 1993; Hochstadt et al., 1987), we have substantial data to indicate domains that will be useful in shaping our ability to meet the goals of the year 2010.

Figure 5.2 presents the ways factors at multiple levels influence an individual child's access, utilization, quality, outcome, and cost of receiving mental health services. In the proposed theoretical framework, state, county, local community, and family factors affect children's need for mental health services. For example, states that mandate individualized educational plans for children with learning disabilities are more likely to address the needs of young people with these problems compared to states without such mandates. Communities with preventive programs for all students transitioning to middle schools are likely to reduce the number of children needing mental health interventions at these developmental points.

Communities with a low socioeconomic base and high unemployment are likely to have a higher percentage of children with mental health problems compared to more economically privileged communities. The higher percentage of mental health problems emerge not only because of higher rates of family problems but also because of reduced access and lower levels of funding provided in impoverished settings. In addition to influencing the level of need, both family and structural factors enable or inhibit children's access to mental health care. A non-English-speaking Vietnamese family, for example, may want to seek mental health services, but the community may have no service providers who speak Vietnamese. Even if the family had resources or insurance to pay for services, family (e.g., ethnicity) and community (e.g., percentage of youth receiving care) factors may constrain the delivery of care.

Access. Most of our knowledge of children's access and use comes from studies of adults, but because parents determine their children's use (Rotheram-Borus, Miller, Piacentini, Graae, & Castro-Blanco, 1994), adult data may be informative (Baekeland & Lundwall, 1975). For example, families' insurance significantly influences their access to mental health care; more generous insurance promotes use (Leibowitz, 1986; Manning, Wells, Duan, Newhouse, & Ware, 1984; Miranda et al., 1994) particularly for children and adolescents (Padgett, Patrick, Burns, Schlesinger, & Cohen, 1993). For example, when coverage was free, 8.8% used outpatient services, twice the rate of those who paid for their own care. Use of formal mental health providers was low, but was twice as common when service was free (5% vs. 2.4%), a consistent finding (Frank & McGuire, 1985; McGuire, 1989; Miranda et al., 1994). Despite the large differences in use, there were no significant differences in mental health outcomes (Brook et al., 1983). Private insurance increases the demand for mental health services. This demand can then be satisfied by private providers, unless a family is trying to obtain Medicaid-reimbursed services. Few private providers may be willing to accept the low Medicaid reimbursement rates. The uninsured face even greater constraints on their supply of mental health services because they must depend on the limited supply of public mental health providers. Less is known about how those with public health insurance or no insurance are affected by the difficulty in finding adequate services, or how private providers substitute for public providers. We do not currently know to what extent families use private insurance or pay out of pocket if they cannot use public mental health services, nor do we know how Medicaid providers' willingness to accept low reimbursement levels affects access to care for poor children.

Managed Care. Prior studies have found that costs of outpatient mental health care for enrollees in health maintenance organizations (HMOs) are lower than for fee-for-service (FFS) enrollees (Wells, Manning, & Benjamin, 1986), despite similar referral rates. Pediatricians diagnose mental health problems at similar rates in HMOs and in FFS, but rates in both were low relative to case findings in psychiatric interviews (Costello, 1986). The number of visits for users is lower in capitated systems (Kessler, 1984; Mc-Guire & Fairbank, 1988). Comparing individuals with free FFS care and those randomly assigned to an HMO, the FFS system provides much more intensive therapy per user (about three times as many visits) (Miranda et al., 1994), provides more individual rather than group therapy, and is more likely to use psychotropic drugs. However, outcomes did not differ by type of payment (Wells, Manning, & Valdez, 1990). Most studies have focused on staff or group model HMOs. In a study that included individual practice associations (IPAs), Rogers, Wells, Meredith, Sturm, and Burnam (1993) found that depressed HMO patients (particularly those in IPAs) tended to acquire new limitations in role/physical functioning and decreased medications over time, while depressed FFS patients did not. Most of the existing findings relate to adults and to staff or group model HMOs. Little is known about outcomes of care or pathways to receiving care for children enrolled in HMOs, particularly IPAs and Medicaid-funded HMOs.

Understanding such pathways is critical, however, because managed care has been increasingly instituted in the nation's public mental health system. Over the previous 10 years, government cost cuts have shifted the burden of treating disturbed children to the private sector (Wolch, Kim, & Lee, 1992). Recently, an increasingly competitive insurance environment (Melnick & Lyter, 1987) has led HMOs to shift the burden back to the public sector. The effect of sector shifting on the public system of mental health care for children is not understood at this time.

Sector Shifting. Managed care refers only to services delivered in health care settings; as we noted above, most mental health services will be delivered in other sectors. In addition to shifts associated with managed care, fiscal practices of sector shifting for the delivery of care to psychiatrically disturbed youth is of fundamental concern. When policymakers think in a categorical manner, the chances that the burden for providing mental health services will shift from one public sector to another increase. For example, the state of California has recently passed a "three strikes" criminal sentencing law that requires 25-year-to-life-term incarceration after three felony convictions. Financial resources are likely to be reallocated from service sectors such as mental health, primary health care, and transportation to the criminal justice system to meet its legal responsibilities. Similarly, if a youth needs out-of-home placement for mental health problems, Los Angeles County must pay up to $3,200 per month for foster care placements. However, if the same youth has contact with the criminal justice system and then has probation violations, the youth's out-of-home placement can qualify as a criminal justice placement, and the state, not the county, will pay for the youth's placement. Instead of a $3,200/month charge, the county may only pay $50 to the state and the state will absorb the cost. In the crafting of new welfare reform laws, there is a proposed ceiling on the number of families on Aid to Families With Dependent Children (AFDC). However, there is no cap on out-of-home placements. It would not be surprising that this reward structure would be associated with increasing numbers of poor families perceiving a need for out-of-home placement (with relatives) to continue the family's ability to survive financially. The fiscal incentives for a county mental health department, county government, or state government to engage in sector shifting can be substantial.

A similar process occurs at the individual family level. If a child is certified as needing substantial intervention due to learning disabilities, a family can have the costs of such care covered by the school district, rather than the family's health insurance. This becomes particularly important as the family's insurance manages care and places limits on the maximum amount of services that can be obtained in a year. There are substantial differences in the extent to which an individual family is aware of its rights to secure services for the child. For example, Anglo parents are far more likely to

receive mental health services paid for by their children's school
than are Latino or African American parents (Los Angeles County
Board of Education, 1995; McAllister, 1993; Urban Strategies
Council, 1992).

Ethnic Patterns. Children from different ethnic backgrounds vary
dramatically in the distribution of mental health risk factors and
service use (Hu, Snowden, & Jerrell, 1992; Neighbors, Jackson,
Campbell, & Williams, 1989; Sue & McKinney, 1975). By the year
2000, 40% of the service delivery population will consist of ethnic
minority children. Variations in use appear related to specific
community settings (McAllister, 1993; Urban Strategies Council,
1992). For example, Asian and African American children in Los
Angeles are on AFDC at about the same levels. However, Asian
children are far less likely to use county emergency services and
mental health resources (Sue & McKinney, 1975). Asian children
also are far less likely to enter mental health services than their
cross-ethnic peers in the same community, and when accessing care
they are referred from different sources (other social service providers) compared to African American (family and friends) and
Anglo, non-Latino families (legal and self-referrals) (Uehara,
Takeuchi, & Smukler, 1994). Such differences are typically attributed to differences due to minority status (e.g., discrimination)
and social class, although there has been little research focusing
on how to examine the ways in which cultural differences influence
daily expression and management of children's mental health symptoms. Three alternatives have been suggested to provide more
ethnically sensitive services: (a) Increase training to existing personnel for delivering culturally sensitive services, (b) establish
parallel services that are independent of mainstream organizations
but similar in structure and function, and (c) provide nonparallel
service organizations that have no precedence in the conventional
mental health system. In general, there is support for each of these
alternatives; for example, attending ethnic-specific community
mental health centers is significantly more likely to result in positive
behavioral changes among children who attend general community
mental health centers (Uehara et al., 1994).

Child and Family Factors. Similar to the way in which families
influence need for services, family circumstances affect the course

and outcome of emotional and problem behaviors in children (Gallimore et al., 1989; Rotheram-Borus, Miller, et al., 1994). Families' response to need is to seek services. As noted above, in large urban centers, services are sought from many service sectors, and those with health problems may receive a combination of public and private care (e.g., special education at school, primary health care at an HMO, and medical FFS mental health care). The pathways among these types of services (HMO, public, FFS) and across service sectors (e.g., substance abuse, child welfare) have not been well documented for children and will shift as managed care is increasingly instituted. A child's age and gender are particularly likely to influence the pathways taken through service sectors and types of services. A 6-year-old with behavior problems may be referred for classroom behavioral management interventions, while a 16-year-old with similar behaviors is likely to have contact with the juvenile justice or substance abuse treatment sectors. Children receiving care may or may not receive appropriate treatment for some and not other needs. Which of the child's problems are addressed depends on which service sector is accessed and the integration and quality of care of the services that are provided. Variations in structural and clinical aspects of care lead to important variations in the child's health outcomes and related direct (treatment) and indirect (parents' loss of work) costs. If we are going to set national goals, we need to tailor the goals for children of different ages.

Quality of Care. The process of delivering mental health care, particularly the quality, appropriateness, and integration of care, is likely to influence the outcome of care for the child, his or her family, and society. Researchers typically assess the quality of care along two dimensions: whether a physician uses the most appropriate intervention available and the manner of physician-patient interaction (Brook, Kamberg, & Lohr, 1982)—both are understudied areas of children's services. Basic descriptive data are needed in the area of children's quality of care. While the American Psychiatric Association (1993) and American Academy of Child and Adolescent Psychiatry (1991, 1992, 1993) have outlined very general standards of care for several types of disorders, there has been little evaluation of how often appropriate care is provided or whether positive outcomes are enhanced with conditions of appropriate care (Brook et al., 1982; Sailor et al., 1991). We do not know whether the most basic standards are followed for children's quality of care: For example, do children with ADHD receive appropriate medication? We have almost no data on whether children served in different sectors receive similar types and levels of mental health services. Nor do we know about subjective indexes of quality, for example, families' perceptions of satisfaction and the quality of their relationships with their mental health service providers.

Service Integration. The more problems an individual child experiences, the more mental health services the child is likely to need and the greater will be the importance of coordinating and integrating services across multiple providers in multiple sectors and types of service over time (service integration). Service integration has been a central theme within each of the service sectors (Agranoff, 1991; Beilenson, 1987; Blank et al., 1992; Center for the Study of Social Policy, 1991; Farrow & Joe, 1992; Gardner, 1992; Halpern, 1991; Kagan, Rivera, & Parker, 1991; Mordock, 1990; Ooms & Owen, 1991). While theoretically intuitive, the data that have been collected have not supported the importance of this factor for improving children's outcomes. Service integration, however, does appear to be a strategy for cutting costs of delivering mental health services. For example, Ventura County, California, has been a national leader in providing culturally sensitive, comprehensive services for children with continuity through case management and a primary focus on "integrating" mental health services for over 10 years. This strategy has appeared to cap escalating mental health costs in that county (Attkisson, Dresser, & Rosenblatt, 1991). Over time, the organization and funding of services for children at risk for mental health problems have become integrated across service sectors. For example, in Ventura County all children entering juvenile justice are screened for mental health problems and outpatient therapy is delivered in schools. While Ventura County's programs appear exemplary, the outcomes for children in these programs and untreated children have not been evaluated.

Outcomes. Outcomes define whether a mental health intervention has a positive effect on the child and family or not. Mental health services may not have a uniformly positive effect on children (Weisz, Weiss, Alicke, & Klotz, 1987). Three issues limit our ability to detect positive outcomes in response to the mental health care being delivered in this country: (a) Care may be inadequate at many points: limited access, inappropriate evaluations, inappropriate treatment, high drop-out rates; (b) children with the most severe problems will receive the most treatment and yet are not expected to substantially improve; and (c) child outcomes are complex, including categorical and dimensional indexes of adjustment that vary with age, gender, and ethnicity (Loeber, Brinthaupt, & Green, 1990; Mrazek & Haggerty, 1994). To assess change, complex designs will be needed. The problems associated with access and the process of treatment have been reviewed above. Perhaps the most difficult issue to untangle when evaluating outcomes is that traditionally, most public funds are focused on serving a small number of youth who are in the greatest need of services. The potential improvements for this small group is often limited. More recently, communities have been adopting a variety of different strategies for improving the mental health status of the greatest number of children and families. Given that very few children receive mental health services (1%-4%) and the likelihood that many services are not likely to meet standards of appropriateness and quality of care, a wide gap has developed between the positive effect we know that programs can generate and the findings on the effectiveness of services (Weisz & Weiss, 1989; Weisz, Weiss, & Donenberg, 1992). These problems are heightened in that more than 50% of outpatients are likely to discontinue services without notice. Currently, evaluations of systems of care have not demonstrated that service delivery has a positive effect on children's mental health status (Bickman, 1996; Bickman et al., 1995). Meta-analytic studies have found that treatments for children delivered in controlled settings are highly effective (effect sizes of about .8) (Angst & Hochstrasser, 1994; Weisz et al., 1987); however, these effects are not evident in evaluations of services for children in community clinics (Offord et al., 1987; Weisz & Weiss, 1989; Weisz et al., 1992). A recent review of 19 evaluation studies found half of the current evaluations to have positive results for psychotherapeutic interventions for children with severe mental health problems in community settings (Weisz et al., 1987). However, overall, there was insufficient power in the vast majority of studies to have ever detected positive outcome. Such fundamental problems in the design of evaluations of psychotherapy create political problems for a field attempting to demonstrate its efficacy. Rosenblatt and Attkisson (1993) have suggested that evaluations must (a) include a range of social perspectives in evaluating outcomes (client, family, social, clinician, and scientist); (b) include multiple contexts for assessment (family, school, community); and (c) cover multiple domains (clinical status, functional impairment, quality of life, safety and welfare). Evaluations will be even more complex when theoretical approaches recognize that change may be developmental (Prochaska, DiClemente, & Norcross, 1992) or phased (Howard, Lueger, Maling, & Martinovich, 1993).

Even with relatively positive data, there is a gap in the "believability" of the findings of efficacy of mental health services (Beutler & Clarkin, 1991). This gap will serve to further inhibit the nation's ability to meet the goals of *Healthy Youth 2000* (Fleming, 1996). Increasingly, psychotherapy and psychotherapy research are being held financially and politically accountable, and national and independent health care systems may not cover psychotherapy unless there are demonstrated favorable outcomes (Lambert, 1991). If this were to become a reality, it will be impossible to meet the goals of *Healthy Youth 2000*. It is imperative that we mount rigorous evaluations with sufficient power to detect differences in outcomes of children's mental health services.

Recommendations

Interventions to Assist in Achieving *Healthy People 2010* Goals

Given this review, recommendations for improving the targeted goals for *Healthy People 2010* fall in three major categories: (a) improving the transfer of technology for delivering psychotherapeutic interventions in community-based settings; (b) questioning the current models of delivering psychotherapy by practitioners who are generalists; and (c) examining alternative financing structures for the delivery of care within primary health care, education, and other sectors.

Technology transfer in the context of this chapter refers to the dissemination of innovative and effective psychotherapeutic child interventions in community-based settings. As noted above, most child-focused interventions that have been tested for efficacy generate effect sizes in the range of .3 to .45 (Weisz & Weiss, 1989). However, such effects are not generated in the field settings, that is, the average mental health setting in a local community. In community settings, however, the typical practitioner delivers a psychodynamic, eclectic intervention strategy, while almost all therapies delivered in a research setting are cognitive-behavioral in orientation and delivery. Every research-based intervention is guided by an extensive manual, provides substantial training and monitoring to the therapists, and uses relatively new intervention agency. Research-based studies are not typically delivered by therapists with a caseload of 80 clients, nor do clinical providers receive supervision on a weekly basis for each of their clients.

To secure results similar to those demonstrated in research settings, substantial changes must be implemented in the delivery of mental health care. First, the next generation of therapists must be taught that the affective state of the client during therapy is not an outcome. The targeted outcomes are performance based and only relevant if demonstrated outside of the therapy hour and following the delivery of the intervention. Second, broad-scale dissemination of manualized interventions with demonstrated positive outcomes must occur. Each federal agency (National Institute of Mental Health; National Institute of Allergies and Infectious Diseases; National Institute of Child Health and Human Development; Centers for Disease Control and Prevention; Association for Children, Youth and Families) must undertake the dissemination of programs with demonstrated efficacy. Currently, successful research programs are typically funded from 3 to 5 years and there is no incentive for the research team to disseminate their findings. Third, systems for monitoring the delivery of services must be set at the local level. While there can be substantial variation in how outcomes are monitored, the existence of a monitoring system is fundamental to achieving *Healthy People 2010* goals.

With such revisions, the fundamental staffing and training systems for mental health services must be reconsidered. The field of developmental disabilities shifted many years ago to training paraprofessionals to deliver specific interventions: toilet training, table manners, job interviewing, keeping a checkbook. Many developmentally linked problems do not require extensive intervention (e.g., bedwetting, reactive depressive disorders), but require specialization from a paraprofessional trained in the theory, techniques, and evaluation of the specific disorder. The shift from mental health to primary health care settings for the delivery of care creates the opportunity to begin to identify specific, time-limited interventions for children. A specialist for children with attention deficit disorder could be trained and deliver group-based services to several groups of 8 to 10 children several times a week. This would be likely to result in higher-quality services to youth in need.

Financing structures offer the greatest potential source for reshaping and/or improving the delivery of care. Whether nationally programmed interventions proceed or not, change is occurring rapidly at the local level. States are shifting publicly insured children to managed care programs; the role and level of mental health funding within these programs is yet undetermined. The only advocacy programs to date have been in the area of a mandated option for hospitalization following childbirth. Historically, the National Community Mental Health Association has lobbied most effectively for the severely mentally ill, autistic children, and schizophrenic children. These priorities must be examined in the context of improving the overall health of the community. Identifying potential trade-offs in funding the most severely disabled versus the general population at risk must be examined in a public forum so that priorities can be set.

Strategy to Set Goals for 2010

To set realistic, achievable goals for *Healthy People 2010,* three strategies are suggested for setting the goals: (a) Set goals for communities, rather than at the national levels for specific individuals; (b) set up a national surveillance system to monitor implementation of the goals on an annual basis; and (c) establish an incentive system and a method for automatic intervention when communities fail to achieve targeted goals so that progress will be made toward the targeted outcomes.

Rather than setting national goals, community-level goals may be more appropriate. Mental health services are delivered at the local level, and the complexities and history of the local system will influence each community's ability to reduce the need and unmet need in its local context. As outlined in the theoretical model in Figure 5.2, there are community-level outcomes that are a function of the structural factors, as well as reflections of the service delivery network (specific agencies and office-based practices). Paralleling the movement for national funding of HIV programs (e.g., Bowen et al., 1992; McKinney, Wieland, Bowen, Goosby, & Marconi, 1993), local planning councils and counties could be made account-able for the design and implementation of the local system of care. Linking funding to the delivery of community-level outcomes will provide incentive to local communities to improve their delivery system. With the mounting social problems of inner cities, it will not be possible for us to meet national goals at the same level for all children. As with income, it is possible to have a large subgroup of the middle class whose functioning and mental health status improves, but with a greater gap between the adjustment of the privileged youth in contrast to those at greater disadvantage. This was precisely the situation in the level of substance use in the early 1980s. Substance use was declining nationally; however, admissions to emergency rooms for drug overdoses was rising dramatically, and a far greater percentage of minority youth were using high levels of drugs. To decrease the gap between disenfranchised and middle-class youth, community targets and outcomes would offer an ad-vantage.

Paradoxically, when local control is given to communities, it is critical to establish a national monitoring system. A prime example of this strategy has been the program of the Division of Adolescent and School Health of the Centers for Disease Control and Preven-tion (CDC, 1995). Over the past 6 years, a system for monitoring sexual-risk acts of the nation's youth has been established. While this system took several years to implement, within 7 years, more than 85% of communities will have participated in the CDC survey. Two years ago, the same division initiated a system for monitoring school districts' implementation of HIV prevention. When setting national goals, the surveillance mechanism must be established several years in advance of the targeted goal to monitor the nation's progress. In the midcourse correction for the year 2000 goals, Fleming (1996) looks to the National Institute of Mental Health UNOCCAP study that is currently in progress to monitor the nation's ability to meet its mental health goals. There is no ongoing surveillance system established for monitoring mental health outcomes, similar to those established for AIDS by the CDC, substance use (National Institute on Drug Abuse), or health (National Institutes of Health). If UNOCCAP is to provide the base rate for the mental health status of the nation's children, perhaps this survey should be established as the ongoing surveillance system for mental health outcomes.

Communities will have great problems in meeting the challenge of achieving national goals for children's positive health outcomes. Some communities will demonstrate such massive failures in achieving the goals that a national intervention policy must be established. Currently, the federal government is funding empowerment zones for a set of inner cities believed to need significant, radical interventions to provide for the health of their community members. Simultaneously, the CDC is experimenting with a strategy of designing fiscal incentives for achieving health goals. For example, with the recognition that taking zidovudine during pregnancy has a positive effect on lowering the probability of HIV transmissions to newborns (CDC, 1994), Congress has given each state until the year 2000 to ensure either that the rate of HIV/AIDS among newborns decreases by 50% or that 95% of pregnant women are voluntarily tested for HIV. If neither of these targets is met, the state runs the risk of losing HIV funding, and a potential policy of mandatory testing of newborns will be revisited (Dewar, 1996). While controversial, a threshold must be set for identifying communities where the majority of children are at severe risk for negative mental health outcomes. A process of identifying and implementing community intervention strategies that are automatically triggered when a substantial percentage of the population is identified at high risk will be needed to ensure that national mental health outcomes are achieved.

Summary

To improve the nation's health, policymakers are faced with multiple challenges. To be able to set the goals for 2010, plans must be designed immediately to identify the level at which the goals will be defined, implement national monitoring systems, and identify strategies for inducing communities to provide for the health and mental health of their citizens. With these tools in hand, addressing the dissemination, training, and financing of mental health care at the local level will be likely to improve our chances of meeting our mental health goals by the year 2010.

References

Aday, L. A., & Anderson, R. M. (1981). Equity of access to medical care: A conceptual and empirical overview. *Medical Care, 19*(Suppl.), 4-27.

Agranoff, R. (1991). Human services integration: Past and present challenges in public administration. *Public Administration Review, 51,* 533-542.

American Academy of Child and Adolescent Psychiatry. (1991). Practice parameters for the assessment and treatment of attention-deficit hyperactivity disorder. *Journal of the American Academy of Child and Adolescent Psychiatry, 30,* i-iii.

American Academy of Child and Adolescent Psychiatry. (1992). Practice parameters for the assessment and treatment of conduct disorders. *Journal of the American Academy of Child and Adolescent Psychiatry, 31,* iv-vii.

American Academy of Child and Adolescent Psychiatry. (1993). Practice parameters for the assessment and treatment of anxiety disorders. *Journal of the American Academy of Child and Adolescent Psychiatry, 32,* 1091-1096.

American Psychiatric Association. (1993). Treatment principles and alternatives. *American Journal of Psychiatry, 150,* 4-10.

Anderson, J., Williams, S., McGee, R., & Silva, P. (1989). Cognitive and social correlates of DSM-III disorders in preadolescent children. *Journal of the American Academy of Child and Adolescent Psychiatry, 28,* 842-846.

Angst, J., & Hochstrasser, B. (1994). Recurrent brief depression: The Zurich study. *Journal of Clinical Psychiatry, 55*(4)(Suppl.), 3-9.

Artiles, A., & Trent, S. C. (1994). Over-representation of minority students in special education: A continuing debate. *Journal of Special Education, 27,* 410-437.

Attkisson, C., Dresser, L., & Rosenblatt, A. (1991). Service systems for youths with severe emotional disorder: Systems of care research in California. In *Close to home: "Community-based mental health services for children": Hearing before the Select Committee on Children, Youth, and Families, House of Representatives, April 19, 1991.* Washington, DC: U.S. Government Printing Office.

Baekeland, F., & Lundwall, L. (1975). Dropping out of treatment: A critical review. *Psychological Bulletin, 82,* 738-783.

Beilenson, J. (1987). *Balancing custody and care: A resource book for case management in juvenile detention systems* (2nd ed.). New York: City of New York, Department of Juvenile Justice.

Berman, A. L., & Jobes, D. A. (1995). Suicide prevention in adolescents (age 12-18). *Suicide & Life-Threatening Behavior, 25,* 143-154.

Berman, A. L., & Schwartz, R. T. (1990). Suicide attempts among adolescent drug users. *American Journal of Diseases of Children, 144,* 310-314.

Beutler, L. E., & Clarkin, J. (1991). Future research directions. In L. E. Beutler & M. Crago (Eds.), *Psychotherapy research: An international review of programmatic studies* (pp. 329-334). Washington, DC: American Psychological Association.

Bickman, L. (1996). A continuum of care—More is not always better. *American Psychologist, 51,* 689-701.

Bickman, L., Guthrie, P. R., Foster, E. M., Lambert, E. W., et al. (1995). *Evaluating managed mental health services: The Fort Bragg experiment.* New York: Plenum.

Biederman, J., Faraone, S. V., Doyle, A., Lehman, B. K., Kraus, I., Perrin, J., & Tsuang, M. T. (1993). Convergence of the Child Behavior Checklist with structured interview-based psychiatric diagnoses of ADHD children with and without comorbidity. *Journal of Child Psychology and Psychiatry, 34,* 1241-1251.

Bird, H. R., Canino, G., Rubio-Stipec, M., Gould, M. S., Ribera, J., Sesman, M., Woodbury, M., Huertas-Goldman, S., Pagan, A., Sanchez-Lacay, A., & Mocoso, M. (1988). Estimates of the prevalence of childhood maladjustment in a community survey in Puerto Rico. *Archives of General Psychiatry, 45,* 1120-1126.

Bird, H. R., Gould, M. S., Yager, T., Staghezza, B., & Canino, G. (1989). Risk factors for maladjustment in Puerto Rican children. *Journal of the American Academy of Child and Adolescent Psychiatry, 28,* 847-850.

Blank, M. J., Melaville, A. I., & Asayesh, G. (1992). *Together we can: A guide to crafting community-based family-centered strategies for integrating education and human services.* Washington, DC: Institute for Educational Leadership.

Borus, J. F., Olendzki, M. C., Kessler, L., Burns, B. J., Brandt, U. C., Broverman, C. A., & Henderson, P. R. (1985). The "offset effect" of mental health treatment on ambulatory medical care utilization and changes. *Archives of General Psychiatry, 42,* 573-588.

Bowen, G. S., Marconi, K., Kohn, S., Bailey, D. M., Goosby, E. P., Shorter, S., & Niemcryk, S. (1992). First year of AIDS services delivery under Title I of the Ryan White CARE Act. *Public Health Reports, 107,* 491-499.

Brandenburg, N. A., & Friedman, R. M. (1990). The epidemiology of childhood psychiatric disorders: Prevalence findings from recent studies. *Journal of the American Academy of Child and Adolescent Psychiatry, 29,* 76-83.

Brook, R. H., Kamberg, C. J., & Lohr, K. N. (1982). Quality assessment in mental health. *Professional Psychology, 13*(1), 34-39.

Brook, R. H., Ware, J. E., Rogers, W. H., Keeler, E. B., Davies, A. R., Donald, C. A., Goldberg, G. A., Lohr, K. N., Masthay, P. C., & Newhouse, J. P. (1983). Does free care improve adults' health? Results from a randomized controlled trial. *New England Journal of Medicine, 309,* 1426-1434.

Brunswick, A. J., & Menzel, C. R. (1988). Health through three life stages: A longitudinal study of urban Black adolescents. *Social Science and Medicine, 27,* 1207-1214.

Center for the Study of Social Policy. (1991). *Leveraging dollars, leveraging change: Refinancing and restructuring children's services in five sites.* Washington, DC: Center for the Study of Social Policy.

Centers for Disease Control and Prevention. (1994). Recommendations of the U.S. Public Health Service task force on the use of zidovudine to reduce perinatal transmission of human immunodeficiency virus. *Morbidity and Mortality Weekly Report, 43*(RR-11).

Centers for Disease Control and Prevention. (1995). Youth risk behavior surveillance—United States, 1993. *Morbidity and Mortality Weekly Report, 14*(SS-1).

Cohen, R., Parmelee, D. X., Irwin, L., Weisz, J. R., Howard, P., Purcell, P., & Best, A. L. (1990). Characteristics of children and adolescents in a psychiatric hospital and a correction facility. *Journal of the American Academy of Child and Adolescent Psychiatry, 29,* 909-913.

Coie, J. D., Watt, N. F., West, S. G., Hawkins, J. D., Asarnow, J. R., Markman, H. J., Ramey, S. L., Shure, M. B., & Long, B. (1993). The science of prevention: A conceptual framework and some directions for a national research program. *American Psychologist, 48,* 1013-1022.

Costello, E. J. (1986). Primary care pediatrics and child psychopathology: A review of diagnostic, treatment and referral practices. *Pediatrics, 78,* 1044-1051.

Costello, E. J. (1989). Child psychiatric disorders and their correlates: A primary care pediatric sample. *Journal of the American Academy of Child and Adolescent Psychiatry, 28,* 851-855.

Costello, E. J., Costello, A. J., Edelbrock, G., Burns, B. J., Dulcan, M. K., Brent, D., & Janiszewski, S. (1988). Psychiatric disorders in pediatric primary care. *Archives of General Psychiatry, 45,* 1107-1116.

Dewar, H. (1996, May 2). AIDS testing compromise is reached. *Washington Post,* p. A9.

Dishion, T. J., & Loeber, R. (1985). Adolescent marijuana and alcohol use: The role of parents and peers revisited. *American Journal of Drug & Alcohol Abuse, 11*(1-2), 11-25.

Donabedian, A. (1980). *Explanations in quality assessment and monitoring.* Ann Arbor, MI: Health Administration Press.

Elliott, D. S., Huizinga, D., & Menard, D. (1989). *Multiple problem youth: Delinquency, substance use and mental health problems.* New York: Springer-Verlag.

Farrow, F., & Joe, T. (1992). Financing school-linked, integrated services. *Future of Children, 2*(1), 56-67.

Fleming, M. (1996). *Healthy youth 2000: A mid-decade review.* Chicago: American Medical Association, Department of Adolescent Health.

Frank, G. (1980). Treatment needs of children in foster care. *American Journal of Orthopsychiatry, 50,* 256-263.

Frank, R. O., & McGuire, T. G. (1985). A review of studies of the impact of insurance on the demand and utilization of specialty mental health services. *Health Services Research, 21,* 241-265.

Friedman, A. S., Utada, A. T., Glickman, N. W., & Morrissey, M. R. (1987). Psychopathology as an antecedent to, and as a consequence of substance use in adolescence. *Journal of Drug Education, 12,* 233-244.

Gallimore, R., Goldenberg, C. N., & Weisner, T. S. (1993). The social construction and subjective reality of activity settings: Implications for community psychology. *American Journal of Community Psychology, 21,* 537-559.

Gallimore, R., Tharp, R. G., & Rueda, R. (1989). The social context of cognitive functioning in the lives of mildly handicapped persons. In D. Sugden (Ed.), *Cognitive approaches in special education* (pp. 51-81). London: Falmer.

Gardner, S. L. (1992). Key issues in developing school-linked, integrated services. *Future of Children, 2*(1), 85-94.

Gillespie, D., & Marten, S. (1978). Assessing service accessibility. *Administration in Social Work, 2,* 183-197.

Goldenberg, C. N., & Gallimore, R. (1991). Local knowledge, research knowledge, and educational change: A case study of early Spanish reading improvement. *Educational Researcher, 20*(8), 2-14.

Halfon, N. (1992). Children in foster care in California: An examination of Medicaid reimbursed health services utilization. *Pediatrics, 89,* 1230-1237.

Halfon, N., English, A., Allen, M., & DeWoody, M. (1994). National health care reform, Medicaid, and children in foster care. *Child Welfare, 73,* 99-115.

Halfon, N., & Klee, L. (1987). Health services for California's foster children: Current practices and policy recommendations. *Pediatrics, 80,* 183-191.

Halpern, R. (1991). Supportive services for families in poverty: Dilemmas of reform. *Social Service Review, 65,* 343-364.

Hawkins, J. D., Catalano, R. F., & Miller, J. Y. (1992). Risk and protective factors for alcohol and other drug problems in adolescence and early adulthood: Implications for substance abuse prevention. *Psychological Bulletin, 112,* 64-105.

Hetherington, E. M. (1989). Coping with family transitions: Winners, losers, and survivors. *Child Development, 60*(1), 1-14.

Hoagwood, K., Hibbs, E., Brent, D., & Jensen, P. (1995). Efficacy and effectiveness in studies of child and adolescent psychotherapy. *Journal of Consulting and Clinical Psychology, 63,* 683-687.

Hochstadt, N. J., Jaudes, P. K., Zimo, D. A., & Schachter, J. (1987). The medical and psychological needs of children entering foster care. *Child Abuse & Neglect, 11*(1), 53-62.

Horwitz, S. M., Leaf, P. J., Leventhal, J. M., Forsyth, B., & Speechley, K. N. (1992). Identification and management of psychosocial and developmental problems in community-based, primary care pediatric practices. *Pediatrics, 89,* 1-6.

Howard, K. I., Lueger, R. J., Maling, M. S., & Martinovich, Z. (1993). A phase model of psychotherapy outcome: Causal mediation of change. *Journal of Consulting and Clinical Psychology, 61,* 678-685.

Hu, T., Snowden, L. R., & Jerrell, J. M. (1992). Costs and use of public mental health and substance abuse services. *Journal of Mental Health Administration, 19,* 273-277.

Hughes, C. W., Preskorn, S. H., Wrona, M., Hassanein, R., et al. (1990). Follow-up of adolescents initially treated for prepubertal onset of major depressive disorder with Imipramine. *Psychopharmacology Bulletin, 26,* 244-248.

Institute of Medicine. (1994). *Reducing risks for mental disorders: Frontiers for preventive intervention research.* Washington, DC: National Academy Press.

Judd, L. L., Rapaport, M. H., Paulus, M. P., & Brown, J. L. (1994). Subsyndromal symptomatic depression: A new mood disorder? *Journal of Clinical Psychiatry, 55*(4)(Suppl.), 13-28.

Kagan, S. L., Rivera, A. M., & Parker, F. L. (1991). *Collaborations in action: Reshaping services for young children and their families.* New Haven, CT: Yale University.

Kelly, J. G. (Ed.). (1979). *Adolescent boys in high school: A psychological study of coping and adaptation.* Hillsdale, NJ: Lawrence Erlbaum.

Kessler, L. G. (1984). Treated incidence of mental disorders in a prepaid group practice setting. *American Journal of Public Health, 74,* 154-164.

Klee, L., & Halfon, N. (1987). Mental health care for foster children in California. *Child Abuse & Neglect, 11*(1), 63-74.

Knoff, H. M., & Batsche, G. M. (1990). The place of the school in community mental health services for children: A necessary interdependence. *Journal of Mental Health Administration, 17*(1), 122-130.

Lahey, B. B., Flagg, E. W., Bird, H. R., Schwab-Stone, M., Canino, G., Dulcan, M. K., et al. (1994). *The NIMH methods for the epidemiology of child and adolescent mental disorders (MECA) study: Background and methodology.* Unpublished manuscript.

Lambert, M. J. (1991). Introduction to psychotherapy research. In L. E. Beutler & M. Crago (Eds.), *Psychotherapy research: An international review of programmatic studies* (pp. 1-11). Washington, DC: American Psychological Association.

Leibowitz, A. (1986). Use of medical care in the RAND Health Insurance Experiment: Diagnosis- and service-specific analyses in a randomized controlled trial. *Medical Care, 24*(9), S1-S87.

Lewinsohn, P. M., Rohde, P., & Seeley, J. R. (1995). Adolescent psychopathology: Vol. 3. The clinical consequences of comorbidity. *Journal of the American Academy of Child and Adolescent Psychiatry, 34,* 510-519.

Loeber, R., Brinthaupt, V. P., & Green, S. M. (1990). Attention deficits, impulsivity, and hyperactivity with or without conduct problems: Relationship to delinquency and unique contextual factors. In R. J. McMahon & R. D. Peters (Eds.), *Behavior disorders of adolescence: Research, intervention and policy in clinical and school settings* (pp. 39-61). New York: Plenum.

Los Angeles County Board of Education. (1995). *Annual report of the Los Angeles County Board of Education.* Los Angeles: Author.

Manderscheid, R. W., Rae, D. S., Narrow, W. E., Locke, B. Z., et al. (1993). Congruence of service utilization estimates from the Epidemiologic Catchment Area Project and other sources. *Archives of General Psychiatry, 50,* 108-114.

Manning, W. G., Wells, K. B., Duan, N., Newhouse, J. P., & Ware, J. E. (1984). Cost sharing and the use of ambulatory mental health services. *American Psychologist, 39,* 1077-1089.

Manning, W. G., Wells, K. B., Duan, N., Newhouse, J. P., & Ware, J. E. (1986). How cost sharing affects the use of ambulatory mental health services. *Journal of the American Medical Association, 256,* 1930-1934.

Mannuzza, S., Klein, R. G., Bonagura, N., Konig, P. H., & Shenker, R. (1988). Hyperactive boys almost grown up: Vol. 2. State of subjects without a mental disorder. *Archives of General Psychiatry, 45,* 13-18.

McAllister, D. R. (1993). *AB3632 information* [Report]. Los Angeles: Los Angeles County Department of Mental Health, Children and Youth Services Bureau.

McGlynn, E. A., Norquist, G. S., Wells, K. B., Sullivan, G., & Libernian, R. P. (1983). Quality-of-care research in mental health: Responding to the challenge. *Inquiry, 25,* 157-170.

McGuire, T. G. (1989). Financing and reimbursement for mental health services. In C. A. Taube, D. Mechanic, & A. A. Hohmann (Eds.), *Future of mental health services.* Washington, DC: U.S. Government Printing Office.

McGuire, T. G., & Fairbank, A. (1988). Patterns of mental health utilization over time in a fee-for-service population. *American Journal of Public Health, 78,* 134-136.

McKinney, M. M., Wieland, M. K., Bowen, G. S., Goosby, E. P., & Marconi, K. M. (1993). States' responses to Title II of the Ryan White CARE Act. *Public Health Reports, 108*(1), 4-11.

Melnick, S. D., & Lyter, L. L. (1987). The negative impacts of increased concurrent review of psychiatric inpatient care. *Hospital and Community Psychiatry, 38,* 300-303.

Miranda, J., Hohmann, A. A., Attkisson, C. A., & Larson, D. (1994). *Mental disorders in primary care.* San Francisco: Jossey-Bass.

Mordock, J. B. (1990). Funding children's mental health services in an underfunded climate: Collaborative efforts. *Journal of Mental Health Administration, 17*(1), 108-114.

Mrazek, P. J., & Haggerty, R. J. (Eds.). (1994). *Reducing risks for mental disorders: Frontiers for preventive intervention research.* Washington, DC: National Academy Press.

National Institute of Child Health and Human Development. (1990). *Children's mental health.* Washington, DC: Author.

Neighbors, H. W., Jackson, J. S., Campbell, L., & Williams, D. (1989). The influence of racial factors on psychiatric diagnosis: A review and suggestion for research. *Community Mental Health Journal, 25,* 301-311.

Offord, D. R., Boyle, M. H., Szatmari, P., Rae-Grant, N. I., Links, P. S., Cadman, D. T., Byles, J. A., Crawford, J. W., Blum, H. M., Byrne, C., Thomas, H., & Woodward, C. A. (1987). Ontario Child Health Study: Vol. 2. Six-month prevalence of disorder and rates of service utilization. *Archives of General Psychiatry, 44,* 832-836.

Ooms, T., & Owen, T. (1991). *Coordination, collaboration, integration: Strategies for serving families more effectively, Part 1: The federal role, background briefing report and meeting highlights.* Washington, DC: Research and Education Foundation, American Association for Marriage and Family Therapy, Family Impact Seminar.

Padgett, D. K., Patrick, C., Burns, B. J., Schlesinger, H. J., & Cohen, J. (1993). The effects of insurance benefit changes on use of child and adolescent outpatient mental health services. *Medical Care, 31*(2), 96-110.

Paulson, M. J., Coombs, R. H., & Landsverk, J. (1990). Youth who physically assault their parents. *Journal of Family Violence, 5,* 121-133.

Prochaska, J. O., DiClemente, C. C., & Norcross, J. C. (1992). In search of how people change: Applications to addictive behaviors. *American Psychologist, 47,* 1102-1114.

Reynolds, W. M., & Graves, A. (1989). Reliability of children's reports of depressive symptomatology. *Journal of Abnormal Child Psychology, 17*(6), 647-655.

Rogers, W. H., Wells, K. B., Meredith, L. S., Sturm, R., & Burnam, M. A. (1993). Outcomes for adult outpatients with depression under prepaid or fee-for-service financing. *Archives of General Psychiatry, 50,* 517-525.

Rogoff, B. (1995). Observing sociocultural activity on three planes: Participatory appropriation, guided participation, apprenticeship. In J. V. Wertsch, P. del Rio, & A. Alvarez, (Eds.), *Sociocultural studies of mind: Learning in doing: Social, cognitive, and computational aspects* (pp. 139-164). New York: Cambridge University Press.

Rogoff, B., Baker-Sennett, J., Lacasa, P., & Goldsmith, D. (1995). Development through participation in sociocultural activity. In J. Goodnow, P. Miller, & F. Kessel (Eds.), *Cultural practices as contexts for development* (pp. 45-65). San Francisco: Jossey-Bass.

Rosenblatt, A., & Attkisson, C. C. (1993). Assessing outcomes for sufferers of severe mental disorder: A conceptual framework and review. *Evaluation and Program Planning, 16,* 347-363.

Rotheram-Borus, M. J., Leibowitz, A., Wells, K., Duan, N., Burnam, A., & Weisz, J. (1994). *Utilization, needs, outcomes, and costs for child and adolescent psychopathology* (National Institute of Mental Health Grant No. U01-MH54278). Los Angeles: University of California, Los Angeles, Department of Psychiatry, Division of Social and Community Psychiatry.

Rotheram-Borus, M. J., Miller, S., Piacentini, J., Graae, F., & Castro-Blanco, D. (1994). Brief cognitive-behavioral treatment for adolescent suicide attempters and their families. *Journal of the American Academy of Child and Adolescent Psychiatry, 33,* 508-517.

Rutter, M. (1985). Resilience in the face of adversity. *British Journal of Psychiatry, 147,* 596.

Rutter, M., & Giller, H. (1983). *Juvenile delinquency: Trends and perspectives.* New York: Guilford.

Rutter, M., Maughan, B., Mortimore, P., Ouston, J., & Smith, A. (1979). *Fifteen thousand hours: Secondary schools and their effects on children.* Cambridge, MA: Harvard University Press.

Sailor, W., Gerry, M., & Wilson, W. C. (1991). Policy implications of emergent full inclusion models for the education of students with severe disabilities. In M. C. Wang, M. C. Reynolds, & H. J. Walberg (Eds.), *Handbook of special education: Research and practice. Vol. 4: Emerging programs. Advances in education* (pp. 175-193). Oxford: Pergamon.

Schorr, L., Both, D., & Copple, C. (Eds.). (1991). *Effective services for young children—Report of a workshop.* Washington, DC: National Academy Press.

Sue, S., & McKinney, H. (1975). Asian Americans in the community mental health care system. *American Journal of Orthopsychiatry, 45,* 111-118.

Swanson, J. W., Holzer, C. E., & Ganju, V. (1993). Hispanic Americans and the state mental hospitals in Texas: Ethnic parity as a latent function of a fiscal incentive policy. *Social Science and Medicine, 37,* 917-926.

Takayama, J. I., Bergman, A. B., & Connell, F. A. (1994). Children in foster care in the state of Washington. *Journal of the American Medical Association, 271,* 1850-1855.

Uehara, E., Takeuchi, D., & Smukler, M. (1994). Effects of combining disparate groups in the analysis of ethnic differences: Variations among Asian-American mental health service consumers in level of community functioning. *American Journal of Community Psychology, 22,* 83-99.

U.S. Congress, Office of Technology Assessment. (1986). *Children's mental health: Problems and services—Background paper* (OTA BP-HH-33). Washington, DC: Author.

U.S. Department of Health and Human Services, Public Health Service. (1991). *Healthy people 2000: National health promotion and disease prevention objectives* (DHHS Publication No. PHS 91-50212). Washington, DC: U.S. Government Printing Office.

U.S. Department of Health and Human Services, Public Health Service. (1995). *Healthy people 2000: Midcourse review and 1995 revisions.* Washington, DC: U.S. Government Printing Office.

Urban Strategies Council. (1992). *Partnership for change: Linking schools, services and the community to serve Oakland youth* [Report by the Urban Strategies Council in consultation with the Oakland Interagency Group for School-Linked Services]. Oakland, CA: Author.

Velez, C. N., Johnson, J., & Cohen, P. (1989). A longitudinal analysis of selected risk factors for childhood psychopathology. *Journal of the American Academy of Child and Adolescent Psychiatry, 28,* 861-864.

Weinstein, J., & LaFleur, J. (1990). Caring for our children: An examination of health care services for foster children. *California Western Law Review, 26,* 319-349.

Weisner, T. (1984). A cross-cultural perspective: Ecocultural niches of middle childhood. In A. Collins (Ed.), *The elementary school years: Understanding development during middle childhood* (pp. 335-369). Washington, DC: National Academy Press.

Weisner, T., Gallimore, R., & Jordan, C. (1988). Unpackaging cultural effects on classroom learning: Hawaiian peer assistance and child-generated activity. *Anthropology and Education Quarterly, 19,* 327-353.

Weisz, J. R., & Weiss, B. (1989). Assessing the effects of clinic-based psychotherapy with children and adolescents. *Journal of Consulting and Clinical Psychology, 57,* 741-746.

Weisz, J. R., Weiss, B., Alicke, M. D., & Klotz, M. L. (1987). Effectiveness of psychotherapy with children and adolescents: A meta-analysis for clinicians. *Journal of Consulting and Clinical Psychology, 55,* 542-549.

Weisz, J. R., Weiss, B., & Donenberg, G. R. (1992). The lab versus the clinic. *American Psychologist, 47,* 1578-1585.

Wells, K. B., Manning, W., & Benjamin, B. (1986). A comparison of the effects of sociodemographic factors and health status on use of outpatient mental health services in HMO and fee-for-service plans. *Medical Care, 24,* 949-960.

Wells, K. B., Manning, W. G., & Valdez, R. B. (1990). The effects of a prepaid group practice on mental health outcomes. *Health Services Research, 25,* 615-625.

Werner, E. E. (1986). The concept of risk from a developmental perspective. *Advances in Special Education, 5,* 1-23.

Williams, S., Anderson, J., McGee, R., & Silva, P. A. (1990). Risk factors for behavioral and emotional disorder in preadolescent children. *Journal of the American Academy of Child and Adolescent Psychiatry, 29,* 413-419.

Windle, M. (1990). Longitudinal study of antisocial behavior in early adolescence as predictors of late adolescent substance use: Gender and ethnic group differences. *Journal of Abnormal Psychology, 99,* 36-91.

Wolch, J. R., Kim, M. H., & Lee, J. O. (1992). *A geography of children's services in Los Angeles County* [Report prepared for the Los Angeles Roundtable for Children]. Los Angeles: Los Angeles Roundtable for Children.

Wordes, M., Bynum, T. S., & Corley, C. J. (1994). Locking up youth: The impact of race on detention decisions. *Journal of Research in Crime and Delinquency, 31,* 149-165.

CHAPTER 6

Improving Access to Health Care: School-Based Health Centers

SHAUNA L. DOWDEN

RICHARD D. CALVERT

LISA DAVIS

THOMAS P. GULLOTTA

It is one thing to imagine a healthier people. It is quite another to undertake the necessary steps to turn those thoughts into reality. *Healthy People 2000* and this volume are testaments to the reality that business as usual will not suffice. Improving the health of children and families in this country will require that we care for people differently. The current health care system (including every level responsible for the nation's health from policymakers, to federal and state regulators, to those in research, public health, and direct practice) can lay claim to having improved the general health of the populace since the turn of the century. But the cost of that care, focusing as it does on remediation, has become cost prohibitive and forced millions of Americans to go without care. These circumstances have caused the United States to reexamine its health care system and explore different models of care to not only control cost but to extend care to those in need.

AUTHORS' NOTE: We wish to acknowledge the helpful assistance of JoAnn Eaccarino, APRN, Jean Enderle, APRN, Nancy Grant, APRN, Susanne Hamblen, APRN, and Rebecca Murray, APRN, in the preparation of this chapter.

We believe that this desire to improve the nation's health stems from the following premises. First, it is not acceptable for children to lack a medical home, as millions do. Similarly, it is not acceptable that the working poor cannot afford health care insurance, as millions cannot. It is not acceptable for insurers to discriminate between physical and behavioral health benefits, depriving individuals of the care necessary to improve their quality of life and denying society fully productive citizens, as they do. It is not acceptable for preventable habits that form early in life, such as the use of alcohol, tobacco, and other drugs, to remain unprevented, resulting in monstrous costs to both the individual later in life and the larger society.

In this chapter, we explore one approach to better serving the complete health care needs of children. We examine the promise of school-based health centers (SBHCs) to deliver such health care. SBHCs represent a service delivery mechanism capable of functioning as a medical home for children, providing primary care for both their physical and behavioral health care needs. This service delivery model has the capacity to promote health and prevent illness. Presently, there are a mere handful of these centers nationwide, with most operating on shoestring budgets and unbeknown to third-party payers. Unfortunately, although anecdotal and single-case studies abound, little experimental data exist on the effectiveness of the services they provide. Rather than disparaging SBHCs, this lack of data may be more reflective of a lack of proper evaluations.

SBHCs appear to be a promising delivery mechanism. They are equipped to fill the gaps created by the changing topography of today's workforce and neighborhoods. As the percentage of women in the workforce with children under the age of 18 increases to and exceeds 65%, and as welfare reform limiting the duration of benefits becomes instituted, we believe schools will be called on to extend their child care hours and facilities. Evidence for this extension of services can already be found in programs such as after-school latchkey programs, extended-day kindergarten, and school breakfast programs. Additionally, given that the decision on where individuals work, live, and send their children to school is no longer based on neighborhood proximity, securing primary health care has grown increasingly complicated. Because of conflicting work and family demands, parents are frequently forced to break health care appointments. This likely does not represent intentional child medical negligence, but rather the inability of many in our labor force, particularly those in the lowest-paid service sector, to alter their work schedules. Conflicts between work and child health care become more difficult to manage as incomes decline and work responsibilities become more fixed. For example, "no show" and cancellation rates approach 25% for many health care providers serving the working poor. Thus, the use of existing school sites as health care delivery sites is appealing from both the service delivery and cost containment perspectives.

In the sections that follow, we examine the need for SBHCs. We look at the planning process by which such centers are developed and services are made available, as well as using data on a state level. Finally, we conclude with a series of recommendations for the future development of these services.

Adolescent Access to Health Care

In 1993, more than 17% of the U.S. population under the age of 65 had no health insurance. Of 40 million uninsured Americans, 8.4 million were children under 15 years of age (U.S. Department of Health and Human Services [DHHS], 1995b). This number of uninsured individuals represents an increase in uninsured individuals among all age groups except children under the age of 5 (DHHS, 1995b). Access to health insurance is often related to family income. In 1993, 35% of individuals with family incomes less than $14,000 were uninsured, compared with only 5% of those with family incomes of $50,000 or more. Even though those with lower family incomes were much more likely to be uninsured, a higher family income does not guarantee adequate coverage. For example, 32% of all uninsured individuals in 1993 had family incomes ranging from $14,000 to $24,999 and 24% of the uninsured had incomes ranging from $25,000 to $49,000. In 1993, nearly 66% of youth resided with family able to afford private insurance or whose employers provided medical insurance. Nearly 19% of young people lived in families who, because of poverty, qualify for Medicaid. The remaining 15% of children live in families unable to afford health insurance and whose employers either do not offer medical insurance or offer it with copayments the employees cannot afford (DHHS, 1995b).

Family income not only affects health insurance status but also the amount and types of medical services received. During 1991-1993, nonpoor children with good to excellent health status had approximately 30% more physician contacts on average than poor or near-poor children with good to excellent health, whereas nonpoor children with fair to poor health status had 86% more physician contacts than poor children and 46% more than near-poor children with similar health status (DHHS, 1995b). Newacheck, Hughes, and Stoddard (1996) found that approximately 17% of children living in poverty and 20% of uninsured children reported not having usual sources for obtaining routine care, whereas only about 7% of nonpoor, insured, White children did not have usual sources of care. Among children reporting usual sources of care, children living in poverty and uninsured children were three times more likely to name a hospital setting as the site of their usual care than nonpoor, insured children. Both uninsured children and children living in poverty were more likely to travel and wait longer to obtain care. Children living in poverty with usual sources of care were three times more likely to wait 60 minutes or more to see a doctor and twice as likely to have traveled 30 minutes or more to obtain care. Uninsured children were similarly more than twice as likely to wait 60 minutes or more. Uninsured children and insured children living in poverty seem to face similar barriers to adequate care. For example, as many as 18% of uninsured children and 23% of children living in poverty were reported to be inadequately immunized, and these children were less likely to see a physician for symptoms that warranted care (Newacheck et al., 1996). The difference in utilization rates and patterns are not, unfortunately, indicative of poorer and uninsured children being healthier than their more affluent and insured counterparts. Newacheck, Jameson, and Halfon (1994) concluded that poor children not only experience a disproportionately high number of health problems, but they also tend to experience these health problems more severely than more affluent children. For example, children from families with incomes below $10,000 were six times more likely than children from families with incomes of $35,000 or more to be described as having fair or poor health. Similarly, poor children were more likely to experience an array of health problems, including an increased incidence of middle ear disease, a three times greater likelihood of tooth decay, 50% more nonacne-related skin conditions, and higher blood lead levels.

As the preceding data indicate, universal coverage would not necessarily increase children's and adolescents' access to and use of primary care services. Himmelstein and Woodhandler (1995) pointed out that although the uninsured were more than twice as likely to be unable to obtain needed care, three quarters of those not receiving needed services were insured. Similarly, Medicaid-covered individuals were as likely to not receive care as uninsured individuals. There are, therefore, additional factors that limit young people's access to adequate health care. Halfon, Inkelas, and Wood (1995) cited a number of nonfinancial barriers to care for adolescents, including low parental education levels, larger family size, family social support, communication difficulties between family and providers, and lack of regular sources of primary care. They concluded that a disparity between children's needs and the current organization of the health delivery system exists.

Children and Adolescents Need to Be Served

A fair number of adolescents experience significant health needs and an even larger portion of adolescents are increasingly becoming involved in unhealthy lifestyles. An estimated 2 million youth suffer from chronic conditions that impede activity, including chronic respiratory illness such as asthma and bronchitis (21%); muscle and skeletal disorders such as arthritis (15%); illness of the nervous system such as multiple sclerosis, epilepsy, and cerebral palsy (6%); and hearing impairments (4%) (Starfield, 1992). Another 32% of the 2 million suffer from mental disorders. *Healthy Youth 2000* has targeted 10 health-related areas of concern for adolescents by developing objectives to monitor and assuage the effect these problems have on youth (Fleming, 1996). Although there has been progress in some areas, the overall picture remains one in which adolescents continue to experience significant health risks. For instance, by 1993 *Healthy Youth 2000*'s target for adolescent smoking had not been met. An estimated 25% of high school students reported smoking 20 or more cigarettes daily (Fleming, 1996). Similarly, data from the 1992 National Health Interview

Survey revealed that 27.6% of males and 25% of females had smoked cigarettes in the past 30 days (DHHS, 1995a). Adolescent consumption of alcohol follows a similar disturbing pattern, where present consumption rates exceed targeted goals by *Healthy Youth 2000*.

During the 30 days preceding the survey, almost half of all high school students had drunk at least one alcoholic beverage, and approximately one third had drunk five or more alcoholic beverages on one occasion (Fleming, 1996). Perhaps even more alarming is the fact that 25% of 12- to 13-year-olds had drunk alcohol and that among young adults who had had at least one drink of alcohol, 15.8% reported having had their first drink by age 12 (DHHS, 1995a). Similarly, 38.1% had their first drink of alcohol by age 14. Although some of this early drinking may be experimental, for a substantial number of adolescents it is not. In 1992, almost 14% of 14- to 17-year-olds reported having drunk alcohol on 40 or more days (DHHS, 1995a). Use of illegal drugs is not far behind alcohol use, with 25.9% of youth 14 to 17 years of age having used some type of illegal drug (DHHS, 1995a). Marijuana use among adolescents has increased from 4.0% in 1992 to 7.2% in 1994 (Fleming, 1996). Marijuana use followed a similar pattern for age of initiation as alcohol in the 1992 National Health Interview Survey, with 13% first using the drug by age 12 and more than one third by age 14 (DHHS, 1995a). Although the rates for cocaine use were lower (5.9% of all youth had tried some form of cocaine in their lifetime), 12.6% of youth reported having used some other illegal drug, including LSD, PCP, Ecstasy, mushrooms, speed, ice, and heroin.

Another increasingly predominant health concern for adolescents involves sexual experimentation and the ensuing consequences. Approximately 30% of adolescents 14 to 15 years of age had experienced sexual intercourse (DHHS, 1995a). More than 50% of all high school students have reported having experienced sexual intercourse, with 20% having had four or more partners (Fleming, 1996). Again, this is a behavior that often first occurs at very young ages, with 12% of males reporting their first experience with intercourse by age 12. The interplay between sexual experiences and drug use is illustrated by the 17.1% of sexually experienced adolescents reporting drug or alcohol use before their last sexual intercourse experience (DHHS, 1995a). Only 50% of adolescents reported condom use during their last sexual intercourse experience; 12.5% used the withdrawal method and 15.8% used no form of birth control (DHHS, 1995a). *Healthy Youth 2000*'s target of 50 pregnancies per 1,000 adolescent girls has not been met. The rate in 1991 was 75 pregnancies per 1,000 girls aged 15 to 17 (Fleming, 1996). Increasingly, these pregnancies are more likely to be carried to term rather than being terminated. In 1987, the ratio of abortions per 100 live births was 72.6, whereas in 1992 that number dropped to 42.7 (DHHS, 1995b) for adolescents aged 15 to 19. As these young women are less likely to place their infants for adoption and more likely to be unmarried without financial support from the child's father than previous cohort groups, they experience poverty and a host of other difficulties (such as poorer health, school failure, and higher career dissatisfaction than nonpregnant youth; Jorgensen, 1993).

Another consequence of unprotected sexual intercourse is sexually transmitted diseases (STDs). In 1994, gonorrhea rates for males aged 15 to 19 years were below *Healthy Youth 2000*'s target of 750 per 100,000 at 606, but the rates for females aged 15 to 19 years were much higher at 927 (Fleming, 1996). In 1990, 5,507 cases of syphilis were reported for young people 10 to 19 years of age (Leukefeld & Haverkos, 1993). In 1992, 19,872 young people aged 13 to 19 suffered with AIDS (DHHS, 1993). Although 60% of HIV-positive White youth were infected by tainted blood products, more than 60% of Black and Hispanic youth were infected as a result of sexual activity (DHHS, 1993). For that same period of time, 91% of AIDS cases in young adults aged 20 to 24 could be traced to homosexual activity (63%), heterosexual activity (11%), and injecting drug use (17%) (DHHS, 1993). Given that a several-year delay exists between exposure to the HIV retrovirus and the onset of AIDS, it is likely that these youth were infected as adolescents (Adams, Gullotta, & Markstrom-Adams, 1994).

Two other areas of health concern targeted in *Healthy Youth 2000* are eating and exercise patterns in adolescents. In 1992, 50.5% of female adolescents were trying to lose weight, and 22.7% of male adolescents were (DHHS, 1995a). Those trying to lose weight are not necessarily overweight. The *Healthy Youth 2000* report revealed that a smaller percentage of male (21%) and female (34%) adolescents were actually overweight. Among those attempting to lose weight, 4.3% of female and 3.3% of male adolescents had used vomiting as a method of losing weight (DHHS, 1995a). Among adolescent females who thought that they were overweight, 24% had attempted to control their weight in the last week (DHHS, 1995a). Both overweight adolescents and those who are not overweight but who attempt to lose weight are at risk for health-related problems.

Another area of concern for adolescents involves their mental health. One outcome of the distress that some adolescents feel is suicide. *Healthy Youth 2000* set a target of reducing the rate of suicide among youth aged 15 to 19 to no more that 8.2 per 100,000. It also set a goal to reduce the prevalence of mental disorders among children and adolescents to less than 10%. Unfortunately, in 1992 suicide remained the third leading cause of death for those aged 15 to 24 and seventh for children 5 to 14 (DHHS, 1995b). The rate of suicide for youth aged 15 to 19 was 10.8, above the *Healthy Youth 2000* target. In addition, nearly 25% of high school students had seriously considered attempting suicide in the previous year.

The problems of accessibility and cost of health care, coupled with increasing rates of unhealthy behaviors among youth, indicate the need for systematic changes in service delivery. Different health care approaches are required to reach youth who find it difficult to access care, whose families cannot afford care, and who are experimenting with behaviors that could have deleterious consequences. In the next section, we offer the SBHC as a service model that addresses accessibility and cost and may promote the health status of all youth.

School-Based Health Centers

What does an SBHC look like? The typical center's medical service component is staffed with a physical health care professional able to diagnose and prescribe appropriate care including medications for routine medical issues. Those issues can include the treatment of minor episodic illnesses, the provision of well care services, treatment for chronic ailments, reproductive health care, and STD treatment. This health care professional, whether a nurse practitioner or physician's assistant, relates to a supervising physician and a larger health care establishment, ensuring that young people who need additional medical services will receive them.

The behavioral health component of these centers is staffed with one or more master's-level professionals. Their services are primarily group and prevention focused for problems involving substances, family, peer, and school relationships. Intervention services (crisis intervention and short-term focused therapy) are also offered. As with their medical colleagues, these mental health professionals relate to a supervisory structure that enables a troubled youth to move to more intensive outpatient and pharmacological treatments should that be necessary.

SBHCs are intended to improve accessibility to health care with an emphasis on health promotion and the early identification and treatment of illnesses. To achieve these objectives, the staff of these centers are expected to involve themselves in the life of the school. They are expected to be visible in the school hallways and lunch areas, to initiate health promotion efforts, and to make frequent classroom presentations. This high visibility is intended to encourage student health promotion through information, personal role modeling, and social support.

Other benefits include opportunities to establish an ongoing relationship with one health care provider in times of both sickness and health and a way to avoid appointment cancellations and costly visits to hospital emergency rooms.

Are Programs Within School-Based Health Centers Effective?

As noted earlier, the services SBHCs offer have not been adequately evaluated. In this statement we draw an important distinction between the SBHC as a location for service delivery and the particular services it offers. For example, virtually no one disputes the wisdom of schools as places to effectively educate groups of young people, but many would disagree about the methods used to achieve that education. We contend that SBHCs offer an ideal setting for parent-enrolled youth to receive primary health care. What is at issue is the most effective means to deliver that care to achieve the objectives found in *Healthy People 2000*. What curricula, interventions, and practice techniques for whom, when, and how are they administered are subjects that remain unexplored.

In the few published studies, these issues are not adequately addressed. For example, the data on the effectiveness of school-based interventions for reducing unwanted pregnancies are mixed. A widely cited study by Edwards, Steinman, Arnold, and Hakanson (1980) reported widespread use of St. Paul school-based centers for reproductive health services. This use resulted in reported high contraceptive usage by students and corresponding declines in unwanted births to adolescents. More recently, Kirby and his associates reexamined the supposed success of the St. Paul program (Kirby et al., 1993). By matching the names of female students from academic records to the mothers' names on health department birth records, this research group was able to more accurately assess the birthrates for students attending schools with health centers between 1971 and 1986 in St. Paul. The authors conclude that "the school-based clinics in St. Paul did not significantly reduce birthrates in their respective schools" (Kirby et al., 1993, p. 15).

Zabin and her colleagues (Zabin, Hirsch, Smith, Streett, & Hardy, 1986) undertook a study of four Baltimore SBHCs and the efforts of those centers to reduce unwanted adolescent births. The intervention consisting of "sexuality and contraceptive education, individual and group counseling, and medical and contraceptive services," was delivered by a multidisciplinary team consisting of a social worker and nurse practitioner, and lasted nearly 3 years (Zabin et al., 1986, p. 119). The contraceptive services were delivered off-site. The results of this intervention demonstrated an increase in sexual knowledge among students, little change in attitudes, and a statistically significant delay in the age of first intercourse for youth involved in the full program.

Finally, the Bureau of Primary Health Care (1994) in a document titled *School Based Health Centers That Work* reported that although "evaluation studies have not been performed on any of the [school-based centers found in this document] because they simply do not have adequate resources . . . most clinics were able to supply some statistical data about changes observed over time in clinic registration, service utilization, teen pregnancy, school dropouts, and several other measures" (p. 11). That material combined with anecdotal information suggested that SBHC programs have (a) improved young people's access to health care, (b) decreased adolescent pregnancies, (c) ensured that pregnant adolescents received appropriate and timely prenatal care, (d) reduced drop-out rates, (e) reduced school absenteeism (due to minor illnesses), (f) provided early detection and intervention for physical and behavioral health problems, and (g) improved self-esteem and communication skills. These subjective impressions are echoed by Joy Dryfoos (1994) in her visits to centers across the country.

There are legitimate reasons for the inability of SBHCs to evaluate the effectiveness of their interventions. They include a lack of funding to undertake this research; the difficulty of tracking youth whose mobility between schools, classes, and communities is staggering; and securing the community/school support necessary to undertake these studies. Nevertheless, the need to determine what works best, in what way, and for whom is a challenge that must be successfully addressed if SBHCs are to fulfill their mission.

Planning, Producing, and Preserving School-Based Health Centers

There are numerous issues that need to be addressed within an SBHC's lifespan. The first involves the activities of a community planning group interested in starting a program. Ideally, this group should combine expertise from the health care community (school nurses, local hospitals, and private medical and mental health practitioners), the school community (school administrators and parents), and the larger community (local politicians, clergy, community activists, professional fund-raisers). To be successful, group members need to be aware of national, local, and historical data on SBHCs, as well as information regarding previous efforts to implement SBHCs in their community.

History suggests that initial community opposition to opening a program is likely. Media or other groups may misconstrue the purpose of SBHCs, fueling community misconceptions. It is important that early in the planning process a program spokesperson be chosen who can effectively communicate the purpose and goals of the group and respond to requests for information. Experience suggests that an effective way to handle community concerns is to clearly establish the need for services. One effective way of accomplishing this is via a community needs assessment.

The needs assessment should identify problems, concerns, risk behaviors, and perceived needs (both medical and psychosocial) of the target population, and identify which services and resources are already available to address these needs. The district where the SBHC services are needed most, presumably with the highest concentration of medically underserved children and adolescents, should be determined as well. Information regarding the community's willingness and readiness to implement an SBHC is vital. Strategies for distributing the results of the needs assessment to the community should include clarification of the scope of services planned to be delivered by the program and demonstration that these services will fill the gap between what is needed and what is available.

Implementation, the next phase, involves several issues, including securing a community organization with the resources available to support an SBHC. Next, a governing board, if not already in existence and separate from the administrative organization, should be established to develop the policies and procedures that govern the operation of the SBHC. Funding for SBHCs can be obtained in a number of ways, including federal, state, local city funds, private corporations, foundations, and individual private donors. Though many communities have started to bill third parties for services provided by SBHCs, to date this process recoups only a fraction of the expenses incurred. The location of the SBHC should reflect the results of the needs assessment, as well as meet additional specifications. The site should be in a school with a supportive school administration and one able to accommodate the physical needs of the SBHC, including enough space to ensure the confidentiality of services received by the students.

With an Advisory/Governing Board, funds, and a site secured, the next step becomes staffing the SBHC. Most SBHC staff are directly employed by the parent organization. Salary savings can be achieved if the parent organization is willing to provide staff on an in-kind basis. In the process of recruiting potential candidates, highlighting the benefits of working school hours (summers free, periodic vacations) has been helpful, if this potential benefit can be offered in a fashion that maintains year-round programmatic coverage. Local universities with midlevel medical practitioner training programs are a potential source for recruitment of SBHC medical personnel, as well as other professional networking organizations. Finally, a Community Advisory Board should be developed with the purpose of advising from the community at large and channeling suggestions to administration and the Governing Board. Its composition should mirror that of the planning group and may in fact be a continuation of the planning group.

Ongoing communication and maintenance of political, community, and school support are important components to continued success of the SBHC. Internally, much of the marketing to students will be by word of mouth as students obtain services. Externally, there are a number of strategies that the SBHC can employ to increase student enrollment, use, and awareness. These include maintaining a column in the school newsletter, participating in community events such as awareness days and local health fairs, registering with the local Info-Line or other community referral sources that provide information on child and adolescent health issues, involving local media during special health promotion events sponsored by the SBHC, and providing students, parents, and school personnel with satisfaction questionnaires.

SBHC maintenance should also include monthly or bimonthly meetings between SBHC staff and school administrators and personnel to strengthen the collaborative efforts between the SBHC and school health services personnel and decrease duplication of services and share current medical and mental health issues. Once the SBHC becomes operational, there is still the likelihood of community opposition. Frequent informational sessions for the community can provide opportunities to market the positive influences the SBHC has had on the school and community. The SBHC should develop culturally sensitive materials to be distributed that describe services rendered, hours of operation, how students access services, and other basic information.

Possible School-Based
Health Center Organizational Structures

Although not the first state to develop SBHCs, Connecticut has been one of the most innovative in developing this service. In this section, we examine the various organizational structures the state has funded, their strengths and their limitations.

Even though Connecticut's 41 operational SBHCs provide many of the same services as their counterparts across the country, their structures are markedly different. In Connecticut, local communities, and not counties or the state, hold the primary responsibility for designing each SBHC. Thus, each SBHC reflects the local community's identified needs and level of comfort with the services to be offered. As a state-level strategy for extending services to needy young people, the Connecticut experience is worthy of study as it illustrates one way in which local opposition can be turned into support. The key to this process is local involvement, participation, and a role in decision making. In Connecticut, this experiment in local control has resulted in the emergence of seven distinct organizational models.

Hospitals

Hospitals have considerable experience in providing health care to local communities. There are advantages for SBHC sponsorship by hospitals. Hospitals can provide the financial stability that SBHCs need to sustain themselves while waiting for grant money, which can be delayed within federal and state agencies. In addition, hospitals can provide SBHCs with medical staff. With their competitive salaries, equitable benefits, and stable environments, these institutions have traditionally been able to find highly skilled candidates.

Being hospital employed yet school based also permits SBHC staff to rotate through the hospital's other outpatient facilities during nonoperational periods of the SBHC (i.e., school vacations, summers). A partnership is created where the SBHC is assured access to hospital services, such as including laboratory testing and referrals to specialty clinics, needed to ensure the provision of quality, comprehensive services to the students. These services can include 24-hour coverage for the SBHC through the hospital's on-call schedule. Hospitals are also able to provide continuing medical and nursing education that medical staff need to maintain proficient skills. Similarly, SBHC staff have access to the administrative services of the hospital, such as human services, billing, and legal counsel.

There are, however, disadvantages to this type of organizational structure. There is the possibility that the hospital will view the SBHC as a "minor player." The hospital and SBHC may have different views about important issues. Issues that may be important for SBHC staff but not necessarily hospital management can include contracting with Medicaid managed care organizations, grant submission, and approval of budget revisions. Another disadvantage can involve the hospital's lack of experience in working with grant funds and, therefore, their lack of understanding about payment delays, completion of applications, reporting requirements, and other obligations to funding sources. In addition, SBHCs may encounter difficulty with hospital administrative procedures, such as committee approval, internal postings, disciplinary process, and termination procedures, when attempting to adopt or revise policies and when hiring or terminating personnel.

Community Health Centers

Community health centers (CHCs) are licensed outpatient health care facilities that historically have provided services to the medically uninsured and underinsured. CHCs typically provide services for the entire age spectrum, promote access and accessibility, and strive to eliminate barriers to care. All of these factors make CHCs qualified candidates for sponsoring SBHCs.

CHCs have additional advantages, including their knowledge about and experience in providing health services to children and adolescents. They are likely to have experience with grant writing and the grant implementation process, as well as reporting requirements and delays in receiving funding. They have the ability to provide summer employment for the SBHC staff. In addition, SBHCs can refer students to the CHC for services that may not be offered by the SBHC, such as dental, nutritional, and Ob-Gyn care. Because SBHC staff may be the clinicians providing services at the CHC during evening hours, weekends, and vacations, this referral process helps to maintain a continuity of care.

Advantages of sponsorship by a CHC also include the opportunity for SBHC staff to network and interact with CHC staff of the same discipline. This allows intradisciplinary quality assurance activities to occur (e.g., peer review for social workers, chart review for medical providers). These interactions can also provide the opportunity for SBHC staff to participate in workshops, in-service programs, and mandatory training sponsored by the CHC. Support with implementation of the billing process is also likely to be available to SBHCs, given CHCs' billing experience with Medicaid and Medicare programs.

Unfortunately, CHCs have difficulty recruiting health care providers due to their poor salaries, the unfavorable location of many facilities, and a lack of interest by some health care providers in working with indigent populations. Additionally, given delays in disbursements of grant funds, large volumes of uncollectibles, and decreasing amounts of available funding, CHCs may not be financially equipped to support SBHCs. CHCs have historically not been effective fund-raisers. They have typically relied on federal and state funding, revenues generated from third-party billing, and public and private donations. Should the SBHC need to engage in fundraising activities, the CHC may not be a viable source of support.

Private, Not-for-Profit Boards of Directors

A private, not-for-profit board of directors is the sponsoring entity in one Connecticut community. The board was formed solely out of the necessity to maintain SBHC operations in that community. This board has effectively executed the responsibilities of a sponsoring organization despite model obstacles. It is not a preferred model, but with the correct mélange of committed and responsive board members, it can be successfully instituted. This model does have some advantages, namely, its freedom and flexibility. Policy changes can be implemented within a short period of time, without the bureaucracy that often characterizes larger sponsoring organizations. The organization has the freedom and ability to design and customize programs to its own specifications. It can conduct fundraising activities without limits imposed on it, freeing it to pursue private and public funding sources that might otherwise be restricted.

A private, not-for-profit board of directors, however, has no financial stability of its own. Because it has no other sources of revenue outside of the SBHC, it may have to seek out short-term financing to meet payroll and cover unexpected expenses. Another concern for this type of organization is whether to employ SBHC staff directly. Financial constraints and an inability to provide direct clinical support may necessitate a subcontractual agreement for the provision of health services at SBHCs. Finally, given the model's disadvantages, there is a strong possibility for failure if cohesive links are not secured and maintained with health care providers and agencies within the community.

Human Service Agencies

A not-for-profit human service agency operates two SBHCs in Connecticut. This agency is viewed as an umbrella organization that houses many community programs and operates under the philosophy of "spinning off" programs when they become self-sustaining. This is an organization that has experience in grant writing, grant implementation, and fund procurement, as well as in organizing and establishing community programs. Implemented programs are more likely to garner credibility and community support because they are presumably generated by community needs. Finally, human service agencies are likely to be experienced in implementing programs for children and adolescents.

Not-for-profit human service agencies often encounter the same difficulties mentioned for not-for-profit boards of directors, because they, too, have no independent financial stability. The SBHC is viewed as a separate program sponsored by an agency that manages multiple, yet independent, programs. Revenues and funding from other programs cannot be used to support the SBHC. Additionally, because the nature of the boards' responsibilities includes responding to a spectrum of programs that can vary immensely, board composition may lack sufficient representation from the medical community. The parent organization is not a direct provider of services; therefore, it must subcontract with community health care providers for the provision of health services and is thus not able to directly provide clinical support activities required by the SBHC staff.

Boards of Education

The function of the local board of education has been that of assuring appropriate educational programs and resources for students. Although they have not historically been involved in providing comprehensive health care beyond mandated health services, several communities in Connecticut have opted to employ this model. Advocacy for SBHCs at the board level is likely to grow into support at the school and parent levels. Because the board of education obtains financial support from the town council, it provides a strong financial base for SBHCs. Opportunities for augmentation of services and the development of new sites are enhanced by the ability of the board to channel funds from the school system into SBHCs. Another advantage of this model involves the fact that SBHCs sponsored by a municipality are waived from the Certificate of Need (CON) process in Connecticut.

Boards of education are often not experienced in providing comprehensive health care services to students and must contract out services if they do not wish to employ staff directly. Disadvantages to subcontracting medical staff have been mentioned previously. In addition, negotiating within the constraints of local politics unmistakably affects funding. As such, SBHCs under this model may have to endure the local bureaucracy when adopting or revising policies, and renewing applications for continued funding. In Connecticut, this is the most costly model to fund because medical providers employed by the boards of education are required to become union members. These salaries are typically higher than nonunion medical practitioners.

City Health Departments

In Connecticut, city health departments have reduced the number of services they provide to local communities. They have developed into a resource for assessing health services by focusing on data collection and the availability of health care within the community. This administrative model is able to connect SBHCs with other services concurrently being provided in the community by the local health department, such as HIV testing, WIC, and Healthy Start programs. These additional services can be easily integrated into those being provided by the SBHC, promoting comprehensive, "one-stop shopping" health care. SBHCs operating under city health departments may be able to access more readily other city services necessary for the evolution and operation of the SBHC (including renovations, weights and measures for calibration of medical equipment, etc.). Advantages to this model also seen in other types of administrative models include SBHC staff having the opportunity for summer employment in other areas of the health department (well child care and family planning clinics), sponsorship by a municipality waiving the SBHC from the CON process in Connecticut, and the ability of the local health department to provide financial support while the SBHC waits for grant funds.

Disadvantages to this model also mirror some of the previous models. Local bureaucracy may hamper the timeliness of adopting and revising policies and renewing application for continued funding. In addition, the health department may not have resources to directly provide mental health services, and it thus may have to subcontract with a mental health or social service agency.

Social Service/Mental Health Agencies

There are 11 SBHCs and an expanded school health program in the New London and Groton communities that are sponsored by a social service/mental health agency, Child and Family Agency. A unique advantage to this type of model is its ability to offer an impressive mental health component to its SBHCs. In addition, because the parent organization provides numerous outside mental health programs, it enjoys enhanced financial stability, which it can share with SBHCs. It is also able to offer experience and assistance with billing processes and negotiating with the myriad managed care organizations that exist and their individual requirements (e.g., periodic updates of clinical assessments, treatment plans, and obtaining prior authorization for services). SBHC staff have the opportunity to be employed during evening, weekend, and summer periods, allowing for continuity of care for students who require additional services during summer and vacations. This arrangement also provides staff with peer review, clinical supervision, and in-service training. Close cooperation with the parent organization allows students and their families to access services at hours more convenient for working parents. Additionally, SBHCs' services can be augmented by 24-hour on-call services staffed by mental health clinicians able to properly assess and triage students, reducing unnecessary emergency room visits.

The strong mental health and nurse practitioner component of this type of parent organization lacks a complementary physician component, requiring the mental health agency to subcontract the private physician community for supervisory services.

Each of the models offered in this section has limitations, but they are limitations that each of the applicant communities has chosen to live with. And in this statement lies an insight: Permit a local community to design its own service delivery mechanism, and it is likely that services will be developed; impose a fixed structure on a community, and it is just as likely that the proposed service will be swamped by opposition.

School-Based Health Centers
Functioning in Connecticut

In Connecticut, nearly 40% of the children and adolescents registered for care by SBHCs had no regular source of medical care outside of this resource. This percentage highlights SBHCs' ability to offer an avenue for care that might otherwise not be received.

In 1995, there were 40 SBHCs funded by the Connecticut Department of Public Health. The greatest concentration are housed in high schools (17), followed by middle schools (12) and elementary schools (9). The remaining two SBHCs were housed in an early childhood care center and a school that catered to students in prekindergarten through eighth grade. An additional eight SBHCs operated in Connecticut in 1995 without state funding.

Throughout Connecticut, utilization rates for 1995 in Department of Public Health-funded SBHCs increased from 1994. The total number of students receiving services reached 12,117, a 36% increase from 1994. These students visited SBHCs 60,441 times to receive a total of 224,767 services, reflecting a 44% increase in total number of visits and a 60% increase in total number of youth provided with services from 1994. The 10 most frequently provided medical services by Department of Public Health-funded SBHCs are listed in Table 6.1. The increased number of young people provided with services is also clear from these data.

In comparing this list of services with the *Healthy People 2000* objectives for adolescents and young adults, it would appear that SBHCs in this Connecticut sample are providing reproductive health care education and services to parent-enrolled youth. The development of additional SBHCs would enable this nation to make

Table 6.1 Medical Services Most Frequently Provided by Department of
Public Health-Funded School-Based Health Centers in SFY 1995

		No. of Youth Services Provided to Students	
Rank	Service Type	SFY 1995	SFY 1994 (rank)
1	Medical history taken	22,138	14,094 (1)
2	General health education	21,528	11,816 (3)
3	Reproductive health education	20,013	13,092 (2)
4	Physical exam	18,036	11,062 (4)
5	Health screening	9,082	4,774 (6)
6	Medicine administered or dispensed	8,932	5,513 (5)
7	Reproductive health services[a]	3,746	2,342 (8)
8	Prescription given	2,966	1,554 (9)
9	Tuberculosis testing	1,314	1,047 (10)
10	Emergency treatment	930	n/a[b]

NOTE: SFY = state fiscal year.
a. Includes pelvic exams, Pap smears, sexually transmitted disease diagnosis and treatment, and
methods check.
b. n/a = not applicable; service type not ranked in SFY 1994.

greater strides in extending information to young people on
reproduction matters and STDs. It would extend an "awareness
of the risks of sexual behavior and of sexually transmitted diseases [that] is particularly crucial for adolescents. Through school-
based education on family life and human sexuality, youth can be
offered the knowledge and skills they need to reduce their
risk" of unwanted pregnancies and STDs (DHHS, 1990, p. 505).
The provision of preventive educational services can be done in
partnership with the health education staff of the educational institution. The diagnosis and treatment of STDs can be done at the
SBHC in a supportive role with the young person's primary care
physician.

In another area, that of tuberculosis identification, the data found
in Table 6.1 suggest that SBHCs are ideal locations for testing and
meeting *Healthy People*'s goal in this regard and others involving
providing "information and counseling about immunizations and
offer[ing] immunizations as appropriate for their patients" (DHHS,
1990, p. 523).

Table 6.2 Dental Services Most Frequently Provided by Department of Public Health-Funded School-Based Health Centers in SFY 1995

		No. of Youth Services Provided to Students	
Rank	Service Type	SFY 1995	SFY 1994
1	Fillings	673	n/a[a]
2	Prophylactic treatment	639	n/a
3	Preventive care training	601	n/a
4	Periodic exam	573	n/a
5	Complete X ray	472	n/a
6	Emergency treatment	246	n/a
7	Single X ray	236	n/a
8	Fluoride application	211	n/a
9	Dental scaling	200	n/a
10	Extraction	84	n/a

NOTE: Dental services provided only in Bridgeport (two elementary schools and three high schools) and Stamford (one high school). SFY = state fiscal year.
a. n/a = not applicable; service type not ranked in SFY 1994.

Six Connecticut SBHCs also provide dental services, ranging from preventive care training to fillings and emergency dental treatment. The top 10 dental services provided are displayed in Table 6.2. These services are in keeping with the objectives of *Healthy People 2000* (DHHS, 1990, p. 353) to "reduce untreated dental caries" among adolescents. As *Healthy People* notes:

Dental caries is a unique microbial infection. Once established, it is progressive, does not heal without treatment, and leaves visible evidence of past infection. Because early diagnosis and prompt treatment of caries can halt tooth destruction and prevent tooth loss, low prevalence of untreated caries should be attainable. (p. 353)

The location of dental services within SBHCs provides opportunities for the early diagnosis and treatment necessary to stop tooth decay and tooth loss.

Psychological services were also a valuable resource offered to students. Utilization rates for the 10 most frequently provided

Table 6.3   Psychosocial Services Most Frequently Provided by Department of Public Health-Funded School-Based Health Centers in SFY 1995

		No. of Youth Provided With Services	
Rank	Service Type	SFY 1995	SFY 1994 (rank)
1	Psychological counseling/support	21,528	10,159 (1)
2	Referral/advocacy	12,784	6,079 (3)
3	Family problem counseling	10,354	6,730 (2)
4	Peer problem counseling	7,012	5,910 (4)
5	School problem counseling	6,833	4,814 (5)
6	Stress management counseling	5,405	2,762 (6)
7	Substance abuse counseling	3,106	2,141 (7)
8	Depression counseling	3,031	1,427 (8)
9	Violence counseling	2,989	1,353 (10)
10	Parenting counseling	2,796	n/a[a]

NOTE: SFY = state fiscal year.
a. n/a = not applicable; service type not ranked in SFY 1994.

psychosocial services also increased from 1994 to 1995, as displayed in Table 6.3. Psychosocial services remain an important piece of SBHC operation, with students using counseling services to deal with family, peer, and school-related issues, as well as more personal issues such as depression and substance abuse.

Healthy People 2000 identifies violence, depression, and the use of alcohol, tobacco, and illicit drugs as major health impediments for adolescents and young adults:

> Although the 1980s brought some improvements in the health status of adolescents and young adults, many other young people still must confront a constellation of problems, including alcohol and other drug abuse, school failure, delinquency, peer group violence, and unwanted pregnancy. Although education about risks is important, programs for adolescents and young adults must go beyond education to include in-depth counseling and support. (DHHS, 1990, p. 18)

Clearly, the behavioral health care staff at these SBHCs provided significant care to youth in need in areas identified by *Healthy*

People 2000. What is not known by this utilization data is whether the specific interventions used by those staff made a difference. Furthermore, the authors of this chapter have concerns that a very small number of young people needing significant behavioral health services could inhibit population-focused efforts directed at health promotion. While not ignoring the need of the individual, group needs must be attended to.

Summary

It is apparent that young people do not have access to adequate health services, and similarly apparent that many of these children and adolescents have a crucial need for such services. By not addressing this disparity between the health needs of young people and the services available to them, those responsible for the nation's health have created a situation in which the treatment of preventable health concerns costs much more than their prevention. Prevention efforts have been shown to affect adolescent tobacco use, drug and alcohol abuse, and sexual behaviors (Pentz et al., 1989; Vincent, Clearie, & Schluchter, 1987; Zabin et al., 1986) and to cost less than the treatments for the health-related outcomes of such behaviors (National Adolescent Health Information Center, 1994). To institute prevention services cost-effectively, all young people need to be tracked. The National Adolescent Health Information Center (1994) notes that because adolescent behavior changes dramatically from year to year, to ensure successful primary prevention efforts, yearly contacts with youth are needed. SBHCs have the ability to follow the majority of students from year to year and therefore represent a potential source for closing the gap between needed and available services for young people.

Because SBHCs offer barrier-free access to students, insurance status, costs, and parental availability do not affect adolescents' ability to obtain needed services. SBHCs offer comprehensive and accessible care to all students. Gullotta and Noyes (1995) note that SBHCs are also able to promote the integration of services and continuity of care within a community focus. That is, SBHCs function within a community paradigm, where, as seen in Connecticut, the community embraces the planning and implementation of health services for its youth. SBHC services are often linked to area hospitals and mental and social service agencies, and they thus offer students access to additional needed services. Students develop relationships with SBHC staff not only within the school setting but also outside of the school setting within the larger community because SBHC staff are likely to be allied with other community service agencies. These extensive staff relationships and community partnerships have the ability to promote healthy lifestyle choices by young people.

Issues for designing and preserving SBHCs develop out of this community focus, and they include both confronting community opposition and creating avenues for financial and structural community support and service expansion. Connecticut can serve as an example of successful SBHC implementation where local communities retain control. Although perfection has not necessarily been achieved by the seven organizational models in existence in Connecticut, their success in delivering community-tailored services to children and adolescents flourishes. An examination of service delivery data reveals that utilization and enrollment rates rise from year to year throughout the state and across various organizational models.

Unfortunately, the data provided here do not allow for definitive statements regarding the lasting effects of SBHC services on children's and adolescents' health. Such service analysis is needed to fully assess what SBHC interventions will have a positive effect on children's and adolescents' health. Presently, however, it can be successfully argued that SBHCs offer a unique ability to reach many youth, potentially almost all youth, cost-effectively in a manner that places them in a position to be qualified and effective gatekeepers for managed care organizations. Through SBHCs' comprehensive, barrier-free access and emphasis on prevention through early identification and treatment, appears their ability to reduce adolescent health concerns while not squandering available funds.

Recommendations for *Healthy People 2010*

1. Our first recommendation is to provide the necessary financial support to increase the number of SBHCs from the current 600 nationwide to 6,000 by the year 2010. Currently, there are 29,120 secondary schools in the United States. The U.S. Census Bureau

(1995, p. 141) reports that 4,688 have 1,000 or more students. Each of these schools should have an SBHC. The remaining 1,312 new sites should be apportioned between elementary, middle, and smaller high schools across the country.

2. Next, the focus of SBHCs should remain preventive care including assessments and referral. SBHCs offer an ideal site for population-focused interventions. They provide unique opportunities for the staff to become acquainted with the students while they are healthy. These opportunities provide teaching and role modeling instances for the development of healthy lifestyles. These opportunities should not be lost to providing intensive treatment to a very small number of youth needing intensive service.

3. Our third recommendation focuses on the type of preventive services that SBHCs should offer. By the year 2010, dental care should be added to the existing primary health care and behavioral health care services that are presently offered.

4. The fourth recommendation is that in the behavioral health area these school-based services should encompass prevention's available technology (Gullotta, 1994) (i.e., knowledge enhancement, the promotion of caring groups, the enhancement of resiliency and interpersonal competencies, and advocacy for the change of identified institutional practices that contribute to dysfunctional patterns of living among young people).

5. Next, SBHCs should be the center for population-focused interventions to promote physical and behavioral health. It has been our experience that many school-based educational programs with intentions of reducing drug, alcohol, and tobacco use or preventing STDs or decreasing interpersonal violence soon become lost in schools. The initial enthusiasm that launched these educational efforts rarely penetrates the day-to-day operation of the system such that most of these programs fail from neglect within a few years of their introduction. The home for these group preventive interventions can and should be the SBHC.

6. The sixth recommendation supports a staffing pattern that is able to address the physical and mental health concerns of young people. For too long, medical, dental, and behavioral health services to young people have operated in isolation from each other. Within a school and under the auspices of an SBHC, a nurse practitioner, social worker, and dental hygienist can offer the preventive services so necessary to ensuring good health. With

linkages to public institutions and private practitioners, these health care professionals working in partnership can improve the health of youth in need.

7. Acknowledging that health care professions operate in isolation from one another, attention must be given to providing the necessary graduate training to encourage disciplinary integration. Ideally, these cross-disciplinary collaborations should occur in graduate school and residency. The federal government should encourage these collaborations by including SBHCs as acceptable sites for students in the health professions to perform their postgraduate externships.

8. It is vitally important that at an undergraduate level, college students have an opportunity to gain a greater understanding of how health can be promoted and illness prevented. For example, given the strife and tension found in many schools across the United States, it is difficult to understand why schools of education have not developed courses that would equip new teachers at all grade levels with abilities in conflict resolution and social problem solving.

9. Much interest has been expressed in recent years for strengthening ties between parents and educators. In many communities, parents are only peripherally involved, and residents without children have no involvement whatsoever with their local school system. Child and family SBHCs offer one opportunity to increase broad community involvement with the school community while increasing family access to affordable medical care. This family-child model of SBHC care should be piloted.

10. Federal and state law should require third-party payers to include school-based health services in their benefit package. Presently, most SBHCs are funded by grants. To develop viability, it is essential that these centers be able to bill and collect for their services.

11. We do not believe that there is one, two, or even three ideal operational models for administering SBHCs. We recommend that experiments in sponsorship continue.

12. Priority funding should be given to organizations and school systems that are willing to engage in community research to determine what services are most effectively offered through this delivery mechanism. This research initiative should be designed within the Public Health Service and carried out across the country with volunteer SBHC sites.

References

Adams, G. R., Gullotta, T. P., & Markstrom-Adams, C. (1994). *Adolescent life experiences* (3rd ed.). Pacific Grove, CA: Brooks/Cole.

Bureau of Primary Health Care. (1994). *School based health centers that work.* Washington, DC: U.S. Government Printing Office.

Dryfoos, J. (1994). *Full-service schools: A revolution in health and social services for children, youth, and families.* San Francisco: Jossey-Bass.

Edwards, L., Steinman, M., Arnold, K., & Hakanson, E. (1980). Adolescent prevention services in high school clinics. *Family Planning Perspectives, 12*(1), 6-14.

Fleming, M. (1996). *Healthy youth 2000: A mid-decade review.* Chicago: American Medical Association, Department of Adolescent Health.

Gullotta, T. P. (1994). The what, who, why, where, when, and how of primary prevention. *Journal of Primary Prevention, 15*(1), 5-14.

Gullotta, T. P., & Noyes, L. (1995). The changing paradigm of community health: The role of school-based health centers. *Adolescence, 30*(117), 107-115.

Halfon, N., Inkelas, M., & Wood, D. (1995). Nonfinancial barriers to care for children and youth. *Annual Review of Public Health, 16,* 447-472.

Himmelstein, D. U., & Woodhandler, S. (1995). Care denied: U.S. residents who are unable to obtain needed medical services. *American Journal of Public Health, 85,* 341-344.

Jorgensen, S. R. (1993). Adolescent pregnancy and parenting. In T. P. Gullotta, G. R. Adams, & R. Montemayor (Eds.), *Adolescent sexuality* (pp. 130-140). Newbury Park, CA: Sage.

Kirby, D., Resnick, M. D., Downes, B., Kocher, T., Gunderson, P., Potthoff, S., Zelterman, D., & Blum, R. W. (1993). The effects of school-based health clinics in St. Paul on school-wide birthrates. *Family Planning Perspectives, 25*(12), 12-16.

Leukefeld, C. G., & Haverkos, H. W. (1993). Sexually transmitted diseases. In T. P. Gullotta, G. R. Adams, & R. Montemayor (Eds.), *Adolescent sexuality* (pp. 161-180). Thousand Oaks, CA: Sage.

National Adolescent Health Information Center. (1994). *Fact sheet on investing in preventive health services for adolescents.* San Francisco: University of California National Adolescent Health Information Center.

Newacheck, P. W., Hughes, D. C., & Stoddard, J. J. (1996). Children's access to primary care: Differences by race, income, and insurance status. *Pediatrics, 97,* 26-32.

Newacheck, P. W., Jameson, W. J., & Halfon, N. (1994). Health status and income: The impact of poverty on child health. *Journal of School Health, 64,* 229-233.

Pentz, M. A., Dwyer, J. H., MacKinnon, D. P., Flay, B. R., Hansen, W. B., Wang, E. Y., & Johnson, C. A. (1989). A multicommunity trial for primary prevention of adolescent drug abuse. *Journal of the American Medical Association, 261,* 3259-3266.

Starfield, B. (1992). Child and adolescent health status measures. *Future of Children, 2*(2), 25-39. [Special issue: U.S. Health Care for Children]

U.S. Census Bureau. (1995). *Statistical abstract of the United States, 155th edition.* Washington, DC: U.S. Government Printing Office.

U.S. Department of Health and Human Services. (1990). *Healthy people 2000: National health promotion and disease prevention objectives.* Washington, DC: U.S. Government Printing Office.

U.S. Department of Health and Human Services. (1993). *Child health USA '92* (HRSA No. MCH-92-6). Washington, DC: U.S. Government Printing Office.

U.S. Department of Health and Human Services. (1995a). *Health-risk behaviors among our nation's youth: United States, 1992* (Vital and Health Statistics, Series 10, No. 192). Washington, DC: U.S. Government Printing Office.

U.S. Department of Health and Human Services. (1995b). *Health, United States 1994.* Washington, DC: U.S. Government Printing Office.

Vincent, M. L., Clearie, A. F., & Schluchter, M. D. (1987). Reducing adolescent pregnancy through school and community-based education. *Journal of the American Medical Association, 257,* 3382-3386.

Zabin, L. S., Hirsch, M. B., Smith, E. A., Streett, R., & Hardy, J. B. (1986). Evaluation of a pregnancy prevention program for urban teenagers. *Family Planning Perspectives, 18*(3), 119-126.

• CHAPTER 7 •

Evaluation of Prevention Programs for Children

ERNEST VALENTE, JR.

KENNETH A. DODGE

A mid-decade review of the national policy plan that was begun 5 years ago (called *Healthy People 2000*; U.S. Department of Health and Human Services, Public Health Service [DHHS], 1991b) expresses some optimism that lives of children in the United States are improving. The report also indicates that despite this good progress, significant challenges remain, especially in the prevention of behavioral maladjustment, mental disorder, and violence (DHHS, 1995; Fleming, 1996). One important challenge is the long-term prevention of these problems. In 1994, the Institute of Medicine (IOM) issued a guide for the next decade of research in preventive intervention (IOM, 1994). This guide suggested that research in prevention in any domain follows a five-stage sequence, with a feedback loop from the last stage to the first stage indicating that the process is iterative. The five stages are (a) identification of the problem, its prevalence, and lifecourse; (b) identification of risk and protective factors for the problem so that

AUTHORS' NOTE: We acknowledge support from the following sources: NIMH Grants R18MH48083, R18MH50951, R18MH50952, and R18MH50953 awarded to the Conduct Problems Prevention Research Group (Karen L. Bierman, John D. Coie, Kenneth A. Dodge, Mark T. Greenberg, John E. Lochman, and Robert J. McMahon); Department of Education Grant BS184430002; the Center for Substance Abuse Prevention; and Research Scientist Award K05MH01027.

its development can be understood; (c) design and analysis of innovative pilot interventions to prevent the problem; (d) the design, implementation, and analysis of large-scale trials of a preventive intervention program; and (e) large-scale implementation and dissemination of the program to society. This chapter is directed toward the fourth stage in this sequence, that is, the formal evaluation of large-scale preventive interventions promoting positive mental health in children and adolescents.

Although the concepts in this chapter apply to a broad array of substantive problems (Stage 1 of the IOM model), we will cite examples in the domain of conduct problems, clearly one of the most pressing issues facing society. Young children with conduct problems disrupt school learning environments. Untreated, early conduct problems can evolve into more serious, sometimes criminal, behaviors. Some children with conduct problems evolve into habitual, violent criminals. Homicide is already the major cause of death for young African American males, and all projections suggest that this trend will spread to young members of all demographic groups over the next decade. The treatment of violent behavior in adults is complicated by its intractability. Once established firmly in childhood and adolescence, it is resistant to change. It appears that long-term prevention attempts begun in early childhood hold the most potential for reducing violent crime (Yoshikawa, 1994).

It is a difficult task to design violence prevention programs that can be refined, established, and accepted in the relatively short period of time between now and 2010. Successful programs will incorporate cutting-edge theoretical advances into their design (at Stage 2 of the IOM model). Several recent papers have summarized the theoretical advancements in the field of conduct disorder (e.g., Coie & Dodge, in press; Hinshaw, 1994). Current theory suggests that adolescent conduct disorder is predictable from the time of early childhood, and that multiple factors play roles in its development, including biological predisposition, the sociocultural context in which a child lives, parenting quality, peer relationships, social cognitive skills, academic performance, and adult role models. These theoretical advancements have led to the design of interventions in diverse areas (Stage 3 of the IOM model), including parent training, academic tutoring, social cognitive skills training, classroom curricula, mentoring, and peer relationships enhancement

(Conduct Problems Prevention Research Group [CPPRG], 1992). Although each of these intervention targets has proven to lead to short-term positive changes in child functioning, the long-term preventive efficacy of any single intervention has not yet been proven. The most parsimonious explanation of this set of findings is that conduct problems development is overdetermined and can be perpetuated by influences in any one of the domains cited above. The time is ripe for comprehensive prevention efforts that incorporate interventions from all of the relevant developmental domains. Such a large-scale prevention trial is what the IOM calls the fourth stage of prevention research. Several prototypes are now undergoing field trials, including the Metropolitan Area Child Study (Guerra, Huesmann, Tolan, Van Acker, & Eron, 1995), the FAST Track Study (CPPRG, 1992), and the Baltimore preventive trial (Kellam, Rebok, Ialongo, & Mayer, 1994).

Program quality must be demonstrated if effective programs are to be recognized, accepted, and used. It is our intention to argue for the utility of program evaluation, in the context of field trials of candidate programs, in providing the information needed to achieve these goals. Although conducting a high-quality evaluation is a difficult task, the information gathered in evaluation research is critically important in the creation and dissemination of innovative programs (Weiss, 1995).

Our contribution in this chapter is to outline what we consider to be the state of the art in program evaluation and to discuss recent advances. Much can be written about evaluation, and we must decide on some organizing principles to present a coherent discussion. We have selected organizing principles that reflect both the purpose of this volume and our own beliefs about evaluation. Our discussion will therefore be limited to theory-based experimental or quasi-experimental quantitative evaluations of mental illness prevention programs for children and adolescents.

We have chosen to focus on theory-based evaluations because of their potential to provide both high-quality program effectiveness data and substantive information about the illness process that is the target of the treatment program. Theory-based evaluation designs are guided by the expectations about how and why the prevention program should work. These expectations are formed through causal beliefs, informed by contemporary basic theory, about the underlying illness processes. This close relation between causal theory and evaluation design improves the validity of the evaluation findings (Chen & Rossi, 1987) and generates evaluation designs that can provide important information about the underlying causal processes (Cook, Anson, & Walchli, 1993).

We have a strong preference for randomized experimental or nonrandomized quasi-experimental quantitative evaluation research designs (Boruch & Wothke, 1985; Campbell & Stanley, 1963; Cook & Campbell, 1979). We do recognize the view that qualitative designs are useful in evaluation research (Cronbach, 1982; Guba & Lincoln, 1981; Lincoln & Guba, 1985; Pearsol, 1987), but this chapter reflects our bias toward quantitative studies. The advantages of randomized experiments are obvious in their potential for more definitive conclusions regarding the causal effectiveness of the intervention itself without the potential confounds and alternate explanations that are inherent in nonexperimental demonstrations. We believe that such demonstrations have tremendous value in publicizing and disseminating programs, which constitutes the last stage of the IOM model of prevention research strategy. A well-conducted experiment affords the high level of confidence in outcomes that is necessary to make a convincing case for wide acceptance and use of an innovative program.

We focus on the evaluation of prevention programs (rather than other intervention efforts) for several important reasons. The DHHS has emphasized prevention as a national health improvement strategy for adults (DHHS, 1991b) and children (*Healthy Children 2000*; DHHS, 1991a), making prevention programs the focus of much current research. The evaluation of theoretically derived prevention efforts is an important step in the refinement of subsequent prevention efforts (IOM, 1994; Price & Smith, 1985), and theoretically guided evaluations of prevention programs can help advance substantive knowledge about the underlying causal mechanisms that result in the illness that is the target of the prevention effort (Kellam & Rebok, 1992). Thus, the proliferation of prevention research and the role of evaluation in advancing knowledge of illness processes point to the need for evaluation in the prevention research process.

We are psychologists with experience in evaluation of mental illness prevention programs, so we will focus on mental health programs rather than physical health programs. Our examples will be drawn from the mental illness prevention literature. We believe, however, that the concepts presented here will generalize to the evaluation of any kind of prevention effort.

It is our belief that theory-based evaluations of prevention efforts provide a unique opportunity both to improve subsequent intervention efforts and to advance substantive knowledge about illness etiology. Issues in theory-based evaluation of prevention programs also subsume issues common to evaluation in general, so this perspective provides a good framework to present recent advances in the broader field of evaluation science. It is therefore our goal to make a case for the benefit of theory-based evaluations of mental health prevention programs and to discuss some important technical and methodological aspects of this type of evaluation process.

The present chapter reviews current thinking in three related areas of evaluation of health improvement programs for children. First, we will make a brief case for the necessity of evaluations of mental health improvement programs, and we will discuss recent trends in evaluation research in general. Next, we will focus more specifically on prevention research, arguing for the dual role of evaluation in the prevention context as both testing efficacy and informing theory. Finally, we will discuss specifics about design and statistical issues raised by this perspective.

The Emerging Field of Prevention Science

Evaluation has long been considered an important, but neglected, part of the process of designing effective preventive interventions (Bickman, 1983; Lorion, 1983; Lorion & Lounsbury, 1981). Evaluation in this context has been historically viewed primarily as a way to provide information about the efficacy of programs—an important way to determine program utility and to argue for the potential economic benefit of preventive efforts (Lorion, 1983). One example is the early evaluations of Project Head Start (House Select Committee on Children, Youth, and Families, 1988), which assessed the effectiveness of this early intervention in helping children from poverty backgrounds achieve success in early elementary school.

Recent advances in evaluation science in general, and evaluation of prevention programs in particular, have broadened the scope of information that can be provided by evaluation research. Theory-based evaluation (Bickman, 1987b; Chen, 1991) can provide theoretically informative data, making evaluation an even more useful and pervasive part of the program design and dissemination process. In their critical review, Cook et al. (1993) concluded that high-quality theory-based evaluation research provides both efficacy information and theoretical information about the target of the program.

Concomitant with these advances in evaluation science, the role of evaluation has been more completely integrated into the overall prevention research process. In their guide to evaluating prevention programs, Price and Smith (1985) presented a model for the conduct of prevention research that is a useful framework for understanding the various activities required in the development of a prevention program. Their model shows how developing a useful prevention program requires the integration of several activities: exploration, theory development, evaluation, dissemination, and revision. In this view, evaluation is not only a way to demonstrate program efficacy but a central and important feature of program development.

Price and Smith (1985) described the conduct of prevention research as a process that encompasses four major domains of activity: (a) problem analysis, where the problem to be prevented is defined and described; (b) design innovation, where the knowledge of the underlying illness process is studied, and a suitable prevention is designed; (c) field trials, where the proposed prevention programs are evaluated; and (d) dissemination of successful prevention programs (or successful intervention components) to users. The more recent IOM model further subclassifies the first stage as involving separable stages of problem identification and theory development.

Price and Smith explain that each of the domains is within itself cyclical, so that each stage may be repeated until enough information is gathered to warrant progressing to the next stage. Information gathered at each stage is used at the next stage of the process. For example, information gathered at the problem analysis stage should provide information about the target population and risk factors that will guide the design of the prevention program.

Another important feature of the process is that the product of a successfully completed field trial cycle should be a treatment innovation or project prototype described in sufficient detail to be carried out by other agencies or groups. This ties the research process to application, defining realistic parameters for the provisional prevention program.

Findings from the evaluation of a proposed prevention program can feed back to the beginning of the process, informing substantive understanding of the illness process and the design of subsequent prevention programs. The importance of this feedback loop was further emphasized in a recent IOM report (1994) concerning the prevention of mental disorders.

The need for high-quality evaluation is also driven by the fact that many diverse intervention programs have been proposed to prevent identical mental health problems. Some of these programs are complementary (such as parent training and child social cognitive skills training), but other sets of programs may seem (especially to the public) contradictory. Consider, for example, juvenile diversion programs versus stricter sentencing laws as interventions for adolescent conduct problems, or mainstreaming behavior-disordered children versus alternative schools and pull-out programs. The sheer number of alternative programs necessitates the availability of sound evaluative data to determine which prevention programs should be used. This point is even more important in a climate of public skepticism about the cost-effectiveness of prevention in general and a time of federal cutbacks in budgets for social programs.

Past failures of prevention programs implemented on a large scale (such as some aspects of the community mental health movement), and even rare deleterious intervention effects (McCord, 1978, 1992), point to the need to determine that programs are effective before they are implemented on a large scale. Prevention programs are often very expensive, and ineffective programs can hinder the broader cause of prevention by deflating public confidence in the concept. Because of the long time lag between program implementation and observation of outcomes, program advocates may be unaware of deleterious effects and may unknowingly disseminate ineffective, or even iatrogenic, interventions.

It seems clear that the role of evaluation is critically important in the development and assessment of preventive interventions. As evaluation data play an increasingly central role in theory development, and as the number of programs competing for adoption and use skyrockets, the need for high-quality evaluation data is more pressing than ever.

Theory-Based Evaluation

Until about 15 years ago, evaluation science was concerned primarily with improving the validity of evaluation research via methodological improvements (Chen & Rossi, 1987). This focus was driven by the view that the development and use of adequate research methods was a necessary foundation for the science. Evaluators focused on design issues rather than theory development, and they were not necessarily even aware of how and why programs were expected to work (Wortman, 1983). The primary goal of evaluation was to conduct a methodologically rigorous study that provided internally valid information about whether the evaluated programs led to particular outcomes. This traditional orientation, while advancing evaluation science through methodological improvements, tended to produce atheoretical "black box" evaluations. Such studies are referred to as black box evaluations because they were conducted to determine the success or failure of the programs in their entirety (Bickman, 1987a; Chen & Rossi, 1983).

The reduction of programs to "black boxes" simplifies the use of experimental and quasi-experimental design methods (Lipsey & Pollard, 1989), but the black box design is not elaborate enough to answer questions about the specific effects of the evaluated programs (Cordray, 1986). For example, it is sometimes of interest to know whether some program components are more effective than others, or whether program effects increase with exposure ("dosage"). These issues become even more important when the black box method yields weak, null, or mixed results, because the evaluator cannot determine whether the poor results are due to theory failure or because the program has a mixture of effective and ineffective components (Chen & Rossi, 1980). As the development of effective research methods matured, theoretical concerns assumed a more central focus in evaluation science. Theory-based evaluation (Bickman, 1987b; Chen, 1989, 1991; Chen & Rossi, 1980, 1983, 1987, 1989) addresses the problems inherent in black box evaluation by linking the evaluation design to the program theory. Bickman (1987a) defines program theory as "the construction of a plausible and sensible model of how a program is supposed to work." Understanding program theory requires opening up the black box and completely understanding the various functions of the program. Theory-based evaluation is designed to test multiple aspects of the program theory and to provide information about program specifics. This evaluation process is necessarily more complex than the traditional black box design and requires a thorough understanding of the program processes.

Theory-based evaluation is a relatively new process. As recently as a decade ago, fewer than 10% of the evaluation studies reviewed by Lipsey, Crosse, Dunkle, Pollard, and Stobart (1985) fully integrated program theory into the evaluation design. In addition to enhancing the quality and scope of evaluation efforts, articulation of a theory of prevention of a particular outcome forces program designers to think more clearly about the intervention. Crucial features of intervention can get prioritized. Expectations about when intervention effects should occur can heighten awareness among interventionists so that midstream modifications in intervention can occur.

Chen (1991) described six major domains of program theory. These domains provide a framework for understanding program functioning and facilitate the application of program theory to evaluation design. Analysis of each domain in the context of a specific program yields a component of the program theory for each domain. Each domain theory can then be used to formulate theory-based evaluation components corresponding to each domain. The evaluation is designed by selecting those evaluation components that will provide the desired information.

The *treatment domain* concerns understanding and documenting the conceptualization and design of the program treatment. Questions about the meaning, functioning, planning, and organization of the treatment are part of this domain. Social programs are often complex and difficult to deliver, so treatment that is planned may not be completely successfully implemented. For this reason, it is important that evaluations include strategies for documenting the treatment as actually implemented in addition to the treatment as planned. *Treatment theory* describes what the specific treatment should be; that is, what should be done to achieve the desired proximal results. *Treatment evaluation* describes the actual treatment as planned, measures the treatment as implemented, and examines their congruence.

The *implementation environment domain* describes the environment in which the treatment should be implemented to be successful. Questions in this domain include logistic aspects of the program, such as whether the targeted group is actually exposed to the program, staff training, and delivery atmosphere (e.g., group sessions or individual training sessions). *Implementation environment theory* describes the atmosphere in which the specific treatment should be delivered to be effective. Accordingly, *implementation environment evaluation* describes the planned implementation environment, measures the actual implementation environment, and examines their congruence.

The *outcome domain* concerns the changes that occur as a function of the treatment program, both intended and unintended. Intended outcomes are those that the treatment was specifically designed to achieve, and they are typically measured and used to gauge program effectiveness. Unintended outcomes are effects of the treatment program that were not anticipated or predicted by treatment theory. They may be beneficial, benign, or detrimental. Theory-driven evaluations place a higher priority on measuring unintended outcomes than has been typical in traditional evaluation (Sherrill, 1984). A comprehensive *outcome theory* will explore both the types of outcomes suggested by the specific program treatment theory and any likely unintended outcomes. *Outcome evaluation* clearly identifies both types of outcomes in the specific program context.

The *impact domain* concerns assessing the impact of the treatment on the outcome. This domain involves a complete understanding of the relation between the treatment program and the outcome. Issues of causal inference and internal validity are also subsumed by this domain. Impact assessment is a primary focus of both traditional and theory-based evaluation designs, although theory-based evaluations may involve multiple treatment-outcome assessments. The hypothesized causal process in a specific program is specified in the *impact theory* of program functioning. The theory-based *impact evaluation* assesses the effect of the treatment on the outcomes, and differs from traditional impact assessments by employing a large evidence base for demonstrating program efficacy. Causal inference is strengthened by using randomized experiments or multiple-method quasi-experimental designs (e.g., nonequivalent control group combined with interrupted time series pretests) where experiments are not possible. More evidence for program efficacy is obtained through the use of broader outcome definitions (including unintended outcomes) and the specification of intervening causal mechanisms.

The underlying causal processes that lead to treatment effects are the subject of consideration in the *intervening mechanism domain*. Program treatments are rarely expected to affect outcomes directly—more commonly the treatment effects operate through some intervening mechanism. *Intervening mechanism theory* specifies how these intervening mechanisms operate in the specific program, and *intervening mechanism evaluation* empirically confirms the hypothesized underlying causal process.

Finally, the *generalization domain* concerns how the results of the evaluation might be used in populations and settings in the future. *Generalization theory* explores how the specific program might operate in different populations or settings (e.g., in a different implementation environment). Assessing the function of the treatment program in different populations and environments is one way to perform a *generalization evaluation* of the specific program.

Theory-based evaluations have an emphasis on measuring program implementation and clearly specifying the causal mechanisms responsible for treatment impact. More information about causal explanation can be gathered in theory-based evaluations because they carefully identify and measure implementation, intervening mechanisms, and broader outcomes (Cook et al., 1993). Because of this emphasis, theory-based evaluations have the potential to provide additional information about the causal mechanisms operating in the illness process that is the target of the intervention.

The amount of information gathered in theory-based evaluations is much greater than in traditional evaluations, but the information comes at the cost of greater methodological complexity. The additional complexity of the theory-based evaluation process increases the need for varied research designs and analytical strategies (Lipsey & Pollard, 1989). A benefit of this complexity is that it has focused more attention on elaborating important components of the process, such as implementation (Palumbo & Oliverio, 1989) and strength of treatment (Scott & Sechrest, 1989).

It is important to note that although there are numerous potential advantages to using theory-based evaluation, it may not be possible in all evaluation environments. Bickman (1989) explains that increased costs and inadequate knowledge may sometimes preclude the use of theory-based evaluation. Compared to traditional evaluations, theory-based evaluations require more planning, a greater amount of measurement development, more extensive data collection, more complex data storage and analysis, and additional report writing activities. All are expensive, and the resulting increase in costs may exceed the available resources. Lack of technical knowledge (how to develop a program theory) and content knowledge (about the evaluated program) may also be a barrier to the use of theory-based evaluation. Lipsey and Pollard (1989) also note that the complex research designs and statistical analyses required for some theory-based evaluations may daunt some evaluators. Cordray (1989) discusses some limitations of theory-based evaluations in the policy context and proposes some alternative ways of achieving similar evaluation goals (e.g., multiple methodologies, meta-analysis).

Developmental Theory and Evaluation in the Prevention Context

The prevailing theory of prevention holds that the inhibition of physical or mental illness is accomplished by reducing risk factors and increasing protective factors that are associated with disease or mental disorder (Robins, 1992). Risk factors increase the likelihood, and protective factors decrease the likelihood, that a disease or disorder will occur in a given individual relative to the general population. Accordingly, prevention research is largely concerned with the identification and elaboration of risk and protective factors, and preventive intervention efforts seek to decrease risk factors and increase protective factors that will inhibit the development of disease or mental disorder in individuals.

This view of prevention theory leads to two major theoretical and methodological implications for prevention research. First, theories of prevention must include causal chains where background risk and protective factors affect subsequent individual and environmental factors that ultimately lead to the occurrence or prevention of a disorder. The effects of the background variables operate through the intervening variables to affect disorder outcomes. Prevention evaluation methods must allow for the formulation and testing of such mediated models of causality. Second, this ordering of events in the prevention process implies a temporally serial process where early risk and protective factors affect later mediators and even later disorder outcomes. Prevention evaluation must employ longitudinal methods where prevention processes can be followed through time to determine their impact on the ultimate development of the disorder. The demands of prevention evaluation are well served by a theory-based evaluation approach.

The need for increased theoretical and methodological precision in prevention research is acknowledged in the 1994 IOM report on preventive intervention. The report lists several obstacles to the progress of the field of mental health prevention, one of which is the lack of an organizing theoretical framework. Understanding the operation of risk and protective factors on proximal and distal mental disorder outcomes is especially underdeveloped. These theoretical gaps can be filled with information generated by well-designed evaluations of prevention programs.

The mediational and longitudinal aspects of prevention theory and research maximize the potential utility of theory-based evaluation of mental illness prevention programs, because theory-based evaluation focuses on intervening variables and multiple outcomes. Additional evidence for the utility of theory-based evaluation in the prevention context can be found in the 1994 IOM report, which lists six types of information needed to assess the quality of published research on preventive intervention programs: (a) a description of the hypothesized risk and protective factors; (b) a description of the targeted group; (c) a description of the intervention program itself; (d) a description of the research design and statistical methods used in the prevention study; (e) a description of the implementation of the preventive intervention; and (f) a description of whether outcomes have been influenced. The authors of the IOM report recommend that researchers, practitioners, and policymakers use these assessment criteria to make critical decisions about the mental illness prevention field. Theory-based evaluations of mental illness prevention programs can provide all six types of information.

Developmental theory has an important role in the establishment of mental illness prevention programs (Cicchetti & Toth, 1992; Sroufe & Rutter, 1984). Theory-based evaluations of prevention programs must also incorporate developmental theory, because designing a theory-based evaluation requires a complete understanding of program functioning. Acquiring such understanding in the prevention context requires taking a developmental theoretical perspective, because prevention theory assumes that early risk and protective factors affect later mental illness outcomes. In addition to providing information about the causal functioning of the prevention effort, theories about the developmental course of mental illness provide information critical to the design of preventive interventions. What characteristics identify the target group? At what age is intervention most effective? What potential preventive factors should be targeted, and when? What are potential short-term and long-term outcomes that can be used to determine the progress of the prevention effort? All of these questions can be informed by well-articulated developmental theories of mental illness etiology. Prevention evaluation research and developmental theory are mutually informative because both are primarily mediational and longitudinal in nature.

For example, Dodge (1986, 1993b) has outlined a model of the development of conduct disorder that includes mediational components. Dodge's model includes several intervening cognitive stages between background risk factors and the ultimate development of conduct disorder. Such intervening variables are important in the development of prevention evaluation because they can serve as targets of intervention and proximal outcomes that can demonstrate the midterm effectiveness of long-term prevention efforts.

Another example is the work of Sroufe and his colleagues (Sroufe, 1989, 1991), who have explored early pathways to psychopathology (such as attention deficit hyperactivity disorder) by comparing normal and pathological development. Such an approach leads to an understanding of where and when during development initial psychological deviations begin, and what characteristics denote the branching of a pathological developmental process from a normal one. This kind of theorizing can help prevention efforts by identifying the temporal sequence of events in the development of the disorder, and potential indicators of incipient mental illness. This information can inform the design of preventive interventions by guiding the early identification of target groups and the timing of the interventions.

There is a wealth of basic research on conduct disorder (Yoshikawa, 1994), including several recent and ongoing longitudinal studies (Lahey et al., 1995; Zoccolillo, Pickles, Quinton, & Rutter, 1992). Enough basic research has been conducted and theoretical understanding has progressed to the point where it is reasonable to design and evaluate conduct disorder prevention programs (CPPRG, 1992; Guerra et al., 1995; Kellam, Rebok, Ialongo, & Mayer, 1994). Consistent with the current state of theoretical understanding of conduct disorder, these preventive interventions include longitudinal designs and focus on intervening developmental mechanisms.

Longitudinal preventive interventions, in addition to their potential for reducing mental illness, can be especially theoretically informative (Dodge, 1993a; Kellam & Rebok, 1992; Robins, 1992). Targeting hypothesized precursors of later illness for intervention can validate the underlying theory if influencing those precursors interrupts or precludes the development of the illness. Because of this, Robins (1992, p. 4) points out that prevention experiments are superior even to treatment experiments in terms of their value in providing information about the causal relation between preventive factors and outcomes. Kellam and Rebok (1992) agree with Robins that preventive trials enhance causal inference, and they identify a further benefit of prevention experiments. Citing the Woodlawn epidemiological studies (Kellam, Brown, Rubin, & Ensminger, 1983), Kellam and Rebok note that the development of mental illnesses is characterized by multiple background variables, multiple intervening variables, and multiple outcomes. There are typically several plausible developmental paths among these groups of variables—single background variables can affect multiple intervening variables, single intervening variables can affect multiple outcome variables, and so on. Prevention evaluations can help clarify the complicated relations among the variables in the developmental process. Specific intervening variables can be targeted by the preventive intervention, and the effects on outcomes evaluated. If the intervention is successful, observing which outcomes are affected by the intervention provides information about which outcomes are caused by the targeted intervening variables.

All of the conduct disorder prevention programs cited above have at least partially employed this developmental theory/prevention evaluation approach. Kellam and his colleagues have used this approach extensively to explore the effects of school achievement and aggressive behavior on the subsequent development of depression and delinquency in the Baltimore preventive trial. They have published many of these results, and the progress of their work to date serves as an excellent example of the developmental theory/ prevention evaluation research process.

Kellam and Rebok (1992) note that the first step in using prevention evaluation results to inform developmental theory is to describe the developmental process the intervention is designed to affect. This understanding of the natural developmental process, what Kellam and Rebok call a *baseline developmental model* of mental illness, is required to get an adequate understanding of the underlying illness process. For example, Kellam et al. (1991) analyzed longitudinal data concerning the natural development of concentration problems, aggressive behaviors, and school achievement for a sample of children who did not receive any treatment or intervention. Using statistical methods sensitive to change over time, they found that in the absence of preventive efforts, concentration problems led to subsequent aggressive behavior and lower achievement. Earlier research (Kellam et al., 1983) had shown that aggressive behavior is a precursor of delinquency and that low achievement results in later depressive symptoms. What emerges from this research program is a picture of how the concentration problem's background variable influences the aggression and achievement intervening variables, that in turn affect the long-term outcomes of depression and delinquency. This baseline developmental model describes potential proximal targets for intervention (conduct problems, aggressive behavior, school achievement) and possible divergent pathways to different outcomes (aggression to delinquency and achievement to depression).

Research of this type has come to be called *developmental epidemiology* (Kellam & Rebok, 1992; Scott, Shaw, & Urbano, 1994), because of its focus on the development of naturally occurring mental illness. Developmental epidemiology is characterized by longitudinal research on untreated populations. Kellam et al.'s (1991) research fits this definition because it employed longitudinal methods to chart the development of delinquency and depression, and because it focused on naturally occurring mental illness processes in untreated children.

The next step in the developmental theory/prevention evaluation process is to conduct an intervention that targets hypothesized risk or protective factors in the developmental model, and confirm that the intervention is successful. Building on their developmental epidemiological results, Kellam and his colleagues conducted and evaluated two preventive interventions designed either to decrease aggressive behavior or increase school achievement. The interventions were delivered to children in the first grade of public school, and each child received one of the interventions but not both. Following from their developmental epidemiological findings, they expected that decreasing the aggressive behavior risk factor or increasing the reading achievement protective factor would indirectly decrease the likelihood that children who participated in the prevention program in first grade would experience subsequent delinquency or depression. Aggressive behavior and reading achievement are the intervening variables in the developmental model. Results indicated that the prevention efforts were successful in affecting the proximal targets in the desired ways—the interventions reduced aggressive behavior and improved reading achievement in first-grade children (Dolan et al., 1993).

The final step in the developmental theory/preventive evaluation process is to confirm that successfully intervening on risk and protective factors has a preventive effect on mental illness outcomes. Kellam and his colleagues have found some preliminary evidence that the impact of the intervention on first-grade aggressive behavior and reading achievement does indeed prevent the later development of delinquency and depression, the outcomes according to the developmental model. Participation in the intervention designed to promote reading achievement was related to reductions in depressive stability and symptoms (Kellam, Rebok, Mayer, Ialongo, & Kalodner, 1994). Participating in the intervention designed to reduce aggressive behaviors in first grade was related to a reduction of aggressive behaviors at the time of transition to middle school, when behavior problems are typically more likely (Kellam, Rebok, Ialongo, & Mayer, 1994). These results suggest that the interventions do indeed have a preventive effect on later outcomes, but further follow-up is yet necessary to prove this definitively.

Taken together, the results generated by this program of research support the efficacy of the intervention and also provide information about the putative developmental model of delinquency and depression. The preventive interventions successfully reduced aggressive behavior and increased reading achievement, which in turn reduced subsequent aggressive behavior and depression. The combination of mediating variables and longitudinal data in this example provides strong support for the hypothesized developmental model of delinquency and depression, especially because the intervening risk and protective factors are shown to operate over time.

Methodological Implications of the Developmental Theory/Prevention Evaluation Approach

Basing an empirical evaluation of a prevention trial on a theoretical model of development and an a priori concept of how intervention should lead to specific outcomes opens numerous methodological issues. Several pertinent issues will be discussed next.

Randomization. In the interest of testing both the effectiveness of an intervention and the veracity of a developmental model, random assignment of participants to prevention and control groups is crucial. Only through randomization can we be confident that the emergent differences between these two groups are due to the intervention and not prior selection factors. In practice, this simple goal turns out to be very difficult to achieve.

The appropriate method for assigning participants to conditions involves first identifying all participants and guaranteeing (as much as possible) their long-term participation. Then, random assignment should be made to prevention versus control conditions (or whatever additional groups are planned, such as partial prevention). However, few participants will react well to expecting to become part of an intervention and then being denied the opportunity. Likewise, some of the prevention group participants might not agree to receive intervention. If the prevention group includes only those persons who are willing to be involved in intervention, but the control group includes all participants, the design becomes biased. It might be that "willing" participants are more likely to improve over time than "nonwilling" participants, even without intervention. Design issues also suggest that it might be biasing to inform participants in the control condition that they are "control subjects" because it could induce a negative expectation for later development. Ethical considerations lead some designers to reject this proposition altogether.

Some designers resolve this dilemma by identifying one group of individuals who would be willing to participate in an intervention and then identifying another group from a separate source who would be willing to participate in a nonintervention longitudinal study (without mentioning the intervention). This design resolves some ethical dilemmas, but it does not constitute random assignment because the two groups come from separate sources and are likely to differ on many dimensions a priori. An improvement would be to identify potential participants from one source, randomly assign them to receive prevention or not, and then approach them about participation. This approach retains the attribute of randomization, but it may lead to differential (or worse, biased) nonparticipation rates and attrition over time. Still a further improvement has been made in the FAST Track program run by the CPPRG (1992). In this program, participants were first approached to participate in a longitudinal study of child development. After consent was confirmed, participants were randomly assigned to prevention versus control conditions. Then, the prevention group participants were approached to participate in the prevention program. This design retains the virtues of random assignment as long as all of the prevention group participants, even those who refuse to participate in the intervention, are considered part of the intervention group sample for later evaluation. Thus, the prevention group condition comes to include both recruitment and intervention as part of its defining features.

Clustering. Another major problem is that interventions are often implemented in the context of an existing classroom, school, or community. The interventions often involve the teacher, the peer group, or the school itself. Random assignment of children within a classroom (or school) to intervention versus control conditions could lead to contamination of the control group children, because they might indirectly benefit from intervention with the teacher or peers. Therefore, random assignment sometimes must occur with the classroom or school as the unit of assignment. The unit of assignment should correspond with the unit of analysis. A major problem that arises is that when the unit of analysis is the classroom or school, the number of cases for analysis is often small. A prevention program might involve hundreds of children but only 10 classrooms (or two schools), so the statistical power to detect differences between the intervention and control groups is often too weak, given the expected magnitude of effects of intervention. Evaluators sometimes try to avoid this problem by assuming that assignment to classroom or schools has been random and that interaction among children is nonexistent, so that the child can be used as the unit of analysis. Unfortunately, these assumptions are rarely met.

Sampling Bias. Even when initial random assignment has been achieved successfully, biases can creep into the samples over time, through differential participation, attrition, and mobility. Attrition is always a problem for longitudinal inquiry, and it is incumbent on the evaluator to test whether those children who leave differ in important substantive ways from those children who remain in the study. If children who leave differ, then the evaluation findings can be generalized only to the populations with characteristics of the remaining participants.

Differential attrition between the intervention and control groups is a second problem. Because of the attraction of receiving help and the development of commitment to interventionists, it might be that families in the intervention group are more likely to remain in the study. The opposite might also occur, if the intervention proves taxing or difficult to complete. In either case, if attrition rates differ for these two groups and if children who leave differ from remaining participants, then differences develop over time between the two groups even when the original groups had been randomly assigned and had not differed. These differences might take the form of systematic selection biases that are confounded with experimental conditions. The result is that the groups could appear to become different as a function of intervention, when the real difference can be attributed to an emergent selection bias.

There are no fully satisfactory ways of counteracting this problem, and evaluators must note this limit in their findings.

Examining Subgroups. Often, a preventive intervention will have different impacts on subgroups of children. For example, a program to prevent conduct problems might be effective with children who have minor behavioral difficulties but might not have any impact at all on children with initially severe behavior problems. Or an intervention might be effective for one gender but not the other, for one ethnic group but not another, or for one age group but not another. Analyses of intervention effects on subgroups are potentially very exciting for the field because they potentiate the matching of different kinds of interventions with different kinds of children.

One common mistake made by evaluators is to determine subgroups within the intervention group and then contrast each subgroup with the entire control group. Thus, the "mild" behavior-problem subgroup within the intervention group might be contrasted with the entire control group (including both "mild" and "severe" behavior-problem control subgroups). This obvious mistake can be avoided by assigning children to subgroups based on preintervention characteristics only, and then contrasting intervention versus control condition within subgroups only.

Another popular analytic technique is to examine subgroups of intervention children who meet different characteristics across the course of intervention. For example, one might examine the effects of intervention only on that subgroup of intervention children who complete every session of intervention (or who show interest in the program). This subgroup is often contrasted with the entire control group of children, a problem that has been noted above. One problem here is that there is no satisfactory way of determining within the control group which children also would have completed every session (or shown interest), so that there is no way to compose an appropriate comparison group. Some attempts might be made to simulate this subgroup by empirically predicting participation (or interest) in the intervention based on preintervention characteristics, and then using this regression-type prediction to form a similar control subgroup based on preintervention characteristics. This approach has merit, but it must be noted that it is never fully adequate because the empirical prediction has been conducted after the fact and might not replicate. Usually, the evaluator's only option is to report findings for subgroups as a nonexperimental and post hoc finding.

How to Evaluate a Long-Term Intervention Before the Long Term Is Over

Many programs aim to prevent long-term maladaptive outcomes, such as adolescent delinquency, drug use, or teen pregnancy, that will not be evident for many years. Other persons and agencies often do not have the luxury to wait many years before deciding whether to implement a promising program. When a prevention program is based on a theoretical developmental model, with both proximal and distal goals, it may be possible to acquire initial evaluation evidence even in the short term.

Intervention program effects can be divided into three categories of implementation, proximal effects, and distal effects. The first level is implementation. Evaluators can determine whether it is possible to implement an intervention as planned by evaluating whether the proposed intervention actually takes place. For example, a program designed to deliver parenting training to high-risk mothers can be evaluated in terms of the percentage of mothers who participate, who attend sessions, and who receive intervention services.

The second level is proximal effects. Most prevention programs attempt to alter some characteristic in the child or environment that, in turn, is hypothesized to lead to later changes in the outcome of interest. For example, the FAST Track program (CPPRG, 1992) is an attempt to alter young children's academic and social skills, based on the hypothesis that proximal changes in these skills will lead to distal changes in adolescent juvenile court adjudication and conduct disorder. Evaluators can determine whether the intervention indeed alters the proximal process as hypothesized. It is unlikely that a program that fails to affect proximal change when this change is hypothesized will show long-term, sleeper effects on the distal outcome. Thus, programs that propose possible implementation and proximal effects should be able to demonstrate those effects even in a short period of time.

Of course, positive implementation and positive proximal effects do not guarantee long-term effects on the distal measures of interest. Thus, the last level of evaluation is the distal, ecologically valid level. This measure is what is being prevented.

Evaluation of Dissemination

The final stage of the prevention research cycle (IOM, 1994) is the wide-scale dissemination of a laboratory-based program into local communities. Instead of a program being designed, implemented, and evaluated by a group of scholars or innovators (as with most prevention research), the program comes to be owned by local communities (as with most interventions). This step is necessary, of course, for the new program to become part of the fabric of the community and to continue to be implemented across time. One important measure of a program's worth is the degree to which it becomes owned by local communities.

An emerging field within prevention research (Weissberg, 1990) concerns the generation and evaluation of theories, strategies, and policies to apply broad-scale dissemination of programs (e.g., how effective are demonstration programs versus advertising in leading to wide-scale implementation of model programs?). A separate question concerns the evaluation of those disseminated programs (e.g., is a program that has been disseminated to a local community as effective in preventing negative outcomes as the model program that spawned the dissemination?). Each of these activities requires sound evaluation efforts.

Evaluation of the Implementation of Disseminated Programs. Weissberg (1990) has noted the debate among community psychologists regarding the best way to implement social innovations in a new context. The profidelity perspective is that the disseminated program should be adopted with all features of the original model being retained. Only by doing so can local officials be confident that the disseminated program will achieve the same outcomes as the model program. The proadaptation perspective is that because each local community has a different set of resources, culture, and needs, a model program must be changed and adapted to serve the local culture. The original program was developed within a context, and the disseminated program must also be implemented within its local context. Weissberg (1990) has argued that optimal disseminations will integrate features of each perspective.

Evaluation of the dissemination process will require program developers to be clear about which features of a model program are crucial to a theory of prevention and which features have been included to meet the needs of a local culture. In the FAST Track program (CPPRG, 1992), for example, training parents in behavior management skills is a crucial part of the prevention theory, but administering this skill training in groups over an evening meal versus administering it in Saturday morning classes is less crucial to the prevention theory and more crucial to local norms and ways of conducting business. Perhaps the crucial feature of the latter question is the more general point that the intervention be administered in a setting that is comfortable for parents. Program developers must be clear about the conceptual features of implementation that are important.

Once program developers are clear about which features must be disseminated rigorously and faithfully, then evaluation of a dissemination effort will follow from this set of guidelines.

Evaluation of the Effectiveness of Disseminated Programs. Because of the differences between original and disseminated programs in participants, staff, and implementation (including both planned and unplanned differences), it is imperative that the effectiveness of disseminated programs also be evaluated. Unfortunately, many model programs lose their effectiveness when disseminated (Haskins, 1989). One of the methodological dilemmas for prevention researchers concerns the strategies that can be used to evaluate a locally owned program.

By definition, disseminated programs are not administered by prevention researchers, so the opportunity for rigorous research designs and data collection may be minimal. Still, local disseminators can conduct important evaluations of their own programs. In fact, we would argue that local disseminators should be required to evaluate their own efforts, in the same way that a local practitioner of health or mental health interventions should be required to evaluate her or his interventions. These evaluations are best conducted with randomized experiments, but, of course, such designs alter the meaning of full dissemination. Alternatives include the use of single-subject case designs, in which a program is implemented for a period of time. Outcome measures, collected by local program owners, are contrasted for the period prior to implementation and afterward. If local disseminators lack confidence that differences are due to the dissemination (rather than secular changes in a measure), then the program could be temporarily stopped and reimplemented to chart changes as a function of the program implementation. At the very minimum, local program administrators should collect outcome measures for a program, to compare performance of a community with performance of its model or other communities.

Statistical Issues in Prevention Evaluation

Cook and Shadish (1994) have noted that social experiments combining theoretical testing with field demonstrations of innovative programs, like the kind of prevention evaluations we are presenting here, are becoming increasingly more common. The increased prevalence of theory-based research has raised a concomitant need for statistical methods capable of appropriately analyzing the data produced in more complicated research designs. It is difficult to review statistical methods for prevention evaluations because the theory-based approach is relatively new, and many statistical techniques that are applicable to prevention evaluations are currently in development. At this point, any review is sure to be out of date by the time it is published. However, several established statistical procedures are useful in prevention evaluation, and a few developing trends are worth watching.

Developmental theory usually specifies a causal chain of variables in the developmental course. Interventions that arise out of developmental theory typically target variables in early stages of the causal chain that are presumed to inhibit the later development of undesired outcomes. Prevention evaluation designs require complex statistical methods that can test the effects of intervening variables, and appropriately model longitudinal outcome processes. The analysis of data generated by preventive interventions is further complicated by the fact that the targeted outcomes often occur infrequently in the general population (i.e., they are *low base-rate* phenomena). An underlying assumption of many statistical techniques is that the measured outcome variable is normally distributed. The distribution of a low base-rate phenomenon in the population is not normal, so an associated sample outcome measure will not be normally distributed. Even when an outcome is normally distributed in the population, sample outcome measures collected in the field tend not to be normally distributed (Micceri, 1989). It is critical for the prevention researcher to be aware of statistical tools that are appropriate for (a) detecting the effects of intervening variables, (b) modeling longitudinal processes, and (c) nonnormally distributed outcome variables.

Intervening Variables. Intervening variables can function as mediators or moderators of the effect of the background variable on the outcome. Mediation occurs when the effect of the background variable on the outcome operates through the intervening variable. Change in the background variable is associated with change in the intervening variable, which in turn is associated with change in the outcome variable. In a fully mediated relationship, there is no direct effect of the background variable on the outcome variable after the intervening variable is accounted for; all of the effect operates through the intervening variable. Moderation occurs when the intervening variable changes the relationship between the background variable and the outcome variable. An intervention effect may operate as a moderating variable by changing the association between a background variable and an undesired outcome.

It is important to note that the relationships involving an intervening variable must be carefully specified on the basis of an appropriate theoretical model before they are statistically tested. It is difficult, if not impossible, to distinguish between mediated and moderated relationships on the basis of statistical results alone. It is especially important to have a clear understanding about any potential moderator effects in the intervention process. If undetected, moderated relationships can obscure the effects of the intervention on the outcome (Bryk & Raudenbush, 1988).

It may be necessary to test both mediated and moderated relations in the context of the same prevention evaluation. For example, recall that Kellam and his colleagues first established a mediated relationship showing that increased concentration problems (the background variable) were associated with increased aggressive behavior (the intervening variable), which was in turn associated with decreased academic achievement. Next, they tested an intervention where the good behavior game was intended to break the causal chain between concentration problems and decreased academic achievement. In this case, the intervention was an intervening variable that moderated the relationship between concentration problems and decreased academic achievement. Increased concentration problems were associated with decreased academic achievement for those who did not receive the intervention, but there was no such relationship for those who did receive the intervention—the intervention changed the relationship between the background variable and the outcome variable.

Hoyle and Smith (1994) point to the utility of structural equation modeling (SEM) in modeling mediated relationships among variables. Bollen's text *Structural Equations With Latent Variables* (1989) is a good reference for understanding SEM techniques. In cases where SEM is not feasible, Baron and Kenny (1986) outline a regression procedure for detecting mediated relationships.

Moderated relationships are tested by detecting the strength of statistical interactions. There are several approaches for investigating statistical interactions, both in the context of the analysis of variance (Judd, McClelland, & Culhane, 1995; Rosnow & Rosenthal, 1989) and regression (Aiken & West, 1991; Jaccard, Turrisi, & Wan, 1990). Be advised that detecting statistical interactions is difficult, and there is disagreement about how best to do it (Meyer, 1991).

Multisample analysis in SEM (Bollen, 1989) is also useful for detecting moderated relations. In multisample analysis, relationships in one subgroup of a defined population (e.g., those who received intervention) are contrasted against the same relationships in another subgroup (those who did not receive intervention).

Longitudinal Data. Preventive interventions are aimed at an early point in the development of an undesired outcome and designed to inhibit the subsequent development of that outcome. Outcomes are measured on the same individuals across time so that differences between the developmental trajectories of the intervention and control groups can be detected. Measurement of the same individuals over time causes errors from a particular measurement occasion to be correlated with the errors from preceding occasions of measurement. The statistical tools used to analyze such data must be sensitive to changes in developmental trajectory, and they must be able to handle data from correlated measurement occasions without generating biased results.

Hierarchical linear modeling (HLM), when used to estimate growth curve models, meets both of these conditions. Growth curve modeling captures information about developmental trajectories because the model estimates a growth curve for each subject. The parameters describing growth curves for individuals in different groups can be tested for differences. The rates of change in the outcome variable among groups are directly compared, allowing a very sensitive test of change over time. Growth curve models also incorporate the correlated errors of multiple-occasion outcome measurements, so the results of growth curve analysis are not biased by correlated measurement error.

The potential of growth curve models for analyzing data from prevention evaluations, where the preventive intervention is designed to alter the developmental trajectory of an illness process, is enormous. The text *Hierarchical Linear Models* (Bryk & Rauden-bush, 1991) is an excellent introduction to the general hierarchical linear model, and it illustrates how HLM can be used to estimate the growth curve model. Some growth curve models can also be estimated in SEM (Farrell, 1994; Muthén, 1991; Willett & Sayer, 1993).

Original conceptualizations of HLM were limited to linear models of growth trends. While linear growth curve models including power terms reasonably approximate several common nonlinear growth trends (Burchinal & Appelbaum, 1991), the development of statistical technologies to estimate growth curve models with nonlinear growth trends is advancing rapidly (Hedeker & Gibbons, 1994; Liang & Zeger, 1986; Lindstrom & Bates, 1990; Zeger & Karim, 1991; Zeger & Liang, 1986).

Nonnormally Distributed Outcome Variables. As noted above, out-come variables in prevention evaluations are sometimes nonnor-mally distributed, and therefore violate the assumptions of many statistical procedures. One way to treat nonnormally distributed variables is to transform them (e.g., by taking their log or square root). Such transformations can normalize the distribution of nonnormally distributed raw variables, making them more appropriate for analysis using statistical methods with normal-distribution assumptions (Judd et al., 1995). Data transformations may not always be possible or advisable, however. The distribution of the transformed variable may not be sufficiently normalized as to be suitable for analysis by normal-distribution methods. Another drawback to transformations is that the scale of a raw variable is changed by transformation, often requiring conversion back to the original metric before the results of the analysis can be interpreted. Such a conversion may not be possible in multivariate models, or in models where both outcome and predictor variables require transformation.

In some cases, it may be more useful to use a statistical technique that is specifically designed to handle nonnormal data, such as generalized linear modeling (McCullagh & Nelder, 1989). Generalized linear models have underlying assumptions just like normal-distribution techniques, and they are not a panacea for analyzing nonnormal outcome variables. The analyst must have a good understanding of the relationship between the mean and variance of the outcome variable to specify an appropriate generalized linear model.

Many well-developed statistical techniques exist for cases where the outcome variables are categorical, such as logistic regression for binary outcomes and Poisson regression of counts (Agresti, 1990; McCullagh & Nelder, 1989; Muthén, 1984). Such models are useful for analyzing data from developmental epidemiological studies (Scott et al., 1994), where the outcome variables are counts of at-risk individuals who do or do not develop the undesired outcome. Models for categorical variables may also be useful for cases where the distribution of a continuous outcome variable is exceedingly difficult to accommodate through transformation or generalization. In general, information is lost when a continuous outcome variable is categorized, but a radical solution for very ill-conditioned continuous data might be to divide the continuous variable into categories, then analyze the resulting categorical variable.

One promising approach to the problem of ill-conditioned data focuses on the measurement of outcomes rather than the statistical modeling of those outcomes. Sum or mean scores composed of groups of items with poor distributions are usually equally poorly distributed. An alternative method of deriving scores is proposed by Thissen (1993), who explains how item-response models can be used to generate comprehensive, stable scores from sets of poorly distributed individual items, or even groups of items on markedly different scales.

Conclusion

The nation's health agenda targets the reduction of several unhealthy behaviors that have proven to be resistant to intervention with adults: alcohol, tobacco, and other drug use; irresponsible sexual behavior; and violent and abusive behavior. While these behaviors are difficult to improve via intervention with adults, much promise exists in the prospect of targeting interventions designed to prevent the development of these behaviors in children. Strategies of prevention require an understanding of not only the static features of unhealthy behaviors but also the way they develop over time. Prevention evaluation methods must test the ability of preventive interventions to interrupt the development of undesired behaviors early, and how well they inhibit the subsequent development of unhealthy behaviors over time. We have described a research approach that is capable of serving both needs—testing prevention program efficacy over the entire course of development, and providing critical information about the specifics and predictions of etiological theories.

Evaluation research can be a useful tool fostering the development and implementation of effective intervention programs. We feel that the approach to the evaluation of prevention programs that we have presented in this chapter can help achieve the nation's public health goals at several stages in the prevention research cycle:

1. *Theory development.* The interplay of developmental theory and evaluation research methods will allow critical tests of specific theoretical predictions in naturalistic settings, helping to develop and refine our theoretical understanding of illness processes.

2. *Implementation clarity.* Rigorous evaluation research demands require that the program implementation strategy be fully articulated and that the actual program delivery be well measured. Such thor-

oughness will promote the feasibility of experimental interventions and the accuracy of disseminated versions, ultimately enhancing the effectiveness of large-scale prevention programs.

3. *Identification of effective programs.* Experimental and quasi-experimental evaluation research designs will provide accurate information about the efficacy of intervention programs, allowing the identification of the most promising of numerous, potential programs. Promoting and implementing only the most effective intervention programs will ensure that public health prevention efforts will have maximum impact.

4. *More effective disseminated programs.* Good evaluative data will allow the practitioner to review a range of options before choosing an effective program that is feasible in his or her implementation environment. Providing objective information that allows practitioners to choose optimum programs will enhance the likelihood of success of those programs. The generalization evaluation component of the theory-based evaluation model specifically emphasizes the testing of intervention programs in various environments, placing emphasis on the evaluation of disseminated interventions.

5. *Grounds for improvement.* An important feature of the prevention research cycle is that it is iterative. High-quality evaluations will accurately document both the successes and the shortcomings of experimental intervention programs. This knowledge will guide the refinement of subsequent preventive interventions that will serve to improve the health of our nation's people.

References

Agresti, A. (1990). *Categorical data analysis.* New York: John Wiley.

Aiken, L. S., & West, S. G. (1991). *Multiple regression: Testing and interpreting interactions.* Newbury Park, CA: Sage.

Baron, R. M., & Kenny, D. A. (1986). The moderator-mediator variable distinction in social psychological research: Conceptual, strategic, and statistical considerations. *Journal of Personality and Social Psychology, 51,* 1173-1182.

Bickman, L. (1983). The evaluation of prevention programs. *Journal of Social Issues, 39,* 181-194.

Bickman, L. (1987a). The functions of program theory. In L. Bickman (Ed.), *Using program theory in evaluation: New directions for program evaluation* (pp. 5-18). San Francisco: Jossey-Bass.

Bickman, L. (Ed.). (1987b). *Using program theory in evaluation: New directions for program evaluation.* San Francisco: Jossey-Bass.

Bickman, L. (1989). Barriers to the use of program theory. *Evaluation and Program Planning, 12,* 387-390.

Bollen, K. A. (1989). *Structural equations with latent variables.* New York: John Wiley.

Boruch, R. F., & Wothke, W. (Eds.). (1985). *Randomization and field experimentation: New directions for program evaluation* (No. 28). San Francisco: Jossey-Bass.

Bryk, A. S., & Raudenbush, S. W. (1988). Heterogeneity of variance in experimental studies: A challenge to conventional interpretations. *Psychological Bulletin, 104,* 396-404.

Bryk, A. S., & Raudenbush, S. W. (1991). *Hierarchical linear models.* Newbury Park, CA: Sage.

Burchinal, M., & Appelbaum, M. I. (1991). Estimating individual developmental functions: Methods and their assumptions. *Child Development, 62,* 23-43.

Campbell, D. T., & Stanley, J. C. (1963). *Experimental and quasi-experimental designs for research.* Boston: Houghton Mifflin.

Chen, H. T. (1989). The conceptual framework of the theory-driven perspective. *Evaluation and Program Planning, 12,* 391-396.

Chen, H. T. (1991). *Theory-driven evaluation.* Newbury Park: Sage.

Chen, H. T., & Rossi, P. H. (1980). The multi-goal, theory-driven approach to evaluation: A model linking basic and applied social science. *Social Forces, 59,* 106-122.

Chen, H. T., & Rossi, P. H. (1983). Evaluating with sense: The theory-driven approach. *Evaluation Review, 7,* 283-302.

Chen, H. T., & Rossi, P. H. (1987). The theory-driven approach to validity. *Evaluation and Program Planning, 10,* 95-103.

Chen, H. T., & Rossi, P. H. (1989). Issues in the theory-driven perspective. *Evaluation and Program Planning, 12,* 299-306.

Cicchetti, D., & Toth, S. L. (1992). The role of developmental theory in prevention and intervention. *Development and Psychopathology, 4,* 489-493.

Coie, J. D., & Dodge, K. A. (in press). Aggression and antisocial behavior. In W. Damon (Series Ed.) & N. Eisenberg (Vol. Ed.), *Handbook of child psychology: Vol. 3. Social, emotional, and personality development.* New York: John Wiley.

Conduct Problems Prevention Research Group. (1992). A developmental and clinical model for the prevention of conduct disorder: The FAST Track program. *Development and Psychopathology, 4,* 509-527.

Cook, T. D., Anson, A. R., & Walchli, S. (1993). From causal description to causal explanation: Improving three already good evaluations of adolescent health problems. In S. G. Millstein, A. C. Petersen, & E. O. Nightingale (Eds.), *Promoting the health of adolescents: New directions for the twenty-first century* (pp. 339-374). Oxford: Oxford University Press.

Cook, T. D., & Campbell, D. T. (1979). *Quasi-experimentation: Design and analysis issues for field settings.* Chicago: Rand-McNally.

Cook, T. D., & Shadish, W. R. (1994). Social experiments: Some developments over the past fifteen years. *Annual Review of Psychology, 45,* 545-580.

Cordray, D. S. (1986). Quasi-experimental analysis: A mixture of methods and judgment. In W. M. K. Trochim (Ed.), *Advances in quasi-experimental design and analysis: New directions for program evaluation* (No. 31, pp. 9-27). San Francisco: Jossey-Bass.

Cordray, D. S. (1989). Optimizing validity in program research: An elaboration of Chen and Rossi's theory-driven approach. *Evaluation and Program Planning, 12,* 379-385.

Cronbach, L. J. (1982). *Designing evaluations of educational and social programs.* San Francisco: Jossey-Bass.

Dodge, K. A. (1986). A social information processing model of social competence in children. In M. Perlmutter (Ed.), *Minnesota Symposia on Child Psychology* (Vol. 18, pp. 77-125). Hillsdale, NJ: Lawrence Erlbaum.

Dodge, K. A. (1993a). The future of research on the treatment of conduct disorder. *Development and Psychopathology, 5,* 311-319.

Dodge, K. A. (1993b). Social-cognitive mechanisms in the development of conduct disorder and depression. *Annual Review of Psychology, 44,* 559-584.

Dolan, L. J., Kellam, S. G., Brown, C. H., Werthamer-Larsson, L., Rebok, G. W., Mayer, L. S., Laudolff, J., Turkkan, J. S., Ford, C., & Wheeler, L. (1993). The short-term impact of two classroom-based preventive interventions on aggressive and shy behaviors and poor achievement. *Journal of Applied Developmental Psychology, 14,* 317-345.

Farrell, A. D. (1994). Structural equation modeling with longitudinal data: Strategies for examining group differences and reciprocal relationships. *Journal of Consulting and Clinical Psychology, 62,* 477-487.

Fleming, M. (1996). *Healthy youth 2000: A mid-decade review.* Chicago: American Medical Association, Department of Adolescent Health.

Guba, E. G., & Lincoln, Y. S. (1981). *Effective evaluation: Improving the usefulness of evaluation results through responsive and naturalistic approaches.* San Francisco: Jossey-Bass.

Guerra, N. G., Huesmann, L. R., Tolan, P. H., Van Acker, R., & Eron, L. D. (1995). Environmental stress and individual beliefs as correlates of economic disadvantage and aggression: Implications for preventive interventions among inner-city children. *Journal of Consulting and Clinical Psychology, 63,* 518-528.

Haskins, R. (1989). Beyond metaphor: The efficacy of early childhood education. *American Psychologist, 44,* 274-282.

Hedeker, D. R., & Gibbons, R. D. (1994). A random-effects ordinal regression model for multilevel analysis. *Biometrics, 50,* 933-944.

Hinshaw, S. P. (1994). Conduct disorder in childhood: Conceptualization, diagnosis, comorbidity, and risk status for antisocial functioning in adulthood. In D. C. Fowles, P. Sutker, & S. H. Goodman (Eds.), *Progress in experimental personality and psychopathology research. Special focus on psychopathology and antisocial personality: A developmental perspective* (pp. 3-41). New York: Springer.

House Select Committee on Children, Youth, and Families. (1988). *Opportunities for success: Effective programs for children, update 1988.* Washington, DC: U.S. Government Printing Office.

Hoyle, R. H., & Smith, G. T. (1994). Formulating clinical research hypotheses as structural equation models: A conceptual overview. *Journal of Consulting and Clinical Psychology, 62,* 429-440.

Institute of Medicine. (1994). *Reducing risks for mental disorders: Frontiers for preventive intervention research.* Washington, DC: National Academy Press.

Jaccard, J., Turrisi, R., & Wan, C. K. (1990). *Interaction effects in multiple regression.* Newbury Park, CA: Sage.

Judd, C. M., McClelland, G. H., & Culhane, S. E. (1995). Data analysis: Continuing issues in the everyday analysis of psychological data. *Annual Review of Psychology, 46,* 433-465.

Kellam, S. G., Brown, C. H., Rubin, B. R., & Ensminger, M. E. (1983). Paths leading to teenage psychiatric symptoms and substance abuse: Developmental epidemiological studies in Woodlawn. In S. B. Guze, F. J. Earls, & J. E. Barrett (Eds.), *Childhood psychopathology and development* (pp. 17-51). New York: Raven.

Kellam, S. G., & Rebok, G. W. (1992). Building developmental theory through epidemiologically based preventive intervention trials. In J. McCord & R. E. Tremblay (Eds.), *Preventing antisocial behavior: Interventions from birth through adolescence* (pp. 162-194). New York: Guilford.

Kellam, S. G., Rebok, G. W., Ialongo, N., & Mayer, L. S. (1994). The course and malleability of aggressive behavior from early first grade into middle school: Results of a developmental epidemiologically-based preventive trial. *Journal of Child Psychology and Psychiatry, 35,* 259-281.

Kellam, S. G., Rebok, G. W., Mayer, L. S., Ialongo, N., & Kalodner, C. R. (1994). Depressive symptoms over first grade and their response to a developmental epidemiologically based preventive trial aimed at improving achievement. *Development and Psychopathology, 6,* 463-481.

Kellam, S. G., Werthamer-Larsson, L., Dolan, L., Brown, C. H., Mayer, L., Rebok, G. W., Anthony, J. C., Laudolff, J., Edelsohn, G., & Wheeler, L. (1991). Developmental epidemiologically based preventive trials: Baseline modeling of early target behaviors and depressive symptoms. *American Journal of Community Psychology, 19,* 563-584.

Lahey, B. B., Loeber, R., Frick, P. J., Hart, E. L., Applegate, B., Zhang, Q., Green, S. M., & Russo, M. F. (1995). Four-year longitudinal study of conduct disorder in boys: Patterns and predictors of persistence. *Journal of Abnormal Psychology, 104*(1), 83-93.

Liang, K. Y., & Zeger, S. L. (1986). Longitudinal data analysis using generalized linear models. *Biometrica, 73,* 13-22.

Lincoln, Y. S., & Guba, E. G. (1985). *Naturalistic inquiry.* Beverly Hills, CA: Sage.

Lindstrom, M. J., & Bates, D. M. (1990). Nonlinear mixed effects models for repeated measures data. *Biometrics, 46,* 673-687.

Lipsey, M. W., Crosse, S., Dunkle, J., Pollard, J., & Stobart, G. (1985). Evaluation: The state of the art and the sorry state of the science. In D. S. Cordray (Ed.), *Utilizing prior research in evaluation planning: New directions for program evaluation* (No. 27, pp. 7-28). San Francisco: Jossey-Bass.

Lipsey, M. W., & Pollard, J. A. (1989). Driving toward theory in program evaluation: More models to choose from. *Evaluation and Program Planning, 12,* 317-328.

Lorion, R. P. (1983). Evaluating preventive interventions: Guidelines for the serious social change agent. In R. D. Felner, L. A. Jason, J. N. Moritsugu, & S. S. Farber (Eds.), *Preventive psychology* (pp. 251-268). Oxford: Pergamon.

Lorion, R. P., & Lounsbury, J. (1981). Conceptual and methodological considerations in evaluating preventive interventions. In W. R. Tash & G. Stahler (Eds.), *Innovative approaches to mental health evaluation.* New York: Academic Press.

McCord, J. (1978). A thirty-year follow-up of treatment effects. *American Psychologist, 33,* 284-291.

McCord, J. (1992). The Cambridge-Somerville study: A pioneering longitudinal experimental study of delinquency prevention. In J. McCord & R. E. Tremblay (Eds.), *Preventing antisocial behavior: Interventions from birth through adolescence* (pp. 196-206). New York: Guilford.

McCullagh, P., & Nelder, J. A. (1989). *Generalized linear models* (2nd ed.). London: Chapman and Hall.

Meyer, D. L. (1991). Misinterpretation of interaction effects: A reply to Rosnow and Rosenthal. *Psychological Bulletin, 110,* 571-573.

Micceri, T. (1989). The unicorn, the normal curve, and other improbable creatures. *Psychological Bulletin, 105,* 156-166.

Muthén, B. (1984). A general structural equation model with dichotomous, ordered categorical, and continuous latent variable indicators. *Psychometrika, 49,* 115-132.

Muthén, B. (1991). Analysis of longitudinal data using latent variable models with varying parameters. In L. Collins & J. Horn (Eds.), *Best methods for the analysis of change: Recent advances, unanswered questions, future directions* (pp. 1-17). Washington, DC: American Psychological Association.

Palumbo, D. J., & Oliverio, A. (1989). Implementation theory and the theory-driven approach to validity. *Evaluation and Program Planning, 12,* 337-344.

Pearsol, J. A. (1987). Justifying conclusions in naturalistic evaluations. *Evaluation and Program Planning, 10,* 307-308.

Price, R. H., & Smith, S. S. (1985). *A guide to evaluating prevention programs in mental health* (DHHS Publication No. ADM 85-1365). Washington, DC: U.S. Government Printing Office.

Robins, L. N. (1992). The role of prevention experiments in discovering causes of children's antisocial behavior. In J. McCord & R. E. Tremblay (Eds.), *Preventing antisocial behavior: Interventions from birth through adolescence* (pp. 3-18). New York: Guilford.

Rosnow, R. L., & Rosenthal, R. (1989). Definition and interpretation of interaction effects. *Psychological Bulletin, 105,* 143-146.

Scott, A. G., & Sechrest, L. (1989). Strength of theory and theory of strength. *Evaluation and Program Planning, 12,* 329-336.

Scott, K. G., Shaw, K. H., & Urbano, J. C. (1994). Developmental epidemiology. In S. L. Friedman & H. C. Haywood (Eds.), *Developmental follow-up* (pp. 351-374). San Diego, CA: Academic Press.

Sherrill, S. (1984). Identifying and measuring unintended outcomes. *Evaluation and Program Planning, 7,* 27-34.

Sroufe, L. A. (1989). Pathways to adaptation and maladaptation: Psychopathology as developmental deviation. In D. Cicchetti (Ed.), *Rochester Symposia on Developmental Psychopathology, 1,* 13-40.

Sroufe, L. A. (1991). Considering normal and abnormal together: The essence of developmental psychopathology. *Development and Psychopathology, 2,* 335-347.

Sroufe, L. A., & Rutter, M. (1984). The domain of developmental psychopathology. *Child Development, 55,* 17-29.

Thissen, D. (1993). Repealing rules that no longer apply to psychological measurement. In N. Frederiksen, R. J. Misleavy, & I. Behar (Eds.), *Test theory for a new generation of tests* (pp. 79-97). Hillsdale, NJ: Lawrence Erlbaum.

U.S. Department of Health and Human Services, Public Health Service. (1991a). *Healthy children 2000*. Washington, DC: U.S. Government Printing Office.

U.S. Department of Health and Human Services, Public Health Service. (1991b). *Healthy people 2000: National health promotion and disease prevention objectives* (DHHS Publication No. PHS 91-50212). Washington, DC: U.S. Government Printing Office.

U.S. Department of Health and Human Services, Public Health Service. (1995). *Healthy people 2000: Midcourse review and 1995 revisions*. Washington, DC: U.S. Government Printing Office.

Weiss, C. H. (1995). Nothing as practical as good theory: Exploring theory-based evaluation for comprehensive community initiatives for children and families. In J. P. Connell, A. C. Kubisch, L. B. Schorr, & C. H. Weiss (Eds.), *New approaches to evaluating community initiatives: Concepts, methods, and contexts* (pp. 65-92). Washington, DC: Aspen.

Weissberg, R. P. (1990). Fidelity and adaptation: Combining the best of both perspectives. In P. Tolan, C. Keys, F. Chertok, & L. Jason (Eds.), *Researching community psychology: Issues of theory and methods* (pp. 186-189). Washington, DC: American Psychological Association.

Willett, J. B., & Sayer, A. G. (1993). Using covariance structure analysis to detect correlates and predictors of individual change over time. *Psychological Bulletin*.

Wortman, P. M. (1983). Evaluation research: A methodological perspective. *Annual Review of Psychology, 34*, 223-260.

Yoshikawa, H. (1994). Prevention as cumulative protection: Effects of early family support and education on chronic delinquency and its risks. *Psychological Bulletin, 115*, 28-54.

Zeger, S. L., & Karim, M. R. (1991). Generalized linear models with random effects; A Gibbs sampling approach. *Journal of the American Statistical Association, 86*(413), 79-86.

Zeger, S. L., & Liang, K. Y. (1986). Longitudinal data analysis for discrete and continuous outcomes. *Biometrics, 42*, 121-130.

Zoccolillo, M., Pickles, A., Quinton, D., & Rutter, M. (1992). The outcome of childhood conduct disorder: Implications for defining antisocial personality disorder and conduct disorder. *Psychological Medicine, 22*, 971-986.

• CHAPTER 8 •

Making Prevention Work

DENISE C. GOTTFREDSON

CAROLYN M. FINK

STACY SKROBAN

GARY D. GOTTFREDSON

Prevention programs seldom work well, primarily because they are not implemented as required by the underlying program theory. This is not a new finding. Twenty years ago, an extensive review of delinquency prevention and treatment programs (Wright & Dixon, 1977) concluded that little evidence of positive effects for prevention programs could be found in the available research, but that implementation quality and quantity helped to explain the success of the relatively few programs that produced positive results. More recently, Lipsey (1992) conducted a meta-analysis of 443 juvenile delinquency prevention and treatment programs to examine the relation of program characteristics, subject characteristics, researcher characteristics, and evaluation design to program effects. Lipsey found that effects overall were small, but his most important finding was that the "dosage" of treatment program and features of the treatment program itself

AUTHORS' NOTE: The preparation of this chapter was funded in part by a grant from the Center for Substance Abuse Prevention, Substance Abuse and Mental Health Services Administration, U.S. Department of Health and Human Services. We wish to thank MaryLane Hunneycutt, Myrna Caldwell, and Judy Ankersen for local support and Nanette Graham for research assistance.

were associated with the size of the effects. More structured, behavioral, and multimodal treatments were more effective. Lipsey's dosage is equivalent to strength of implementation and his findings about implementer characteristics implicates fidelity of implementation. Researcher implementers (who tended to produce more effective programs) presumably hewed closer to the program plan.

Weak program implementation is likely to hinder progress toward the national health improvement goals established in *Healthy People 2000* (U.S. Department of Health and Human Services, Public Health Service [DHHS], 1991). This document calls for widespread dissemination of theory-based, empirically tested innovations to enhance health and reduce risk in children and youth. Policymakers, practitioners, and researchers must recognize that the national dissemination of well-conceptualized, validated programs to settings where they are implemented poorly is unlikely to achieve the ambitious goals expressed in *Healthy People 2000*. In fact, the lack of progress noted by the midcourse reviews (DHHS, 1995; Fleming, 1996) may be attributed in part to the low quality of program implementation.

In this chapter, we summarize literature suggesting that features of the implementing organization and its ecological context are related to the strength and fidelity of implementation. We use schools as a focal point for studying the organizational correlates of implementation strength and summarize evidence about the demographic and geographic location of schools possessing characteristics likely to hinder implementation. We demonstrate how these factors may undermine a potentially strong prevention program using as an example an urban school-based prevention program.

Organizational Factors Related to Level of Implementation

Much of the research on implementation of educational innovations occurred in a flurry of evaluative activity in the late 1970s and early 1980s culminating in an influential report, *A Nation at Risk* (National Commission on Excellence in Education, 1983), which painted a sorry portrait of American education. In general, the research indicated that implementation varies across the country and between individual schools (Berman & McLaughlin, 1978; Liberman & Miller, 1984; McLaughlin, 1990) and that this variance affects outcomes (Loucks, 1975; Stallings, 1985).

Several factors involving program implementation influence program outcomes. Information regarding these factors can be gleaned from quantitative evaluations of school improvement efforts as well as more qualitative research involving interviews and case studies. Several authoritative reviews of implementation shape our discussion (Clark, Lotto, & McCarthy, 1980; Fullan, Miles, & Taylor, 1980; Fullan & Pomfret, 1977; Purkey & Smith, 1983). These reviews have related characteristics of the innovation and of the organization to the strength and integrity of program implementation.

Characteristics of the Innovation

In their review of implementation of curriculum innovations, Fullan and Pomfret (1977) found that successfully implemented curricula were explicit and not confusing to teachers (see also Kennedy, 1978). In addition, Fullan et al. (1980) found implementation of change regarded as "practical" to teachers greater than implementation of change that affected the classroom only indirectly.

Implementation seems to vary with program complexity. In an analysis of 12 case studies, Huberman and Miles (1984) found that the scope of the program predicted the magnitude of change. Projects in the 12 schools tended to be downsized and adapted, resulting in greater change in projects that began more broadly based. The precise point at which programs have sufficient breadth (Berman & McLaughlin, 1978; McLaughlin, 1990; Miles, 1986) and depth (Clark et al., 1980) remains unclear, however. This tendency to narrow the scope of broader-based programs will conflict with the expected trend toward broader, multifaceted programs recommended in recent reviews of effective prevention practices (Elias et al., 1994; Stoil, Hill, & Brounstein, 1994; Tobler, 1986) and with the *Healthy People 2000* objective to increase comprehensive health education programs.

A key to implementing multifaceted innovation may be effective staff training. One study (Wyant, 1974) quantified the length of effective training related to implementation as measured by communication variables on teacher questionnaires. Wyant and colleagues found that training had consistent positive effects on communication, but only after 22 hours of staff involvement. Small amounts of training served to open up communication, but did not allow enough time to progress toward dealing with problems. One of the clearest findings in organizational psychology is that high-ability workers require less training time than less able workers—and they perform better on complex jobs. It comes as no surprise, therefore, that research on effective program implementation in education has found that higher-ability teachers learn to implement programs according to plan more than do lower-ability teachers (Good & Brophy, 1987).

A large-scale evaluation of school health education programs (Connell, Turner, & Mason, 1985) also found evidence that the quality of implementation increased with the amount of staff training. Teachers who received no in-service training were compared with teachers who received full and partial in-service training on measures of the percentage of the program taught and program fidelity. On the average, fully trained teachers delivered a larger percentage of the program with greater fidelity than teachers with partial training, who in turn implemented the programs more fully than teachers with no training. But because the amount of training received was not a manipulated variable, its effects on the level of program implementation may be confounded with the effects of other teacher qualities related to the amount of training received. Also, the study found that even with no training, 70% of the lessons were delivered with 60% fidelity to the program.

Teacher participation in the process of change, training, and planning appears to affect implementation (Berman & McLaughlin, 1978; Liberman & Miller, 1981, 1984; Loucks, 1983; Social Action Research Center, 1979). Berman and McLaughlin (1978) identify teachers as key to the "mutual adaptation" that occurs with successful implementation of innovations in their 4-year, two-phase study of 293 federally funded programs in 18 states. Teachers play an important role in "local input" into planning and can act as "internal change agents" necessary for implementation (Fullan et al., 1980).

At the same time, mere participation is unlikely to be useful or necessary. Research by industrial organizational psychologists

(Jackson, 1983) implies that providing opportunities for worker participation can increase workers' sense of involvement but produce little else. Teacher participation will be useful when they can provide needed information about practical obstacles or potential opportunities for improvement, or when their consent or commitment is needed for a project that they could otherwise sabotage (see Vroom & Yetton, 1975).

Characteristics of the Organization

Characteristics of school personnel and school climate also predict strength and integrity of implementation. Berman and McLaughlin (1978) found that several teacher characteristics affected implementation of innovations in their study of federally funded programs. A questionnaire given to superintendents, program managers and directors, principals, and teachers—supplemented by follow-up site visits—showed that teachers' sense of their own efficacy affects how they carry out changes in their classrooms. Several other studies imply that teacher morale is related to teacher support of innovative projects (Fullan & Pomfret, 1977; Social Action Research Center, 1979). Runkel and Bell (1976) found that teachers' skill at communicating during emotional periods predicted their readiness for collaborative action. Miles (1986) found teachers' skill deficits to be a barrier to change in five extensive case studies of urban high schools. Huberman and Miles (1984) surveyed students and teachers and found that mastery of innovation that occurred over time reinforced implementation of change in programs. Even difficult changes could be mastered with sufficient administrative assistance, which in turn would lead to teacher commitment to the process.

School climate or culture also predict strength and integrity of implementation. Each school's culture is shaped by its community, its central office, its staff and students, and its physical structure. A cultural perspective on schoolwide change (Rossman, Corbett, & Firestone, 1988) views the nature of change at the school level in terms of "sacred" and "profane" norms. Change aimed at changing sacred norms will encounter resistance from the forces that make up the school. Behavior may change, but the norms may remain. Notwithstanding cultural forces, technical elements of change have been identified on which implementation varies between schools.

One of the most consistent findings points to leadership as crucial to implementation of educational change. Fullan et al. (1980) found leadership by school principals a factor in all three phases of implementation: entry, start-up, and maintenance. Berman and McLaughlin (1978) found that principals gave the innovations local legitimacy and acted as gatekeepers. Hall and colleagues (Hall, 1987; Hall, Hord, Huling, Rutherford, & Stiegelbauer, 1983; Hall, Rutherford, Hord, & Huling, 1984) identified three styles of principals and correlated them with degree of implementation. Principals high in initiating style—those who accommodate and become involved in the change process—achieved higher levels of implementation than did the "Responders"—principals who stay behind the scenes and show interest in change only for the short term—or the "Managers"—principals who carry out change when dictated, but do not initiate or add local input.

Leadership is not limited to the principal. Several studies found central office support crucial to implementation (Fullan et al., 1980; Fullan & Pomfret, 1977; Huberman, 1983). Others found teams of central support necessary for change (Louis, 1986; Purkey & Smith, 1983). One study of teams of innovators found that teams accomplished more effective implementation of programs when administrators or principals were members of the planning team.

Another type of support identified with innovation can be generally termed *resources*. Concentrating on urban high schools, Louis (1986) surveyed 248 principals in schools involved in successful effective schools programs for at least 1 year and found that lack of resources, time, and money were most often listed as barriers to implementation. Reviews of research also identified resources, physical and monetary, as limiting to implementation (Fullan et al., 1980; Fullan & Pomfret, 1977). Other evidence implies that resources do not play an important role in the variation of implementation (Berman & McLaughlin, 1978; Clark et al., 1980; McLaughlin, 1990), or that resources affect implementation indirectly through financial support for training (Fullan & Pomfret, 1977; Miles, 1986). Whether resources are externally or locally provided may also affect the implementation and probably has more effect on how innovation is maintained (Holmes, Gottfredson, & Miller, 1992).

Organizational capacity and school climate also affect how implementation occurs. Problem-solving focus, staff morale, perceptions of support, and readiness for change relate to level of organizational development (Derr, 1976; Fullan et al., 1980; Purkey & Smith, 1983). Stability of staff, especially principals, was another element of school climate cited by teachers (Huberman, 1983), in case studies (Mann, 1978), and by studies compiled for review (Purkey & Smith, 1983). Overall, school environments that do not feel "turbulent" or overwhelmed with basic problems have a better chance of implementing "extra" programs. Clinical experience implies that schools with low morale or an impaired infrastructure are difficult places to put innovation in place (Gottfredson, 1984b; Gottfredson & Gottfredson, 1987).

One author (Miles, 1986) noted in his case studies of urban high schools that "improvement happens to those who seek it" (p. 8). Fullan et al. (1980) noted that schools had less implementation when they had a record of previous failures in innovation. Runkel and Bell (1976) surveyed 12 elementary school staffs about the innovations recently attempted and categorized them into five types varying in difficulty of implementation from innovations that barely affect teachers to basic structural changes. The research indicated that teachers perceived their schools as attempting flurries of innovation in descending order of difficulty. Schools failing at one innovation may not try a more difficult change, but may attempt a simpler one.

Local adaptation may be crucial to implementation (Berman & McLaughlin, 1978; Huberman & Miles, 1984; McLaughlin, 1990). Schools with the necessary readiness for innovation seem to be able to adapt an innovation to the local culture, thereby increasing the level of program implementation. Adaptation is a double-edged sword, however. If local adaptation omits key features of an innovation (as often happens) a limited or ineffective adaptation may be all that is put in place.

To summarize, a greater degree of implementation integrity can be expected with explicit, user-friendly innovations for which a great deal of training is offered and when teachers have participated in the planning for the innovation. Greater integrity can be expected in schools that have highly skilled teachers with a high sense of self-efficacy, cultural norms that do not reject the innovation, strong district- and school-level leadership, staff stability, central office support, and a climate supporting change (e.g., problem-solving focus, high staff morale and commitment to change, no history of failed implementation, and a relatively low level of turbulence). Schools seriously deficient in one or more of these features are not yet ready to accept major innovation.

Troubled Schools Less
Capable of Innovation

The distribution of implementation quality across different areas and types of school is not well understood. What little evidence exists points to unequal distribution, with the schools in the most troubled, urban areas having the least capacity for innovation. Gottfredson and Hybl (1989) asked principals in schools in suburban, rural, and urban areas to describe their jobs. Urban and rural principals significantly more than suburban principals responded that dealing with issues of student interaction and social control (e.g. attendance, discipline) is important to their job. With fewer student problems to attend to, suburban principals are allowed more time for planning and action and keeping up to date, both areas that would encourage implementation of change. A survey completed by teachers in all schools in a diverse school district (Gottfredson & Gottfredson, 1989) showed that teachers' perceptions of smooth administration in the school varied with a measure of average student economic status in the expected direction although not significantly in the small sample: Teachers in schools having a larger percentage of students receiving free or reduced lunch saw more problems with the school administration. A large qualitative study of urban high school principals explained some of the difficulties in leadership for innovation as a mismatch of expectations for managing change and the skills of building principals. Beleaguered principals faced expectations for dealing with improving instructional and behavioral outcomes for students, without having enough authority to effect change—and expectations for handling complex reforms, without necessary supervisory or instructional leadership skills (Louis & Miles, 1990).

In addition to a burdened principal, another barrier to change in the urban school may be pervasive school climate problems. The case study of the dangerous and depressing urban high school is a media phenomenon, but one that is supported by research. Teacher morale and orderliness are lower for urban than suburban schools

(Gottfredson & Gottfredson, 1989). A large study of the effectiveness of teams involved in innovations in 89 schools (of which 48% were in large cities and 67% were high schools) found several climate differences by location on questionnaires given to students, teachers, and principals (Social Action Research Center, 1979). It found a relationship between location of school and school crime and disruption. In neighborhoods described by respondents as deteriorated and having problems with drugs, youth gangs, and crime, there was a significantly higher perception of danger. Large city schools had a significantly higher student-to-teacher ratio and a greater security orientation than did suburban schools. These factors affected implementation. A study of working conditions in schools in two large cities found teachers stressed by problems of security, governance, control, and participation (Ginsberg, Schwartz, Olson, & Bennett, 1987).

Implementation is affected by resource availability. In some cases, new programs may have adequate funding, but previous budget cuts may have hurt teachers' ability to provide supplies and curricula. Gottfredson and Gottfredson (1989) found that teachers' perceptions of the resources available for teaching and learning varied with the percentage of students receiving free lunch and the percentage Black students in the school, evidence that those who have the highest need have the least available to them.

Researchers allude to, but have not studied systematically, differences in teacher skills by urban and suburban locations. Teacher skills and mastery of new techniques and technologies facilitate change both directly by increasing the likelihood of strong implementation of a particular technology and indirectly by producing a history of successful innovation in the school, which fuels morale and commitment to future attempts. Perhaps like some urban principals, teachers in urban schools are overburdened and underskilled, at least when faced with innovations. Two studies provide indirect evidence for this. Weiner (1990) studied eight teachers in training and found prospective city teachers discouraged by their student teaching experiences, more so than those who chose to teach in suburban schools. The author concluded that the difficulty in attracting talented young teachers to urban schools requires specialized preparation. A study in Milwaukee looked at why teachers leave urban schools (Haberman & Rickards, 1990).

Most of the 50 teachers surveyed left for "other employment," "the residence requirement," or "personal reasons" but still choose to teach. Lack of discipline and inadequate support from administration were the two top reasons cited, not diverse or underachieving students as the teachers anticipated before they began teaching. Comparative studies would clearly address the issue of teacher ability, but some evidence exists that urban schools may not attract or keep the skilled teachers needed.

The foregoing discussion implies that school characteristics are related to the level of implementation and that some of these school characteristics vary by urban/suburban location of the school. Only one study provides direct evidence that differences in teacher skills, resources, leadership, and environment explain urban/suburban differences in the level of implementation. The Social Action Research Center (1979) quantified the level of implementation of programs initiated by school teams. It found that implementation strength was significantly related to school location ($r = .42$). Large urban schools in poor, crime-ridden neighborhoods also implemented different types of programs. The urban schools, when given a choice about what to implement, concentrated their efforts on discipline, security, and traditional options. Teams in these schools also chose interventions aimed at improving teacher morale rather than more technological and sophisticated innovations. Urban schools planned differently with more administrative participation and equal minority composition on planning teams. The researchers noted that participation in planning decreased teachers' sense of alienation.

Although more definitive research is needed to better understand the distribution of implementation strength and fidelity implementation across different types of schools, it appears that it is precisely those schools whose populations are most in need of prevention and intervention services that are least able to provide those services. The studies summarized above found that leadership, teacher morale, teacher mastery, school climate, and resources are different on average in urban and other schools.

The following section uses a school-based, multicomponent prevention model operating in one troubled urban middle school to illustrate how several of the organizational factors discussed here interfere with the implementation of a potentially powerful prevention effort.

Case Study of a School Not
Ready to Support Change

In the late 1980s, the Gottfredsons (Gottfredson & Gottfredson, 1990) worked with a team of district-level administrators and school-level staff (appointed by the superintendent) in a Southern school district to develop a long-range and comprehensive plan to increase districtwide graduation rates by the year 2001. One of several objectives of the district plan was to reduce counterproductive student behaviors—including drug and alcohol use, delinquent behavior, pregnancy, nonattendance, and misconduct in school—that were seen as precursors of school dropout. The goals and objectives established in the plan mirrored several of the national health improvement goals in *Healthy People 2000*. One *Healthy People* risk reduction objective is to increase the high school graduation rate to at least 90%. Others include reducing physical fighting and weapon carrying, substance use, and pregnancy among adolescents. A subcommittee of the reform task force (consisting of school system administrators, teachers, and the Gottfredsons) supported the development of an application to the Office for Substance Abuse Prevention (later renamed the Center for Substance Abuse Prevention, or CSAP) to demonstrate a substance abuse prevention program in one of the school system's middle schools.

The subcommittee used parts of the program development and evaluation (PDE; Gottfredson, 1984b; Gottfredson, Rickert, Gottfredson, & Advani, 1984) method to develop the proposal for the project. The problems to be addressed in the program were elaborated. A theory about the sources of the problems was articulated, and program components that most directly target the theoretical variables implied by the theory were located. According to the program theory, three intermediate mechanisms—increasing social bonding, increasing social competency skills, and increasing school success—would result in a reduction in problem behaviors, including the use of alcohol, tobacco, and other drugs. This model is supported by an impressive body of research and theory linking each of the intermediate outcomes to problem behavior (see Gottfredson, Gottfredson, & Skroban, 1996, for a summary).

This research-based rationale for preventive intervention was accepted by the district-level educators, and ideas about specific intervention components consistent with the theoretical model were sought. Intervention components that had been demonstrated in prior research to alter the targeted intermediate or ultimate outcomes were preferred. A proposal to implement and test the set of intervention strategies in the context of a schoolwide program was submitted to CSAP.

During the year following the development of the application to CSAP, the assistant principal who had been active on the committee that developed the proposal left the school to become the principal of another school. The superintendent who supported the development of the district-level plan was pressured by the school board to leave town shortly after the proposal was written, and the assistant superintendent for curriculum and instruction who had spearheaded the district reform resigned shortly after it was funded. These events were followed by the demise of the district-level task force. The program was funded for a 5-year period by CSAP after key district leaders were lost.

Program Components

The initial set of intervention strategies, selected by a committee as described above, evolved over the course of the project to take account of local conditions and to strengthen implementation. For example, a community apprenticeship component was dropped when it proved too difficult to find positions for the high-risk youth. Also, several of the components initially delivered in study halls of other classes were combined into an "education and life focus" class into which all students were scheduled during the year. The following paragraphs describe the components that were eventually implemented with any degree of integrity in any year.

Instructional Improvement. Instructional improvement interventions included schoolwide changes in instruction as well as individually targeted tutoring. Cooperative learning (CL) techniques, which make use of small, heterogeneous learning teams to promote learning and school attachment, were to be used schoolwide. A substantial body of research at various grade levels and in numerous content areas has documented the effectiveness of CL for increasing academic achievement. Research has also demonstrated a positive effect of CL on attachment to school, self-esteem, and improved relations among different types of students (Sharan, 1980; Slavin, 1980, 1983a, 1983b). The latter research suggests that CL methods may provide a mechanism for promoting friendships and positive interaction among high- and lower-risk individuals, which may reduce rejection of high-risk students by more prosocial students. Rejection of high-risk youth by their more prosocial peers is a precursor of alcohol, tobacco, and other drug use and other forms of delinquent behavior. According to the implementation plan, all reading teachers and half of the English, math, social studies, and science teachers were to use CL methods consistently in at least one class.

One-on-one tutoring was provided for by adult volunteers and students from local colleges. This instructional strategy has been shown to be effective for increasing academic performance (Glass & Smith, 1979), and some research has shown it to be effective for increasing social competency, as measured by reduced peer rejection (Coie & Krehbiel, 1984). This service was intended only for students identified as being at high risk. About half of the high-risk students were to receive regular tutoring throughout the school year.

Mentoring. A mentoring program was intended to provide prosocial adult models who were supportive and taught appropriate skills and behaviors to the young people. Although relatively little empirical evidence has yet been offered in support of the efficacy of these programs for reducing problem behavior, one recent study of a program that paired elderly mentors with high-risk sixth-grade students demonstrated positive effects of mentoring on attitudes toward school, school attendance, community service, knowledge about and attitudes toward elderly people, and a scale measuring reactions to situations involving drug use (LoSciuto, Rajala, Townsend, & Taylor, 1996). The mentoring program in our study paired high-risk students with teachers in the school who had volunteered as "academic godparents." Mentor-student relationships often involved tutoring, monitoring student progress, and sharing recreational activities. It was anticipated that 50 of these students would receive regular weekly mentoring each school year and that the mentoring contacts would be primarily on a one-on-one basis.

Social Competency Promotion. Several additional components were aimed directly at social competency promotion. These components all focused on developing cognitive-behavioral skills and involved behavioral modeling and cognitive management techniques to help youth recognize potential problems, exercise self-restraint, assess consequences, and make and carry out plans to achieve desired outcomes. While most of the selected social competency modules emphasized social problem solving, two (career and educational decision skills and cognitive self-instruction) emphasized cognitive skills necessary for making good decisions about careers and enhancing academic performance.

Three social competency promotion modules were selected. The life skills training (LST; Botvin, 1989) program was implemented schoolwide. This component provided a 16-session LST course to all sixth graders. LST has been shown in a rigorous test (Botvin, Baker, Dusenbury, Tortu, & Botvin, 1990) to reduce smoking and marijuana use among White youth in Grades 7 to 9. Additional research (Botvin, Batson, et al., 1989; Botvin, Dusenbury, James-Ortiz, & Kerner, 1989) showed that the positive effects generalize to African American and Hispanic American populations. Because Botvin, Renick, and Baker (1983) suggested that the effects of the program are sustained better when booster lessons are delivered in successive years, an eight-session booster for all students in Grade 7 (beginning in 1992-93) and Grade 8 (beginning in 1993-94) was included.

This course was augmented with a 29-session social problem solving (SPS; Weissberg, Caplan, Bennetto, & Jackson, 1990) course for seventh graders. Studies of the efficacy of social competency promotion programs with middle school-aged youth have also demonstrated positive effects on problem-solving skills, prosocial attitudes, teacher ratings of impulse control and sociability, self-reported delinquent behavior, and intentions to use drugs and hard liquor (Caplan et al., 1992; Weissberg & Caplan, 1994; Weissberg, Jackson, & Shriver, 1993). This course was piloted with a few students during Spring 1992. It was initially targeted only at high-risk seventh graders, but was extended to all seventh graders at the beginning of the 1993-94 school year.

A 21-lesson violence prevention curriculum based on Guerra and Slaby's Viewpoints program was also added during the 1993-94 school year for all eighth-grade students. Viewpoints is a social skills training program that teaches youth the skills necessary to successfully resolve problem situations. It focuses on using social skills to avoid alcohol, tobacco, and other drug use; aggression and violence; and other problem behavior. Guerra and Slaby (1990) showed that a 12-session Viewpoints program increased skill in solving problems and identifying problem situations, and it reduced aggressive, impulsive behavior among a delinquent population. This program was adapted for middle school application.

Manning's (1991) model for teaching students skills to regulate their own learning was adapted for use with middle school-aged children. This model (cognitive self-instruction, or CSI) teaches students to define the problem they are supposed to be working on, focus their attention, guide themselves through the activity, cope with negative thoughts, and reinforce themselves for progress. Manning (1988) demonstrated that teaching elementary school-aged students these skills resulted in increased self-efficacy, more on-task behavior, and more positive teacher ratings of classroom behavior. The Manning model and materials were adapted for use with middle school students and implemented beginning in Fall 1993.

A career and educational decision skills (CED) program aimed at introducing careers and requirements for careers and teaching essential career-planning skills was developed initially for all eighth graders. A similar course was developed for all sixth graders for implementation in the third year of the program. The training included sessions on assessing vocational interests, values, understanding the educational requirements of different jobs, gathering occupational information, the pros and cons of career alternatives, developing an educational plan, selecting high school courses, job-seeking skills, and preparing résumés and applications. It is an experimental program developed for implementation in the South Carolina project.

The program taken as a whole corresponded closely to the "quality school health education" called for in *Healthy People 2000*. It was sequential, comprehensive, multimodal, theory driven, empirically tested, and targeted directly at enhancing health and reducing risk. And it was planned in conjunction with local educational leaders to increase local acceptance.

The School

A middle school, Bradley,[1] was selected by district administrators as the site for the demonstration project. The school had worked previously with the researchers on a successful discipline management effort (Gottfredson, Gottfredson, & Hybl, 1993), and its assistant principal had been active on the district subcommittee and was extremely supportive of the project. Bradley had an enrollment of approximately 800 students and served a predominantly residential, lower-middle-class area. The catchment area for the school experienced a major demographic shift beginning in the late 1980s. Its student population began a gradual but steady shift in 1988 from a 50-50 Black-White split to majority Black. During the 1994-95 school year, Bradley's population was 75% Black. A similar shift was seen in the socioeconomic status of the student population during this time period. The percentage of students receiving free or reduced lunch increased from about 60% in 1990-91 to nearly 75% in 1994-95. The student population was exceptionally transient due to a nearby naval base—typically, between 20% and 30% of the students enrolled in a given year either enrolled after the start of the school year or left the school before the end of the year. Students also suffered educational disadvantage: 58% of Bradley's students in 1988-89 were overage for their grade, primarily due to skyrocketing grade retention rates that occurred districtwide after the school board imposed strict promotion standards in response to 1984 state educational reform legislation. Finally, in the 1988-89 school year, Bradley's suspension rate was 99 for every 100 students. The high suspension rate, evidence of unusual discipline problems in the school, was a large factor in Bradley's selection as the demonstration school.

History of Implementation

The program was designed as a schoolwide program. The entire staff was to be involved in the planning and implementation of the program. It was to be implemented in the context of the same organization development method (PDE) that guided the development of the proposal for the project. The method uses continual information feedback and technical assistance to the school staff as they attempt to implement the program. Typically, this method involves the implementing organization in clarifying the rationale (or theory) underlying the program, selecting program components that most directly target the outcomes implied by the theory, setting explicit standards for the strength and fidelity of implementation, monitoring these standards and examining feedback on the quality of implementation, analyzing organizational obstacles to high-quality implementation, and identifying strategies to overcome these obstacles. In this actualization of PDE, the first two steps were accomplished at the district level as part of the task force activity described above. A team consisting of project staff paid by the grant (a counselor and teacher newly hired by the school to implement the program, and eventually three of the school's existing teachers who were directly involved with implementing one or more components) established implementation standards during off-site meetings, and feedback was generally provided only to the team of project personnel. Other school staff were informed of the program, its progress, and any expectations regarding their role in the project in faculty meetings, at one full-faculty in-service training session, at a few more intensive training sessions for specific program components, and by infrequent (two or three times per year) visits to the school by the researchers. The faculty had minimal involvement in planning and revising the program. Data feedback on program implementation was generally presented to the small team consisting of the researchers, the project counselor and teacher, and occasionally one or two other teachers heavily involved with the program. This smaller group was responsible for making programmatic decisions and sharing key information on program implementation with the rest of the school staff.

Gottfredson et al. (1996) summarize data on the number of persons receiving each component during each school year and the integrity of implementation of each component. The first school year, 1991-92, was largely a start-up year for the project. Only three components were attempted, and the level of implementation for each was very low. A small group of teachers was trained to use CL methods, and 13 actually used them. This core of teachers served as peer coaches to teachers trained in subsequent years. The CED course for eighth graders was implemented, but not all lessons were covered. Several teachers were trained to teach the LST course, and teachers taught a portion of the course in health classes. Nine classes received at least some of the course, but only four of these were the intended sixth-grade classes. In short, during this first year the program was not well organized. Most components were not implemented at all, and those that were implemented were implemented inconsistently.

The program was stronger during the 1992-93 school year. CL was implemented by more than half of the teachers, but data on the intensity of the program indicated that it was implemented at less than half the intended strength (i.e., in fewer than half the number of classes intended) by those teachers. Most eighth-grade students received CED at approximately half the intended strength, and students in Grades 6 and 7 received a nearly complete LST course (Grade 6) and booster (Grade 7). In addition, about one third of the high-risk youth received a small amount of tutoring (about five sessions during the year), a reasonable amount of mentoring (contact with a mentor two to three times per month during the school year), and the seventh-grade high-risk students received a reasonably well-implemented SPS skills course. This level of implementation was still well below what was intended. Students in Grade 8, for example, received no intervention aimed at social competency promotion.

A major change in the force field for implementation occurred in the 1993-94 school year. Persistent difficulties in scheduling students into study halls and other classes to receive the various components of the program led to a decision to incorporate all components except for the tutoring and mentoring into an education and life focus (ELF) course. The curriculum for each grade level was varied to include the appropriate components. Approximately one third of the students in the school were to be scheduled into the course during each of the three quarters, so that all students received it by the end of the year. Not all of the intended material was actually covered in each class, however. The CSI, Viewpoints, and Grade 6 CED components were attempted for the first time as part of the ELF class. They reached 26% (Viewpoints), 37% (CSI), and 64% (CED) of the intended populations. The level of integrity ranged from 60% of lessons completed for CED to 96% for CSI. The LST course was implemented with a high degree of integrity, but only between 43% (Grade 7) and 69% (Grade 6) of the students in each grade level received the instruction. The SPS component reached almost three times more students as part of the ELF class than it had the previous year when it was implemented through study halls, but its integrity slipped to about 50%. The CED component for Grade 8 reached a smaller percentage of the eighth-grade population than it had the previous year, but with increased integrity. The high-risk tutoring component weakened from the previous year. This component proved extremely cumbersome to administer because it involved careful scheduling of individual students with individual tutors. The mentoring component reached more students during the 1993-94 school year than it had the previous year, and CL was also implemented more fully: 88% of the teachers used these techniques at about 63% of the expected intensity level. In summary, more components were added with the creation of the ELF class, but by the end of the third year, the program was still not being implemented with the expected strength and integrity.

The same program components were implemented during the 1994-95 school year, the final year. Several components—Viewpoints, SPS, LST for Grade 6, CED for Grade 8, and tutoring—improved over the previous year in terms of the percentage of the population reached. The remaining sixth-grade components (CED and CSI) were de-emphasized to concentrate on LST. The superior level of implementation for Viewpoints appears to have been at the expense of LST for eighth graders, which reached only 31% of the intended students. Generally, the integrity of the components declined in the last year. For example, the CED Grade 8 component slipped from 70% of lessons completed in 1993-94 to 53% completed in 1994-95. The mentoring component remained approximately on par with the previous year, but the schoolwide CL intervention slipped back some. Eighty percent of teachers tried these strategies, but the percentage of intended classes in which the methods were used fell to 42%. The final year of the program was somewhat stronger than the previous year in terms of the number of students reached, but the large boost in implementation strength and integrity expected as the ELF class became routinized was not observed. It seemed to the researchers that program staff were attempting to narrow the program during this last year, perhaps in an attempt to make it more doable.

In summary, the program was never implemented according to the initial expectations of the team that had developed the proposal for the project. While most components of the program were delivered at some point in some way, the program was still in considerable flux by the end of the project period and it appeared to have reached its apex in terms of strength of implementation during the next to the last year.

Outcomes

Gottfredson et al. (1996) reported the results of the outcome evaluation for the project. The study examined change over the 5-year program period on measures of problem behavior and antisocial attitudes, positive school adjustment, and school attendance as a function of (a) membership in the treatment school (as opposed to a neighboring school used as a comparison school) and (b) participation in each of the program components within Bradley. The results showed that the prevention demonstration program, despite its grounding in social science theory and research, failed to reduce substance use, any other form of problem behavior, or any of the measured predictors of these problem behaviors.

Reasons for Failure

The experience described in the previous section is common in school-based prevention, and may be the rule in prevention efforts in troubled schools or school districts. In this section we reflect on the literature on school-based innovation and attempt to isolate the factors most likely responsible for the failure of our program. The following comments are based on observations made by the authors during our 15-year collaboration with the school district, interviews with key school system staff at the end of the project, and a climate survey administered to Bradley teachers before the project began (as part of the evaluation of an earlier project) and during the last month of the project.

Training and Technical Assistance. The review of literature on factors related to implementation quality suggested that effective staff training is a necessary ingredient. One study (Wyant, 1974) suggested that at least 22 hours of training were required to produce positive effects. Another (Connell et al., 1985) suggested that full training produced more and better program implementation than did partial or no training, although 70% of the program lessons were taught even with no training. A comparison of the level of training and technical assistance provided in the demonstration project described in this chapter with the levels provided in original studies supporting each component suggests that the service providers in the original research studies received far more training and technical assistance than the teachers in the case study described here. Guerra and Slaby (1990) reported that graduate students delivered their violence prevention curriculum after receiving extensive formal training (16 hours) provided by the program developer. The students received ongoing (30 minutes per week) face-to-face technical assistance from the developer during the implementation of the program. Caplan et al. (1992) reported master's-level health educators from a university-based community agency cotaught their SPS curriculum with classroom teachers after receiving training (six 2-hour sessions) from the developer. Weekly on-site consultation was also provided by the developers. Weissberg and Caplan (1994) reported that classroom teachers implemented the program with assistance from undergraduate aides and that extensive training (ten 90-minute workshops) was provided by the program developers. On-site consultation and coaching was also provided by the research staff.

Botvin et al. (1983), however, reported positive program effects for the LST program when teachers in suburban New York schools implemented the curriculum after only a 1-day training session. But, in that study, project staff were available to consult with teachers whenever necessary, and extensive implementation-monitoring mechanisms were applied to "assure that the LST program was being properly implemented" (p. 363). It appears that when the program developers are actively involved in the implementation of the program, positive effects are often observed. Lipsey's (1992) extensive meta-analysis of prevention and treatment programs also found that programs delivered by researchers were more effective than those delivered by the typical practitioner, presumably because researchers attended more to issues of strength and integrity of program implementation.

When school-based programs are implemented under less than ideal conditions, results have not been as positive. Botvin, Batson, et al. (1989) reported considerable variation in quality of implementation across teachers in an experiment involving Black students in nine urban schools. In that study, 1 day of training was provided to implementing teachers, with no feedback on the quality of implementation. In a study of Hispanic students in eight urban schools in the New York area, Botvin, Dusenbury, et al. (1989) reported that the amount of the LST program material covered by teachers ranged from 44% to 83%. When the experimental sample was divided into high implementation (with a mean completion rate of 78%) and low implementation (mean of 56%), positive effects of the program were found to be due only to the high-implementation group.

Botvin et al. (1990) compared the effectiveness of two different training mechanisms for teachers implementing the LST program. One involved the 1-day training session described earlier and implementation feedback to teachers. The other involved a 2-hour videotape accompanied by written instructions and curriculum materials. No feedback was provided. The quality of implementation was similar in each condition, with a mean of 67% and 68% of the material covered in each condition. The amount of material covered ranged from 27% to 97%, with only 75% of the students in either experimental condition being exposed to 60% or more of the material. The level of implementation was strongly related to the effectiveness of the program. This study suggests that even the 1-day training for teachers provided in the more intensive condition may not be sufficient to produce high-quality implementation in the absence of ongoing monitoring and consultation to improve the quality of implementation. Ongoing consultation and technical assistance appear more important than initial training in producing high-quality implementation.

It is not possible to compare directly the intensity of implementation of components in our study with the intensity levels reported in previous studies, but comparisons with implementation standards established for each component are possible. For each component, a quantitative standard was set prior to implementation. The standard for SPS, for example, was that 95% of the seventh-grade students would complete at least 80% of the course assignments. The percentage of targeted students actually achieving the standards set for each program component ranged from 0% to 67% (mean = 28%) for the 1993-94 school year, the year in which the program was implemented in its strongest form. If we adopt the 60% fidelity cut point proposed by Botvin et al. (1990), only 1 of the 11 components would be considered strong enough to expect positive outcomes.

Limited initial training, ongoing technical assistance, or both may explain the low level of implementation. The amount of initial training provided for the teacher-implementers was generally less than had been provided in prior research, although it was ample according to customary school district practice. For most components, teachers were initially trained by the component's developers. But in later years, new staff relied on the teacher's manuals and training provided by their peers who had been previously trained. The project leaders in the school had been trained by the developers and felt that additional training was not necessary. They provided training to other teachers in the school. Although inadequate initial training of the providers may be part of the explanation of the subsequent poor level of implementation, the Botvin et al. (1990) finding that the amount of training does not explain variation in program implementation and the Connell et al. (1985) demonstration that reasonable levels of implementation can be achieved without training lead us to speculate that other factors had more influence on the quality of implementation. It is more likely that lack of ongoing technical assistance and support by persons other than the project staff and the general school climate influenced the level of implementation more than the mere number of hours of training received.

Outsiders. A sacred norm among residents of the city in which the demonstration occurred is protecting their history and traditions from pressures for change from the outside. This aspect of the city's culture is documented in history books (Rosen, 1982), is the theme of many novels and films, and is obvious to visitors to the city. The reform effort of which this project was one part came about when the state department of education—an "outsider" organization—declared the cities' schools "educationally impaired" and required the school district to develop an improvement plan. The school district complied reluctantly. A new superintendent from Florida (an outsider) placed in charge of this effort a new assistant superintendent for instruction from New England (an outsider), and the authors (also outsiders) were asked to help. A major focus of the larger reform was redistribution of resources to the schools serving the most disadvantaged students, an idea that met with resistance from guardians of the status quo in the central administration and several school board members who were opposed to most public expenditures on the public schools. (In this city, as in many Southern cities, private schools are the norm for children of well-off citizens.) The reform came to be seen and described by many in the school system as yet another attempt to interfere with local autonomy.

This violation of the most sacred norm of local autonomy was replicated in Bradley, as long-time teachers and counselors resisted attempts by outsiders to change their practices. The literature suggests that school-based change is more likely to succeed when the school staff participate in the planning and implementation of the project—when they feel a sense of ownership and commitment to it. Although it was intended that teachers and administrators would become actively involved in running the project at the school level, the desired level of local participation was never achieved. Teachers instead experienced the program as having been imposed on them from the outside. In interviews with CSAP site visitors (CSR, Inc., 1994) one teacher expressed resentment at having to "change our teaching styles to make some outsiders look good" (p. 23). One person remarked that "this program is more about research and experimenting with cooperative learning than it is about these children" (p. 23). These views of the program were not universal among school personnel. Several veteran teachers and the counselor who managed the effort worked diligently to change the status quo in the school to incorporate the new practices. Their tireless efforts were responsible for the implementation that did occur. But their work was thwarted by those who felt no ownership for the effort, and by the absence of a strong leader.

Leadership. During the period from the inception of the project to its end, Bradley had three different principals and three different assistant principals. Bradley's initial assistant principal was the natural leader for the project. She was organized, respected, and completely knowledgeable about the proposed program, having been a member of the district-level task force. She had been the leader of an earlier successful demonstration project aimed at reducing school disorder and was skilled at generating and maintaining teacher involvement and commitment. Her strengths more than compensated for the weak leadership provided by the woman who was principal during most of the project's implementation— who was known as a strict disciplinarian but not as a strong instructional leader for the school. When the assistant principal left just before the beginning of the project to accept a position as the principal at a different school, the prognosis for the project worsened considerably.

None of the subsequent administrators assigned to the school provided leadership for the project. Interviews conducted at the end of the last year of program implementation showed that the assistant principal lacked understanding about the theory underlying the program, and the school's new principal was described by different teachers as "inexperienced, timid, indecisive, with little follow-through" and "clueless" about the project. Similar observations were made of the person who served as principal for most of the project: She neither undermined nor supported the effort, but was "mostly oblivious" to it. Several teachers and other members of the school staff pointed to lack of administrative support for the program as an obstacle.

This lack of leadership took a toll on the project. Because the project was designed to rely heavily on regular school staff to implement most program components, the support of the principal was crucial. When the principal did not encourage staff involvement, it was not forthcoming. When no consequences resulted from nonparticipation, the status quo was reinforced.

Several key decisions about the program made by the principal seemed not to be based on concern for the effectiveness of the program. The initial project coordinator selected by the high school principal was incapable of doing the job and had to be replaced after getting the project off to a poor start by generating ill will from many of the teachers. The Bradley principal also erred in filling the position for a full-time teacher for the ELF class—a critically important position for the project. Despite strong encouragement from the researchers and direct program staff to use the position to support a well-respected veteran teacher from the school with a real interest in teaching a social competency promotion curriculum, the principal instead placed in the position a new teacher who lacked experience and interest in dealing with troublesome adolescents.

Similarly, district-level leadership for the project diminished once the task force that had created a climate of change for the district was disbanded. In earlier projects conducted with middle schools in the school district, strong central office support was provided by the Supervisor of Middle Schools. The school board eliminated this position just prior to the initiation of the current project. Although the project was technically monitored by the Director of Pupil Personnel Services in the central office, she was already overburdened with other responsibilities and had infrequent contact with the school or the researchers about the project.

Recall that just as the project began, the superintendent who had supported the districtwide planning was replaced for exploring avenues to raise revenue needed for the school. His replacement did not block but did nothing to support the project. He went along with a destructive board decision not to hire 12-month personnel, even with grant funds. He also made it clear that the district reform plan was "not my plan." We know of no visit by the superintendent to the project school during the 5-year period.

We suspect that these problems of weak leadership and incapable staff are common in school-based prevention efforts in troubled schools and school districts. The literature reviewed earlier on uneven distribution of human resources across schools accords with our observations made over the course of many projects and many years of attempting prevention efforts in urban schools. The workforce in large, urban school districts seems to be bimodal, with the highly skilled and committed workers counterbalanced by many unsatisfactory workers. Faculty and administrators who are energetic and capable are recruited and retained in desirable schools. Others migrate to schools with more problems.

Organizational Capacity. Stronger implementation is expected in schools whose climates support innovation. Some of the indicators of a positive climate for change include high staff morale and involvement in problem solving rather than crisis management. Schools overwhelmed with basic problems such as student misbehavior are unlikely to have the capacity to innovate effectively.

Bradley's general organizational incapacity served as a major drag on the program. Bradley operated in a continual state of crisis during the project. The school was overwhelmed by discipline problems, as evidenced by the increasing rates of discipline referrals and suspensions. Teachers reported spending most of their time on discipline problems and that instruction was of secondary importance.

A series of serious incidents occurred in the school over the course of the project. These included mayhem by faculty family members setting themselves on fire, televised accounts of statutory rape in the school, police escorting students to class in handcuffs, and program participants dying in high-speed chases with police while joyriding. The principal was hospitalized for an extended period following a health crisis. These events impaired school spirit.

Project staff saw teacher morale decline and with it, teacher enthusiasm and support for the project. Teachers who taught the project classes reported a general lack of focus in the school. They reported having to conduct project lessons "in haste or not at all" because of interruptions and various unscheduled events. In interviews, teacher after teacher described the student population as "difficult," "challenging," "disrespectful," "rude," and "discourteous." It is not possible to determine the extent to which these unflattering perceptions of the students originated in a true shift in student characteristics or whether the perceived misbehavior resulted from inconsistency in discipline management and a general lack of guardianship at the school. School district administrators described the Bradley staff as "unable to deal with the problems."

Although we had not planned to conduct school climate surveys as part of the evaluation of the project, we asked teachers to complete a survey during the last month of school of the final year to confirm our suspicion that the climate had become less supportive of innovation during the 5-year period. As part of the larger district reform, we had administered the Effective School Battery (Gottfredson, 1984a) to all Bradley teachers during the 1989-90 school year, a year prior to the beginning of the project. The same survey was readministered in Spring 1995. Response rates for the 2 years were 78% and 85%. The 1995 survey showed the school to be average on most dimensions except those related to safety and discipline. Bradley's teachers reported a higher level of victimization experiences (in the top 10th percentile of schools in the normative sample), and their approach to dealing with students was highly authoritarian. Many teachers saw the students as "hoodlums." Also, teacher job satisfaction was low—in the 29th percentile for schools. When the 1995 scores were compared with the earlier scores, significant ($p < .05$) declines were observed in teacher reports of safety and feelings of personal security in the school, and marginally significant ($p < .10$) declines were observed in teacher morale and job satisfaction.

Conclusion
and Recommendations

One of the *Healthy People 2000* objectives is to increase the proportion of the nation's schools that provide comprehensive school health education. The report defined high-quality programs as planned, coordinated, ongoing, including multiple interventions, relying on behavioral science technology, and integrating education, skills development, and motivation on a range of health problems and issues.

By most measures, the program described in this chapter would be counted as a comprehensive school health education program. School and district administrators, if asked to describe their school health program, would certainly have reported that a comprehensive, scientifically tested, sequential program with multiple interventions including education, skills development, and resiliency-enhancement was implemented for several years. They would have reported that local administrators and teachers were involved in the planning of the program, that it was managed and implemented by school staff, that most of the staff in the school were involved with some aspect of the program, and that an enormous amount of time was devoted to the program components. In the final 2 years of the program, students were scheduled into a regular class (for approximately 60 hours of instruction spread over 12 weeks) to receive the program components. An evaluation of national school health programs (Connell et al., 1985) concluded that stable effects on health risk attitudes and behaviors are established at about 40-50 classroom hours of instruction.

Classroom contact hours and educator reports of the quality of the program are not sufficiently sensitive measures of the quality of school health education programs. The program described in the case study in this chapter appeared to be of high quality and consumed large amounts of student time. But lessons were dropped and "reinvented" in ways that reduced the effectiveness of the program, and student absenteeism and nonparticipation further diminished the program's potential to meet its objectives. A mid-course review of progress toward the national health promotion objectives (DHHS, 1995) mentions the inherent difficulties in identifying and establishing meaningful ways to measure the qualitative dimension implied in many of the services and protection objectives in *Healthy People 2000*. Counting the mere number of services provided is likely to be misleading. More programs and services are bound to be located in the most troubled areas, but their effectiveness is likely to be diminished by organizational incapacity. Meaningful measures of quality school health education programs must capture information on the strength and fidelity of these programs. Measures such as those developed by Hall and Loucks (1978) and modified for use in a large-scale study of the fidelity of public sector social programs (Blakely et al., 1987) are required. Without such measures to assess the fidelity and extent of modification of the program components, policymakers are likely to be misled by statistics showing increasing numbers of programs.

How can the strength and integrity of school-based prevention programs be improved? Although research on the "technology" of prevention has advanced in the past decade, we know little about the conditions necessary to apply these advances under real-world conditions. The literature on school innovation reviewed earlier hardly provides a theory of implementation, but it at least provides hints about the organizational barriers to strong implementation. We need more precise information about the causal factors that determine level of implementation, and we need to develop a theory to guide attempts to strengthen intervention practices. We need valid assessment instruments to test schools' readiness for change, and differentiated organization development and technical assistance strategies for providing the necessary support for schools at different stages of readiness. Some schools need substantial capacity-building before they can be expected to innovate success-fully. For some schools, it will be necessary to shore up the organiza-tion to support change and establish problem-solving processes before new practices are attempted. This might be accomplished through an organization development process, essential features of which are the identification and monitoring of clear implementa-tion standards and open analysis and resolution of obstacles that prevent the standards from being met. Most important, school staff must learn how to do this on their own, and they must be provided an environment that supports this kind of problem-solving ap-proach. While mere staff training may be translated into beneficial change in some schools, it will be a drop in the bucket, or even a hindrance or perceived as a waste of precious time, in others. This reality must be confronted if we are to achieve change in those places most in need of change.

Note

1. The name of the school has been changed to protect its confidentiality.

References

Berman, P., & McLaughlin, M. W. (1978). *Federal programs supporting educational change: Vol. 8. Implementing and sustaining innovations* (R-1589/8-HEW). Santa Monica, CA: RAND.

Blakely, C. H., Mayer, J. P., Gottschalk, R. G., Schmitt, N., Davidson, W. S., Roitman, D. B., & Emshoff, J. G. (1987). The fidelity-adaptation debate: Implications for the implementation of public sector social programs. *American Journal of Community Psychology, 15,* 253-268.

Botvin, G. J. (1989). *Life skills training teacher's manual.* New York: Smithfield.

Botvin, G. J., Baker, E., Dusenbury, L., Tortu, S., & Botvin, E. M. (1990). Preventing adolescent drug abuse through a multi-modal cognitive-behavioral approach: Results of a 3-year study. *Journal of Consulting and Clinical Psychology, 58,* 437-446.

Botvin, G. J., Batson, H. W., Witts-Vitale, S., Bess, V., Baker, E., & Dusenbury, L. (1989). A psychosocial approach to smoking prevention for urban Black youth. *Public Health Reports, 12,* 279-296.

Botvin, G. J., Dusenbury, L., James-Ortiz, S., & Kerner, J. (1989). A skills training approach to smoking prevention among Hispanic youth. *Journal of Behavioral Medicine, 12,* 279-296.

Botvin, G. J., Renick, N. L., & Baker, E. (1983). The effects of scheduling format and booster sessions on a broad-spectrum psychosocial approach to smoking prevention. *Journal of Behavioral Medicine, 6,* 359-379.

Caplan, M., Weissberg, R. P., Grober, J. H., Sivo, P. J., Grady, K., & Jacoby, C. (1992). Social competence promotion with inner-city and suburban young adolescents: Effects on social adjustment and alcohol use. *Journal of Consulting and Clinical Psychology, 60,* 56-63.

Clark, D. L., Lotto, L. S., & McCarthy, M. M. (1980). Factors associated with success in urban elementary schools. *Phi Delta Kappan, 61,* 467-470.

Coie, J. D., & Krehbiel, G. (1984). Effects of academic tutoring on the social status of low-achieving, socially rejected children. *Child Development, 55,* 1465-1478.

Connell, D. B., Turner, R. R., & Mason, E. F. (1985). Summary of the findings of the school health education evaluation: Health promotion effectiveness, implementation, and costs. *Journal of School Health, 55,* 316-323.

CSR, Inc. (1994). *CSR cross-site evaluation: Multi-model school-centered prevention demonstration* (CSAP Grant No. 2630). Washington, DC: Author.

Derr, C. B. (1976). "OD" won't work in schools. *Educational and Urban Society, 8,* 227-241.

Elias, M. J., Weissberg, R. P., Hawkins, J. D., Perry, C. A., Zins, J. E., Dodge, K. C., Kendall, P. C., Gottfredson, D. C., Rotheram-Borus, M., Jason, L. A., & Wilson-Brewer, R. (1994). The school-based promotion of social competence: Theory, practice, and policy. In R. J. Haggerty, N. Garmezy, M. Rutter, & L. Sherrod (Eds.), *Risk and resilience in children: Developmental approaches* (pp. 268-316). Cambridge: University of Cambridge Press.

Fleming, M. (1996). *Healthy youth 2000: A mid-decade review.* Chicago: American Medical Association, Department of Adolescent Health.

Fullan, M., Miles, M. B., & Taylor, G. (1980). Organization development in schools: The state of the art. *Review of Educational Research, 50,* 121-183.

Fullan, M., & Pomfret, A. (1977). Research on curriculum and instruction implementation. *Review of Educational Research, 47,* 335-397.

Ginsberg, R., Schwartz, H., Olson, G., & Bennett, A. (1987). Working conditions in urban schools. *Urban Review, 19,* 3-23.

Glass, G., & Smith, M. L. (1979). Meta-analysis of research on the relationship of class-size and achievement. *Educational Evaluation and Policy Analysis, 1,* 2-16.

Good, T. L., & Brophy, T. E. (1987). *Looking in classrooms.* New York: Harper & Row.

Gottfredson, D. C., Gottfredson, G. D., & Hybl, L. G. (1993). Managing adolescent behavior: A multi-year, multi-school experiment. *American Educational Research Journal, 30,* 179-216.

Gottfredson, D. C., Gottfredson, G. D., & Skroban, S. (1996). *A school-based social competency promotion demonstration.* Unpublished technical report, University of Maryland, College Park.

Gottfredson, G. D. (1984a). *Effective School Battery: User's manual.* Odessa, FL: Psychological Assessment Resources.

Gottfredson, G. D. (1984b). A theory-ridden approach to program evaluation: A method for stimulating researcher-implementer collaboration. *American Psychologist, 39,* 1101-1112.

Gottfredson, G. D., & Gottfredson, D. C. (1987). *Using organization development to improve school climate* (Report No. 17). Baltimore: Johns Hopkins University, Center for Research on Elementary and Middle Schools.

Gottfredson, G. D., & Gottfredson, D. C. (1989). *School climate, academic performance, attendance, and dropout* (Report No. 43). Baltimore: Johns Hopkins University, Center for Research on Elementary and Middle Schools.

Gottfredson, G. D., & Gottfredson, D. C. (1990). *Achieving school improvement through school district reform* (Report No. 10). Baltimore: Johns Hopkins University, Center for Research on Effective Schooling for Disadvantaged Students.

Gottfredson, G. D., & Hybl, L. G. (1989). *Some biographical correlates of outstanding performance among school principals* (Report No. 35). Baltimore: Johns Hopkins University, Center for Research on Elementary and Middle Schools.

Gottfredson, G. D., Rickert, D. E., Gottfredson, D. C., & Advani, N. (1984). Standards for program development evaluation plans. *Psychological Documents, 14,* 32 (Ms. No. 2668).

Guerra, N. G., & Slaby, R. G. (1990). Cognitive measures of aggression in adolescent offenders: Vol. 2. Intervention. *Developmental Psychology, 26,* 269-277.

Haberman, M., & Rickards, W. H. (1990). Urban teachers who quit: Why they leave and what they do. *Urban Education, 25,* 297-303.

Hall, G. E. (1987, April). *The principal's role in setting school climate (for school improvement).* Paper presented at the meeting of the American Educational Research Association, Washington, DC.

Hall, G. E., Hord, S. M., Huling, L. L., Rutherford, W. L., & Stiegelbauer, S. M. (1983, April). *Leadership variables associated with successful school improvement* (Report No. 3164). Paper presented at the meeting of the American Educational Research Association, Montreal.

Hall, G. E., & Loucks, S. F. (1978, March). *Innovation configurations: Analyzing the adaptation of innovations.* Paper presented at the meeting of the American Educational Research Association, Toronto.

Hall, G. E., Rutherford, W. L., Hord, S. M., & Huling, L. L. (1984). Effects of three principal styles on school improvement. *Educational Leadership, 42,* 22-29.

Holmes, A. B., Gottfredson, G. D., & Miller, J. (1992). Resources and strategies for findings. In J. D. Hawkins & R. F. Catalano (Eds.), *Communities that care* (pp. 191-210). San Francisco: Jossey-Bass.

Huberman, A. M. (1983). School improvement strategies that work: Some scenarios. *Educational Leadership, 41,* 23-27.

Huberman, A. M., & Miles, M. B. (1984). *Innovation up close: How school improvement works.* New York: Plenum.

Jackson, S. E. (1983). Participation in decision-making as a strategy for reducing job-related strains. *Journal of Applied Psychology, 68,* 3-19.

Kennedy, M. M. (1978). Findings from the follow through planned variation study. *Educational Researcher, 7,* 3-11.

Liberman, A., & Miller, L. (1981). Synthesis of research on improving schools. *Educational Leadership, 39,* 583-586.

Liberman, A., & Miller, L. (1984). School improvement: Themes and variations. *Teachers College Record, 86,* 5-18.

Lipsey, M. W. (1992). Juvenile delinquency treatment: A meta-analytic inquiry into the variability of effects. In T. D. Cook, H. Cooper, D. S. Cordray, H. Hartmann, L. V. Hedges, R. V. Light, T. A. Louis, & F. Mosteller (Eds.), *Meta-analysis for explanation.* Newbury Park, CA: Sage.

Loucks, S. F. (1975). Study of the relationship between teacher level of use of the innovation of individualized instruction and student achievement. *Dissertation Abstracts International, 35,* 3537-A.

Loucks, S. F. (1983). At last: Some good news from a study of school improvement. *Educational Leadership, 41,* 34-35.

Louis, K. S. (1986, April). *A survey of effective school programs in urban high schools.* Paper presented at the meeting of the American Educational Research Association, San Francisco.

Louis, K. S., & Miles, M. B. (1990). *Improving the urban high school: What works and why.* New York: Teachers College Press.

LoSciuto, L., Rajala, A. K., Townsend, T. N., & Taylor, A. S. (1996). An outcome evaluation of across ages: An intergenerational mentoring approach to drug prevention. *Journal of Adolescent Research, 11,* 116-129.

Mann, D. (1978). The politics of training teachers in schools. In D. Mann (Ed.), *Making change happen?* (pp. 3-18). New York: Teachers College Press.

Manning, B. H. (1988). Application of cognitive behavior modification: First and third graders' self-management of classroom behaviors. *American Educational Research Journal, 25,* 193-212.

Manning, B. H. (1991). *Cognitive self-instruction for classroom processes.* Albany: State University of New York Press.

McLaughlin, M. W. (1990). The RAND change agent study revisited: Macro perspectives and micro realities. *Educational Researcher, 19,* 11-16.

Miles, M. B. (1986, April). *Improving the urban high school: Some preliminary news from 5 cases.* Paper presented at the meeting of the American Educational Research Association, San Francisco.

National Commission on Excellence in Education. (1983). *A nation at risk.* Washington, DC: U.S. Department of Education.

Purkey, S. C., & Smith, M. S. (1983). Effective schools: A review. *Elementary School Journal, 83,* 427-452.

Rosen, R. (1982). *A short history of Charleston.* San Francisco: Lexikos.

Rossman, G. B., Corbett, H. D., & Firestone, W. A. (1988). *Change and effectiveness in schools: A cultural perspective.* New York: State University of New York Press.

Runkel, P. J., & Bell, W. E. (1976). Some conditions affecting a school's readiness to profit from OD training. *Education and Urban Society, 8,* 127-144.

Sharan, S. (1980). Cooperative learning in small groups: Recent methods and effects on achievement, attitudes, and ethnic relations. *Review of Educational Research, 10,* 241-271.

Slavin, R. E. (1980). Cooperative learning. *Review of Educational Research, 50,* 315-342.

Slavin, R. E. (1983a). *Cooperative learning.* New York: Longman.

Slavin, R. E. (1983b). When does cooperative learning increase student achievement? *Psychological Bulletin, 94,* 429-445.

Social Action Research Center. (1979). *The school team approach, Phase I evaluation* (Grants No. 77-NI-99-0012 and 78-JN-AX-0016). San Rafael, CA: Author.

Stallings, J. (1985). A study of implementation of Madeline Hunter's model and its effects on students. *Journal of Educational Research, 78,* 325-337.

Stoil, M. J., Hill, G. A., & Brounstein, P. J. (1994, November). *The seven core strategies for ATOD prevention: Findings of the National Structure Evaluation on what is working well where.* Paper presented at the 12th annual meeting of the American Public Health Association, Washington, DC.

Tobler, N. S. (1986). Meta-analysis of 143 adolescent drug prevention programs: Quantitative outcome results of program participants compared to a control or comparison group. *Journal of Drug Issues, 16,* 537-567.

U.S. Department of Health and Human Services, Public Health Service. (1991). *Healthy people 2000: National health promotion and disease prevention objectives* (DHHS Publication No. PHS 91-50212). Washington, DC: U.S. Government Printing Office.

U.S. Department of Health and Human Services, Public Health Service. (1995). *Healthy people 2000: Midcourse review and 1995 revisions.* Washington, DC: U.S. Government Printing Office.

Vroom, V. H., & Yetton, P. W. (1975). *Leadership and decision-making*. Pittsburgh, PA: University of Pittsburgh Press.

Weiner, L. (1990). Preparing the brightest for urban schools. *Urban Education, 25,* 258-273.

Weissberg, R. P., & Caplan, M. (1994). *Promoting social competence and preventing antisocial behavior in young urban adolescents*. Unpublished manuscript. (Available from Roger P. Weissberg, Department of Psychology, University of Illinois at Chicago, 1007 West Harrison St., Chicago, IL 60607-7137)

Weissberg, R. P., Caplan, M., Bennetto, L., & Jackson, A. S. (1990). *The New Haven Social Development Program: Sixth-grade social problem-solving model*. Chicago: University of Illinois at Chicago.

Weissberg, R. P., Jackson, A. S., & Shriver, T. P. (1993). Promoting positive social development and health practices in young urban adolescents. In M. J. Elias (Ed.), *Social decision making and life skills development: Guidelines for middle school educators*. Gaithersburg, MD: Aspen.

Wright, W. E., & Dixon, M. C. (1977). Community prevention and treatment of juvenile delinquency: A review of evaluation studies. *Journal of Research in Crime and Delinquency, 14,* 35-67.

Wyant, S. H. (1974). Effects of organization development training on intra-staff communication in elementary schools. *Dissertation Abstracts International, 34,* 3537-A.

Reinterpreting Dissemination of Prevention Programs as Widespread Implementation With Effectiveness and Fidelity

MAURICE J. ELIAS

The Emperor is not wearing any clothing. The hoopla surrounding large, well-funded prevention demonstration projects and school-based reform efforts must be contrasted with data from the mid-decade review of progress toward achieving national health objectives for youth by the year 2000 (Fleming, 1996) and from *Kids Count* (1995), which monitors indexes of well-being among youth in each of the 50 states as well as within a number of states. These data show clearly that little progress has been made across key areas such as alcohol, tobacco, and other drug use; mental health and mental disorders; violent and abusive behavior; sexually transmitted diseases; and child protective and clinical preventive services. There is a trend toward more youth being caught in the grips of poverty and dangerous environments in their schools and communities. Leaders in the field continue to recognize that the impact of preventive mental health services on public policy and public health has not been substantial, yet must become so if the field is to be viable in the future (Lorion, 1993).

To be most accurate, we might wish to say that the Emperor is wearing one or two socks, perhaps an ascot, even a belt on occasion. There are some areas of progress, and there are some communities that have witnessed profound change in the health of their youth.

But overall—and most certainly for urban youth and those who are minorities—it is best to see the glass as 90% empty rather than 10% full.

Among many reasons for this are shortcomings in the area of dissemination of prevention programs. This can be seen clearly in the structure of perhaps the most critical public document in the health promotion area, *Healthy People 2000* (U.S. Department of Health and Human Services, Public Health Service, 1991). Specifically, there are numerous objectives in the categories of health status, risk reduction, and services. Monitoring the accomplishment of these objectives is addressed in the section on surveillance and data systems. But there is little, if anything, said about the specifics of how these objectives are to be met, or about the dissemination of different programs to reach the services objectives. The absence of such discussions makes it unclear as to how the entire nation's health will be affected in a positive way. Even in a companion document, *Healthy Schools: A Directory of Federal Programs and Activities Related to Health Promotion Through the Schools* (Federal Interagency Ad Hoc Committee on Health Promotion Through the Schools, 1992), there is an extensive listing of programs with virtually no discussion of the conditions of implementation in which those programs had proven themselves effective, nor is there a discussion of parameters of implementation that prospective program adopters might need to consider.

It is becoming clear that those interested in programmatic or systemic efforts to prevent problem behaviors and promote social-emotional competence and good health among our nation's youth must challenge conventional wisdom with regard to dissemination. A realignment toward the concept of implementation and away from the concept of dissemination is needed. In fact, the use of the term *dissemination* both reflects and drives the disappointing rate at which prevention programs spread from their development sites to other sites and retain or exceed their original effectiveness.

Implications of the Language of "Dissemination of Interventions"

It may be surprising how the failure of interventions and programs to disseminate has much to do with the language and conceptual structure that surrounds these very terms. As noted earlier, it serves key public health goals to see that successful preventive *interventions* are effectively *disseminated* or *diffused*. Consider, however, the meanings of these terms. Intervention is from the Latin *intervenire*, meaning "to come between"; *Webster's New World Dictionary* uses the words *interposition* and *interference* in defining intervention. Innovation comes from the Latin *innovare*, "to renew." Improvement is derived from the Latin *probare*, meaning "to approve." *Webster's* defines improvement as making something better, to advance in good qualities. During the 1960s and early 1970s, interventionist language perhaps conveyed the true intention of many professionals who were early adherents to a prevention approach: a disruption from the existing order, an end to social evils, a qualitative change. But social ecology theory (Kelly, 1990) suggests that organizations can support improvement or innovation in the absence of clear crisis more easily than they can support intervention. Indeed, to the extent to which preventive efforts are perceived to be interventions, it is likely that they will be resisted and, on withdrawal of external supports, discontinued (Berman & McLaughlin, 1980; Blumberg, 1980; Commins & Elias, 1991). Entrenched bureaucratic organizations have enormous capacities to assimilate (i.e., to make incoming stimuli conform to already existing structures) and to resist accommodation (i.e., changing structures to allow incorporation and use of valued information contained in incoming stimuli). Interventions, particularly to the extent to which they fail to respect adequately the culture, history, symbols, and rituals of the host setting, are clear candidates for assimilation—if the external boundaries are even allowed to be permeated (Elias & Clabby, 1992; House, 1974; Sarason, 1983).

Dissemination derives from the Latin *disseminatus* or *disseminare*, meaning "to scatter seed," "to spread abroad." Diffusion is a similar word, based on the Latin *diffusus*, "to pour in different directions." In the educational literature, prominent terms include *institutionalization*. The derivation is the Latin *institutum* or *institutus*, meaning "arrangement, plan, intention"; "to set up, erect, construct." *Webster's* defines the word as meaning an established principle of law, custom, or usage. Routinization derives from the French *route*, "the customary way." Dissemination reflects what Stolz (1984) has referred to as a "publish and hope" approach, relying on written communication or one-shot presentations to serve as an adequate medium for generating the organizational change that prevention requires. This is to be contrasted with terms that reflect a process, laborious but planful, of creating a new structure or procedure, a new accepted, "customary way." House (1974), Baldridge (1975), and Berman and McLaughlin (1980) have studied implementation and institutionalization of innovation in literally thousands of schools. They never use the term *prevention,* but their work is certainly preventive. An alternative formulation to typical approaches to dissemination is to work with existing socialization settings to help them become more innovative, dedicated to the continuous improvement of their impact on health and social behavior and the broad fulfillment of their socialization roles. It has been argued that creating such organizational cultures, particularly in the schools, is among the most powerful ways to build and maintain competence in children and adolescents and serve the goal of prevention (Elias & Clabby, 1992; Kelly, 1984).

To accomplish this requires a reexamination of the concept of dissemination. While the broad themes in this chapter may—indeed, should—seem familiar, I will highlight subtle factors that I believe serve as sustaining conditions for the present approach to dissemination of prevention programs. These include the nature of preventive intervention and parameters of effective community-based prevention praxis, aspects of the infrastructure needed for widespread implementation of an innovation, and developmental factors among program developers and implementers. The necessity of carrying out action research in a spirit of continuous improvement and of elaborating on what most models refer to as the dissemination or diffusion stage will be emphasized. Guidelines will be provided for maximizing the likelihood that prevention efforts initiated outside one's setting will be implemented with long-term goal attainment. The Social Decision Making and Problem Solving Project (Elias, 1994; Elias & Clabby, 1992), a school-based prevention initiative closing in on its second decade of operation, will be used as a source of case examples.

Merits of an Action-Research Approach
to Developing Preventive Efforts

There is much consensus that the guiding approach for the operation of social competence promotion and problem behavior prevention programs in school and community settings should be

Lewin's (1951) concept of *action research*. At its essence, action research involves the idea of testing theories and methods by putting them into practice, evaluating their impact, and using the results to refine future theory, method, and practice. Action research is seen as involving ongoing cycles of problem analysis, innovation (intervention) design, field trials, and innovation diffusion (dissemination), leading to ever more precise variations and targeting of programs to recipient populations and settings (Price & Smith, 1985). The entire model is cyclic because ongoing monitoring of problem areas will yield information as to whether the program is having a significant impact, with which populations, and in which settings. Such information then leads to the development of refined or new problem statements, which in turn inspire further cycles of prevention research, development, and evaluation directed toward further problem reduction and health and competence promotion (Mrazek & Haggerty, 1994).

Rossi (1978) added some important elaboration of the idea of evolution or transfer of the control of the program technology—including implementation, evaluation, modification, and extension—to agents other than the developers. He defines three levels through which programs must pass before they can hope to have a policy-level impact.

1. Experimental: A program must demonstrate its effectiveness under small-scale, optimal conditions, compared to a no-treatment or alternative comparison control.
2. Technological: A program must demonstrate that it can be effective under real-world conditions, but still under the guidance of its developers.
3. Diffusional: A program must demonstrate that it can be effective under real-world conditions and when it is not, under the direct scrutiny and guidance of its developers.

When a program successfully passes through Rossi's diffusional stage, it is not automatically diffused; rather, it is capable of widespread use. Implicit at the diffusional or dissemination level is that a program demonstrate experimental and technological effectiveness and that a program undergo a phased generational transfer from the developers to a new cadre of implementers who will take ownership and become agents of effective diffusion and further development, as needed. However, in neither Price and Smith's (1985) nor Rossi's (1978) models is there explication of how broad dissemination of programs—of the kind that would affect statistics for *Healthy Youth 2000* or *Kids Count*—is to take place.

The challenge of dissemination can be concretized by examining cases of a relatively well-publicized and well-supported area that also is related to prevention: school reform. F. James Rutherford, Director of Project 2061 at the American Association for the Advancement of Science, has noted that he gets calls, requests, letters, and the like from all over the country from people who are excited about the work of his project and want his help to implement. He tells them he can't. Why? Because "there are more of you than there are of us" (Rutherford in Olson, 1994, p. 43).

Indeed, those who have created successful demonstration models of school reform, such as Ted Sizer (Coalition of Essential Schools), Robert Slavin (Success for All), Gay Sue Pinnell (Reading Recovery), Henry Levin (Accelerated Schools Project), Joy Dryfoos (Full Service Schools), and James Comer (School Development Program), are among the innovators who have been able to achieve some measure of consensual success in a limited number of settings but have not solved the problem of how to disseminate their work more broadly. Similar tales of woe have been told by those working in the mental health field (Schorr, 1988). This process of "scaling up" goes beyond the diffusional stage described by Rossi and invokes an additional stage, which I refer to as that of "widespread implementation with fidelity and effectiveness."

In a similar way, there is evidence that school-based prevention programs can provide children with skills, supportive environments, and positive life opportunities needed to allow them to cope better with pressure from peers and others to use or abuse drugs and alcohol, engage in delinquent acts, neglect school work, become involved in premature sexual activity, or attempt health-compromising activities (Elias, Gager, & Leon, in press). But these programs are not immune from concerns about scaling up. They have touched far fewer students than those who would appear able to benefit from them. The School Intervention Implementation Study (SIIS) emerged from the realization that there has been little examination of the nature and impact of the dissemination of these programs. In the drive to procure and fund "new programs," the SIIS was an effort to learn about what happens when programs developed and studied under ideal or at least controlled conditions are placed into the schools, typically without systematic evaluation and with the assumption that these programs are going to have a genuine impact on the problem areas that they were designed to affect.

Surveys were sent to the approximately 550 operating school districts in New Jersey, a state that can provide an indication of trends in other parts of the country (Elias, Gager, & Hancock, 1993). New Jersey has metropolitan areas, various types of suburbs, significant rural areas, and shoreline districts. Furthermore, few states in the United States have as many or more school districts than are located in New Jersey; there is a variety of district organizational arrangements and styles that covers the range of what can be found nationally. Finally, New Jersey is a national leader in mandated prevention programs, particularly around substance abuse prevention and AIDS prevention. Thus, the findings from the SIIS were likely to portray the state of the art as contained in the more progressive states, and provide valuable lessons for states that are following down the path of increasing mandated preventive and competence promotion programs. The overall response rate was 65%, highly satisfactory for a study of this kind and scope.

Findings. While the SIIS survey revealed many programs in operation across New Jersey, there was little consistency in their implementation. The vast majority of districts are doing "something" related to the prevention of substance abuse and the promotion of social competence. However, what is taking place is not systematic. In spite of mandates and encouragement for K to 12 programming, only 10% of the districts have a program running throughout the elementary years, 6% have a program throughout middle school, and 12% throughout high school. One third of the districts had at least four grade levels that received no prevention programming. Children receive little continuity in prevention programming within or across communities, and there appears to be an inexplicable neglect of programs for children classified as needing special education services. Furthermore, the programs that are used are not necessarily those supported by a "track record" of empirical evidence for success, or even a documented history of effective use and positive impact in districts similar to those in which they are being carried out locally. But equally distressing is that in districts implementing well-supported programs, instances of implementation success were matched by failure. Thus, even the most promising programs showed an uneven record of dissemination.

Challenges in the Widespread Implementation of Durable Preventive Efforts With Fidelity and Effectiveness

There seems to be a growing recognition that the content of preventive programs and even their passing through Rossi's technological stage is at best a necessary but certainly not sufficient condition for successful replication; what is most important is the nature of the implementation process (Kelly, 1979) and the way it takes place in a variety of implementation contexts.

There are numerous considerations that influence the fate of a prevention program and help explain why Kelly's observation is so astute. The sheer number of factors involved in understanding a phenomenon that one wishes to prevent, or a competency or positive condition one wishes to promote, can seem daunting. As a program or other change effort is contemplated, it becomes necessary to document carefully what is happening in the system so that change pathways can be illuminated and both intended and unintended effects—of both positive and negative types—can be monitored and changes made as needed.

Parameters to consider when one is interested in bringing into a system any innovation in prevention and health promotion can be derived from many sources, especially the orientation of the field toward an ecological approach to research (Vincent & Trickett, 1983) and examinations of community psychology practice by some of its foremost proponents (e.g., Chavis, 1993; Price, Cowen, Lorion, & Ramos-McKay, 1988; Wolff, 1987, 1994). Borrowing from the tradition of Lewin (1951), Rotter (1954), Albee (1982), and Elias (1987), these parameters have been cast in the form of an equation (Elias, 1994). The equation attempts to capture the notion that the greater the value of the terms on the right side, relative to what might be optimal or possible in a setting, the more effective one will be at implementing a preventive innovation, denoted by the term *praxis,* which refers to reflective, action research-oriented prevention practice:

$$Praxis_{D,H,S} = \frac{GITPL + CATP + PEL + ATIS + RAT + AUFM + HOC}{C/R}$$

where
GITPL   =   *grounding in the problem and the literature*
CATP   =   *clarity about theoretical perspectives*
PEL   =   *principles of effective learning*
ATIS   =   *appropriate tailored instructional strategies*
RAT   =   *relevant applicable tactics*
AUFM   =   *available user-friendly materials*
HOC   =   *hospitable organizational contexts*
C   =   *constraints*
R   =   *resources*
D, H, and S refer to the specific *developmental, historical,*
            and *situational* context of the prevention or
            health/competence promotion activity

Change agents interested in prevention must be prepared to immerse themselves into local settings and contexts, to be patient, to build and extend their ranks through participation, collaboration, and explication (O'Donnell, Tharp, & Wilson, 1993). It is a tenet of the field that the energy and direction for solutions for social problems come from the local level (Cowen, 1977; Price & Cherniss, 1977; Tolan, Keys, Chertok, & Jason, 1990). Implicit is that ongoing critical self-awareness is a necessary precursor to lasting change; it also appears to be necessary for effective, enduring collaboration (Elias, 1994). The "praxis equation" outlines the tasks necessary for implementation, based on our current knowledge.

The first two terms reflect the need to be grounded not only in past work but also in the conceptual underpinnings of what one is attempting. The next four terms relate to the mechanics of creating change. Change involves some kind of education, or reeducation, and some corresponding actions. Much has been learned about techniques for accomplishing this kind of education, although remarkably little of it finds its way into the interventions in the literature, in part because of traditional research design and publication-related constraints. To the extent to which effective learning principles, engaging strategies, consonant behavioral tactics, and adequate supportive materials are not available and used, even the most sound intervention or "practice" ideas have only a small chance of coming to fruition as intended.

The seventh term, *HOC,* indicates that consideration must be given to the organization context of the work, and the balance of available resources and constraints in the intervention context. Price and Lorion (1989) and Van de Ven (1986) suggest that members of an organization must be "ready" to accept an innovation, preventive or otherwise. There must be a perception that there is environmental press, or at least support, for the innovation, an awareness and acceptance of a problem by the host organization, and a set of attitudes, beliefs, and practices on the part of staff that is compatible with the preventive effort being proposed. Within the organization, there must be structures and services already in place that will facilitate the preventive approach being planned. Certain types of resources—funds, facilities, and expertise—also must be accessible, and potential implementers will require reassurance that all these supports are in place. These are elements that can be seen as related to the likelihood of success with a preventive innovation. If these are not in place, Price and Lorion would advocate for capacity building before beginning, or continuing to look for the most hospitable site possible. Even a cursory look at the equation makes clear the challenge of intervention in contexts of poverty, violence, distrust, and apathy, and the need for much "groundwork" to be done before embarking on interventions with a hope of lasting success.

Added Challenges of Dissemination

Dissemination of interventions is no less complex. In fact, there often are added challenges. As noted earlier, it is typically the case that innovations are established under demonstration project conditions. This implies that there are special funds, readily available materials, careful training and follow-up consultation, and the presence of evaluators on the scene to observe the work, take measures and give feedback, and involve the host site in modifying the intervention in light of the data. These special conditions create an implementation context that subsequent sites often are hard-pressed to match. The literature is replete with examples of how changes in programs during the dissemination stage led to their demise or to disappointing effectiveness (the way in which the Perry

Preschool Project served as the impetus for a national Head Start program is among the most potent situations in which dissemination took place under conditions highly variant from the original; see Schorr, 1988, for a full discussion of this and other examples).

The developmental aspect of innovations for prevention is fascinating at multiple levels and, though rarely discussed, quite a formidable issue. RMC Research Corporation (1995), which has spent years studying the spread of exemplary education programs through the U.S. Department of Education's National Diffusion Network, reports the following progression since the National Diffusion Network began in the 1970s:

1. Cookbook: Programs had to be thoroughly documented, ideally in "kits" that could be followed precisely.

2. Replication: Model programs were replicated by having staff trained in the methods used by program developers and then bringing these methods back to one's own settings to be carried out as similarly as possible.

3. Adaptation: Models are understood to require adaptation to the unique context of the host site, ideally by having the developer serve as a consultant in making the necessary changes.

4. Invention/innovation: Now models are being seen as sources of ideas and inspiration rather than procedures to replicate or adapt. There is emphasis on creating one's own program, tailored to the unique circumstances at a given time.

Note that these broad trends, played out over three decades, parallel interesting issues in individual development illuminated by Piaget and Erik Erikson. The four approaches above certainly have their parallel in Piaget's stages—sensorimotor, preoperational, and concrete and formal operations. Note, though, that Piaget's theory is an epigenetic theory, a theory about how knowledge develops. The idea of dissemination is based on a model that is at best preoperational, because it is based largely on information distribution, as typically practiced. People obtain materials about a program, perhaps see a brief demonstration or attend a single training session, and then are expected to implement in their home settings.

Erikson (1982) pointed out that the majority of adult learners who will be the targets of dissemination efforts will be in the stage of generativity. Broadly speaking, this stage is one in which development and ownership are key elements. There is a special sense of fulfillment in being generative, as opposed to exact replication of that which others generated. This directly supports RMC's findings, as well as those of the SIIS, and helps explain why so many schools create their own programs out of existing ones rather than adopt or adapt programs developed by others. SIIS and other data indicate that the tendency to invent is greater than the tendency to adapt or adopt.

Thus, successful dissemination really is implementation and institutionalization in a new site that captures the excellence of practice by linking practice to theory. What is "transferred" to others includes not only procedures but an understanding of the principles that undergird and comprise that specific example of practice. From this perspective, it is not only necessary to "talk the talk and walk the walk"; it is necessary to "talk the walk," to explicate practice activities in an articulate and heuristic, generative, instructive, and inspiring manner (Elias, 1994; Fullan, 1994), as the praxis equation attempts to delineate. So doing provides maps of patterns of change, markers for shifts in the terrain, realistic guideposts, and other forms of anticipatory and reactive guidance for work in particular developmental, historical, and situational contexts—the D, H, S in the praxis equation.

Prevention Occurs in Operator-Dependent and Complex Sociotechnical Systems: Limitations and Solutions

Two interrelated factors serve as limiting conditions on the spread of preventive efforts: Prevention and competence promotion involve operator-dependent sociotechnical systems that tend to be characterized by high complexity of their core elements, particularly those that are comprehensive and occur over multiple years and settings. Each of these concepts requires some elaboration.

Operator-Dependent Sociotechnical Systems

Rossi (1978) was able to explain the difficulties in programs reaching the diffusional stage by noting that preventive efforts rely on human beings to carry them out, and typically to exercise many judgments while so doing. Certainly, this is true in any classroom-based prevention program. The teacher or group leader has relatively few guidelines for carrying out the necessary activities in the particular context he or she is facing. From one grade level to the next, sources of implementer-based (operator-dependent) variability abound, a facet of general education that is equally true and underappreciated.

The operator-dependent label, while coined by Rossi, is reflected in the writings of other experts on the spread of innovation. Yin (1979) emphasized the importance of local ownership, early practitioner involvement, and comfort and skill with the innovative technologies. Stolz (1984) indicated that the single largest influence on results seems to be personal interactions between the innovator and key decision makers in the host organization. Rothman, Erlich, and Teresa (1976) elaborated this idea and suggest that what must emerge from these interactions is a combination of leadership, interest, enthusiasm, determination, commitment, aggressiveness, and caring. Without these features—whether they come from a single place, dyadic relationship, or committee—incoming innovations are unlikely to take root.

Tornatzky and Fleischer (1986) suggested that it is important to label preventive innovations, even those that appear to be delimited programs or interventions, as sociotechnical systems. Such systems have several features. First, they are organizationally unbounded, in that they reach into all facets of how an organization operates and require at least some degree of change. This is consistent with Kelly's (1990) ecological concept of interdependence. Second, they are fragile and difficult to specify in detail. Their critical elements are not clearly identifiable, because they cannot be seen easily in independent operation of the kind implied by most experimental or intervention components research designs. Once begun, they take on a unique configuration matched with the host environment. However, there are threads of connectedness, and once aspects of such programs are damaged, diluted, weakened, omitted, or in other ways compromised, the desired results are less likely to be obtained. Hence, sociotechnical systems, by virtue of their complex embeddedness in their host environments, appear fragile.

Third, the operation of sociotechnical systems is longitudinal and developmental. Not only are they intended to last a long time, but they are likely to be operated by a succession of individuals, each of whom enters the system with a different relationship to the history and context. The dissemination of information about a new program or innovation is just the beginning of a process that, to be successful, must permeate the institutional culture.

Price and Lorion (1989) highlighted some additional organizational features of organization life that extend the ideas of Tornatzky and Fleischer (1986), elaborated aspects of the praxis equation, and integrated them with Rossi's caveats about the nature of operator-dependent innovations. They maintained that implementing a model prevention program in a new site is organizational reinvention in several ways. First, bringing in a program is an organizational-level event. Second, a model program can be defined as having core and adaptive features. The former must be replicated as faithfully as possible; the latter must be adjusted to local needs of the setting while still maintaining the overall fidelity of the newly implemented program to the model. The complexities of this process can be at least as daunting as developing a program, a fact that Price and Lorion (1989) indicated is too often lost on prospective implementers.

There are two necessary but not sufficient conditions for such organizational reinvention, conditions that quite clearly reflect the importance of the "human element" in the successful spread of preventive efforts: There must be a focal prevention innovator who possesses key skills, and there must be organizational readiness in the host environment. Among the skills needed by innovation implementation leaders are a strong goal orientation, an orientation toward external networking, the ability to locate and mobilize resources, a collaborative/participatory orientation, negotiation and coalition building, cultural sensitivity, and mastery of elements of the praxis equation.

Ongoing steps also have an impact on potential success. These steps include ongoing environmental scanning, information gathering, team building, and joint planning. The latter function is given particular emphasis, to make sure that stakeholder participation and input are maximized and to foster a greater sense of openness, which in turn should maximize mobilization of available resources. Also at this time, setting benefits—including implementer benefits—should be articulated so that appropriate baseline data and other indicators can be set up and collected as early as possible.

Taken together with the earlier considerations about operator dependence and sociotechnical systems, this explains why school personnel are as likely to modify existing valid programs out of the range of integrity as to modify initially poor programs in ways that might lead them to be successful. It also shows how haphazard the results of such initiatives can be unless managed with exceptional skill, wisdom, and what seems to be an ongoing stream of information that Elias and Clabby (1992) refer to as MEF/MOD—ongoing cycles of monitoring, evaluation, feedback, and program modification. This requires a considerable degree of organizational communication, coordination, and collaboration in an educational or other host setting. It is also worth noting briefly that children who are the recipients of prevention programs—especially over multiple years—also benefit from taking initiative and displaying industry over the course of the programs, rather than being given—disseminated—information from instructors. Adolescents—looking to forge their identity—also are unlikely to simply accept the dictates of a life skills program. Successful implementers report the necessity, for genuine skill acquisition, of some kind of active, creative, discovery, and personal construction of aspects of what a program has to offer, which seem to be fostered by experiential methods.

Complexity

London and MacDuffie (1985) provided a valuable operationalization of the variable of complexity of an innovation. Complexity relates to the scope of change required to carry out an innovation as a sociotechnical system. They identified number and distinctness of goals, perceived benefits and risks to those affected, speed with which change is agreed to and implemented (urgency and suddenness), how well the program and implementation process are grasped by those involved, extent to which the changes can and are implemented the same way in different locations within the setting, costs, impact on job/role performance, and interrelatedness of the changes to various organizational elements and priorities. If a new structure is implemented too rapidly or not communicated clearly, tasks are likely to be ambiguous; this leads people to not be sure of what they are supposed to do, which in turn affects how they behave on their jobs (and there are person, group, and organizational factors that will determine reactions to this ambiguity).

The recipe for ease of implementation is low-complexity innovations that are less time-consuming, slow in occurring, take place in isolated functions, and can be communicated clearly—people understand the purpose, the implementation process, and their role in it. Thus, it is not surprising to find that an intervention program run by outsiders for a delimited period of time that purports to prevent problem behaviors with a minimal role for the teacher will seem quite appealing and is capable of being implemented in many settings. A widespread program of relatively low complexity is the Primary Mental Health Project. However, the broad impact of such approaches—especially in the absence of contiguous, longitudinal, coordinated programming—is quite difficult to establish (Commins & Elias, 1991).

Complexity provides another opportunity to revisit the classic "fidelity versus adaptation" distinction. In complex innovations, it is especially difficult to identify the core elements that are essential to a program's success, particularly through empirical validation. Nevertheless, it is important for innovation developers and those who attempt to bring innovations to new settings to delineate their beliefs about core elements and adaptive characteristics—those features that can be modified with relatively little negative impact. Clearly, bringing a complex innovation to a new setting raises problems related to uncertainty about the former and the latter. Innovation developers such as Slavin who have points on which they will not compromise are implicitly identifying core elements (Olson, 1994). But many of these can be subtle, and it should be assumed that such elements exist for many facets of complex innovations.

In fact, London and MacDuffie (1985) maintained that sociotechnical innovations—and certainly preventive interventions, particularly to the extent to which they are operator dependent—*cannot* be replicated. Users will make changes, whether sanctioned or not, so it makes the most sense to structure that input into the process of innovation diffusion. This raises the following problems: This will prolong the implementation time line; if not managed well, it may dilute the effectiveness of the innovation; and the systemic pace of change is slowed down because there may be a limit to the number of supported change processes that can be undertaken.

Some Solutions to Challenges
in Spreading Innovations

Solutions corresponding to problems related to operator dependence and complexity, although far from simple to carry out, follow from considerations mentioned to this point. First, do not deliver a totally "finished" product; rather, set up an expectation and a process for MEF/MOD. From the beginning, plan ongoing action research based on the principle of starting a "pilot" using the most basic model that has been used in a setting closest to one's own; subsequent modifying through MEF/MOD seems to balance pragmatic, theoretical, and empirical concerns in a systematic manner (Elias & Clabby, 1992). Much can be learned by studying what appears to be "necessary" across diverse sites, what can be modified, what cannot, and so on. It can be expected that after the pilot, the innovation will be reimplemented in modified form. Technical assistance and capacity building are a top priority, along with clear, regular, accessible communication channels among those affected by the innovation.

Agreement on goals must be strong, because these will sustain inevitable ambiguities and obstacles in the process. Strong, clear leadership is essential because hard choices will have to be made and midcourse corrections will be frequent; if an innovation is to spread with adequate support, resources may have to be pooled, concentrated, or channeled in areas or among groups where multiple competing but basically similar innovations are involved. The latter point has special salience in the prevention field, where the tendency is for individual developers to create their own unique and isolated operating systems. This is promulgated by grant mechanisms, pathways for academic advancement, and individual capitalism. There are, of course, exceptions, where investigators have come together to form consortia, work groups, networks, study groups, multisite collaborative projects, and the like (Elias et al., 1996), but these are all too rare, especially given the substantial benefits and impacts that such efforts seem to yield.

Price and Lorion (1989), who are more sanguine about the possibility of specifying the workings and impact of separate components of prevention efforts, urged that regardless of the difficulties of so doing, the spread of innovations benefits from organizational focusing. Even if an intervention has many components and is "complex," it is valuable for it to have a simple profile so that it can be easily recognized. This is also related to the idea of starting in a contained way, with a pilot program. There should be a sense of "We are here to . . . " and "The way we do this is through 1 . . . 2 . . . 3 . . . "—this allows for mobilization of internal resources and overall improved project management. While the reality is more complex, focusing allows communication and key elements to be prioritized planfully (Van de Ven, 1986).

Summary

Dissemination is best conceptualized as a continuous process of implementation and adaptation. To the extent to which an innovation is operator dependent and has fewer technical features, guidelines for making the proper adaptations without rendering key elements of a program ineffective are quite scarce. This validates, among other things, the benefits that derive from having on-site consultants experienced with implementing one's innovation in related settings available to assist with the kinds of configural decision making and anticipations that will be necessary if the effort is to proceed. And it explains why researchers and program developers are loathe to abandon the idea of magic bullet, time-limited, inoculationist, or technology-driven innovations that can be disseminated "informationally," thus minimizing the challenges associated with operator-dependent, sociotechnical systems.

The common denominator appears to be, for operator-dependent or complex sociotechnical programs, limitations in the effectiveness of information-based dissemination as a strategy for training program implementers or for those actually receiving the programs. When dissemination occurs after limited initial trials—even in the context of a single 5-year demonstration project—one often does not have time to delineate the key enduring principles of an intervention in a way that gives less weight to local or idiosyncratic factors. This results in dissemination sites often having to do the equivalent of flying blind in a fog, or trying to play a musical composition while missing some bars or even pages, or else notation about phrasing, tempo, and dynamics of sound. These contexts do not confer automatic failure; indeed, they can produce more limited success, the expected result, or even greater than anticipated success. However, the likelihood of the latter two is not high, and it is greatly dependent on the skills of implementers in the new setting and fortuitous factors, such as obtaining extra resources. Successful dissemination—which implicitly involves some degree of genuine systemic change—represents a collaborative process (Stokols, 1986).

Spreading the Social Decision Making and Problem Solving Project to Many Settings: An Example Still in Progress

The Social Decision Making and Problem Solving Project has been guided by many of the above points as, over a period of 17 years as of this writing, it has spread from a demonstration project in two experimental and three control classrooms to hundreds of classrooms in schools in two dozen states and several countries, as well as nearly 30 school districts in New Jersey. The core of the project involves building the social and emotional skills of students, with a focus on self-control, group participation and social awareness, and a decision-making strategy to use when faced with difficult choices under stress or when planning, toward the goal of promoting successful social and academic performance and preventing problem behaviors (Elias & Clabby, 1992; Elias & Tobias, 1996).

Issues in dissemination that occupied our attention can be gleaned most directly from the praxis equation presented earlier. It is important to note that from the inception of the project, care was taken to make the initial implementation conditions match those likely in the implementation environment. Thus, while there was funding for action research, little of this went into creating ideal training conditions, providing resources and materials to implementing teachers, paying for any training or implementation work, having experts work directly in classrooms, or finding locations with strong receptivity to prior innovations. Furthermore, we were acutely aware of developmental factors and of the need to modify what we were doing for diverse populations, particularly children with special education classifications.

Evolution of the Elementary School-Level Program

The history of much of this effort, as well as the way in which planned and unplanned variations in conditions were addressed, is detailed in Elias and Clabby (1992). Key points, however, can be described here. At the elementary school level, we created a scripted curriculum with extensive accompanying materials, all developed through 9 years of iterations in an action research cycle. Other action research cycles were created to support modifications of the approach for special education and middle and high school populations. In particular, the creation of an acronym for the eight steps of social decision making—"FIG TESPN"—led to dramatic differences in delivering the program to special education students (Elias & Tobias, 1996). Another important finding was the need to take what was originally our third phase of implementation—the application phase, where the skills of the program were systematically applied to academic and social/interpersonal and personal contexts—and begin it much sooner, while the basic social and emotional skills were being learned.

There was also a need to share learnings across implementation sites, and to do so in a systematic way. We created the *Problem Solving Connection Newsletter,* a Resource Exchange Network for those using social problem solving or related interventions; it became a place to ask questions and to share innovations, to incorporate diversity and change into the implementation context. It is where the "Keep Calm Rap" was developed and redeveloped, as well as "Be Your Best," which one class began to sing to the tune of Disney's "Be Our Guest," from *Beauty and the Beast.*

Adaptation to the Middle School

While there is far less uniformity among elementary schools than unsuspecting outsiders might think, there is even greater diversity among middle schools. This means that intervention technologies are not easily transferred from elementary to middle school. But it also means that successful interventions in one middle school context must be transferred to others with much care. In our work attempting to provide follow-up for the elementary school-level Social Decision Making and Problem Solving program into middle school, we found that numerous adaptations had to be made. We found this out by applying the principles of action research, but also by being clear about the essence and intention of the program. Even after creating successful demonstration projects, however, we did not feel as if the work was completed. We needed to provide a well-annotated musical score for others to use. This gave rise to the book *Social Decision Making and Life Skills Development* (Elias, 1993).

The essence of the approach was to provide key principles and specific examples as inspiration, rather than fully scripted materials. Those who made local implementations of social problem solving—local conductors, the first players of different orchestral sections, and some individual musicians—were helped to explicate its phrases and provide others with samples that they can use. Throughout, it was clear that to be successful, we would have to mesh with others' perspectives so that readers could see themselves using the materials, at first, similarly to the examples provided, but soon thereafter, integrated into their own skills and context.

The first part of each innovation presented was a sales pitch—to make the program sound attractive and viable to people working with the kinds of problems the authors were dealing with, but who are less interested and motivated than are the authors. Then came a discussion of the materials—what it is and how to use it—and next was evidence of its effectiveness, accompanied by listings of follow-up and support resources. Finally, there were sample activities, to allow readers to try out specific units, modules, and so on and get a feel not only for the particular details but also get a sense of the flow of the activities with the individuals and groups involved (Elias, 1993). Some examples of modules are the following:

1. A video program that shows children how to watch television and then take it apart, to see people create media programs and then to use social decision making and problem solving to create their own programs, series, documentaries, and public service advertisements.

2. A program to allow students to create school and community service projects.

3. A procedure for creating parent newsletters and other school-home communications; the detail includes such things as what to tell the printer when it comes to reproducing photographs.

4. FIG TESPN, an approach to social decision making and problem solving that takes into account the special learning needs of many children with learning handicaps.

5. Troubleshooting sections, where the practitioners in the field talk about the tough issues and how they have dealt with them, such as getting started, not having enough time, and working with children who seem to place a positive value on aggressive behavior; this moves the state of practice from the basic issues to a more advanced set of concerns.

To support the process of widespread implementation with fidelity and effectiveness in diverse contexts, it was necessary to pay great attention to implementation infrastructure. Using the analogy of music, one can imagine the difficulty in playing a piece of orchestral music one has not heard in its entirety. For this to happen, it is helpful to have ongoing concerts that others can attend, to be able to train master conductors and musicians who will have had experience with the musical work and then can go back and teach it to others, and to have the capacity to send out conductors and musicians to local settings to assist them in learning to play, as well as to help them make modifications in light of their own orchestral strengths and weaknesses and to avoid making modifications that will change the nature of the composition.

A Social Problem Solving Unit was created within the University of Medicine and Dentistry of New Jersey–Community Mental Health Center at Piscataway, in partnership with Rutgers University, especially the Center for Applied Psychology of the Graduate School of Applied and Professional Psychology. This unit has as its mission fostering the implementation of the Social Decision Making and Problem Solving program to school districts across the nation—and internationally—with an action research orientation and high fidelity to parameters of implementation known to be effective for this program. It does so by carrying out the main functions described above with regard to implementation of an orchestral work, as well as the Resource Exchange and other facets described earlier. The program and unit gained approval from the National Mental Health Association (winning the 1988 Lela Rowland Prevention Award and being designated as a model program in the NMHA Prevention Clearinghouse), the National

Diffusion Network of the U.S. Department of Education (which itself is now undergoing a transformation), and the National Education Goals Panel, critical steps in building credibility and opening up contacts with networks of potential and actual implementers from which further refinements in practice and sources of implementation support could be derived.

Data concerning the evaluation of the dissemination of the approaches of the Social Decision Making and Problem Solving Project are available from three major studies. Commins and Elias (1991) undertook an examination of the first four sites to implement the Social Decision Making and Problem Solving program. The methodology involved identifying key conditions empirically found most likely to facilitate long-term program implementation. The two districts showing 10 of 10 conditions were found to have made substantial progress toward institutionalization; the district showing 9 of 10 conditions had made substantial progress; the one showing 4 of 10 conditions showed almost no progress. This study was the first to show that the program was capable of being disseminated effectively and that results of dissemination were a function of implementation parameters. Anecdotally, it is worth noting that of the four districts studied by Commins and Elias in 1987, 9 years later, the Social Decision Making and Problem Solving program has a clear, visible presence in the two "10 of 10" districts, has been integrated into the elementary guidance program in the "9 of 10" district, and is implemented only on a sporadic, individual basis in the remaining district.

Heller and Firestone (1995) conducted a study of the sources of leadership in schools that had implemented long-term social and emotional learning programs. As part of this study, nine elementary schools that had implemented Social Decision Making and Problem Solving for at least 3 years were identified. An interview procedure was set up to determine the degree of institutionalization of the program. They found that five of nine schools had institutionalized the program to a significant degree. Four were deemed "fully institutionalized," meaning that all teachers were using the program with high fidelity. One was designated as "mixed," in that there was a core group of teachers that were high-fidelity users of the program with others using the program less rigorously, and four had a "partial" status, meaning that they maintained affiliation with the Social Decision Making and Problem Solving "experts" and teachers were using the program, although in generally limited, low-fidelity ways.

Detailed analysis of mediating factors indicated that full institutionalization was related primarily to leadership roles being filled consistently and by multiple individuals, usually from varied roles, and to having school-based Social Decision Making and Problem Solving resources or coordinating "committees" of some kind. Relatedly, if there was a critical role in the institutionalization of Social Decision Making and Problem Solving programs, it would have to be teachers, rather than administrators. That is, long-term, high-fidelity institutionalization was more likely when there was an active group consisting of those who implemented the program and who were closest to its impacts. Essential among the activities of such groups were providing a sustained vision of the program, offering encouragement, and setting up in-house procedures to monitor its progress and improve its effectiveness (Heller & Firestone, 1995).

As the Social Decision Making and Problem Solving program expanded through involvement with the National Diffusion Network, trainers were bringing the program to sites inside and outside of its New Jersey base. Beyond a focus on implementation, it became important to examine the extent to which teachers and student recipients of the program were developing their skills to the same degrees as they did in the initial validation sample. In the initial samples, of course, the program was smaller, there were fewer implementation sites, and program management was closer and more intensive. For the more recent study, three new sites in New Jersey plus sites in Arkansas and Oregon were studied.

Results are summarized in Bruene-Butler, Hampson, Elias, Clabby, and Schuyler (1997). Briefly, extent of teacher acquisition of skills in "dialoguing" and "facilitative questioning" met or exceeded those of the original sample in all of the new sites. Comparing Oregon and the original New Jersey site, use of inhibitory questioning strategies declined from pretest to posttest, 53% and 40%, respectively; use of facilitative questioning increased by 117% and 35%, respectively. With regard to acquisition of interpersonal sensitivity, problem analysis, and planning skills, students in all of the recent dissemination sites showed significant pre to post gains, and the effect sizes in all cases were equal to or as much as twice as large as those in the original validation sample. The Bruene-Butler et al. data suggest that the implementation of the Social Decision Making and Problem Solving program in sites assessed in 1994 and 1995 can occur in ways that allow its impact on teachers and students to be as strong as it was in the initial implementation site, where it was begun in 1980.

Technology-Based Applications

The most recent set of innovations relates to the use of technology to deliver social decision making and problem solving. When the opportunity arose to join others who felt that disaffected elementary school-aged children were not receptive to school-based programs, or too often were in school environments that did not value the building of their social competence or the transfer of health and life skills outside the classroom, I began participating with the Hallmark Child Philanthropic Foundation to develop a series of social competence promotion interventions. This exciting project involved the development of a video-based program for 9- to 11-year-olds, to be disseminated by existing networks for training within Boys and Girls Clubs, Girl Scouts, and 4-H Clubs around the nation, a strategy designed to help reach at-risk and disaffected youth who are not responsive to school-based programs. This is an action research project of remarkable scope, centered around the character of TJ, a wheelchair-using African American girl who is the problem-solving DJ for a radio call-in show for kids, along with support characters Jeff, her sort of spaced-out engineer and sound-effects man, and station manager Ray Dio, a former DJ who had his heyday in the '60s and '70s and brings maturity, perspective, and a lot of Latin music and rhythms to the station. The themes for the program are teamwork and cooperation, peaceful conflict resolution, and dealing with anger. Initial data from pilot testing of portions of the program showed meaningful and higher than expected effects on children's self-reported skill knowledge and attitudes and observed behaviors in the clubs (Johnston, Bauman, Milne, & Urdan, 1993). Extensive formative evaluation has taken place to ensure that key aspects of implementation—receptivity and responsiveness of diverse audiences of children, retention of program content and themes, enthusiasm for carrying out activities and follow-up projects based on the videos, and clarity of implementation directions for local group leaders—would be built into the program from the inception. At this point, TJ materials have reached more than 2 million children, making it perhaps the largest systematic program of its kind since Head Start (see Elias & Bartz, 1995; Elias & Tobias, 1996; Hallmark Charitable Foundation, 1994, for details).

To take further advantage of the ways in which video and computers enhance receptivity and effectiveness of social-competence-building efforts among populations that are diverse with regard to culture and learning skills, an organization called Psychological Enterprises Incorporated was developed. Its first activities involved generating a computer software program that provides a tutorial on the steps of social decision making, as well as a vehicle for individual students to work through discipline problems, clinical issues, or even to problem solve preventively (Psychological Enterprises Incorporated, 1993). Action research on this technology and its applications in clinical (Elias, Tobias, & Friedlander, 1994) and school (Elias, Hoover, & Poedubicky, in press; Nigro, 1995) contexts has begun (Elias & Tobias, 1996).

Creating a School-Based Infrastructure for Successful Widespread Efforts at Problem Prevention and Building Social Competence

For preventive innovations to spread and have an impact of the kind that can be incorporated into school settings and detected in statistics such as those recorded by *Healthy People 2000* and *Kids Count,* it will be necessary to create interconnected implementation networks. Documentation and sharing of implementation across different settings, contexts, and types of innovations, as well as variations in the many other relevant implementation parameters, will allow the growth of the field and the improvement of practice. This will require collaborative efforts at many levels, more than can be outlined here and more than has been the tendency to date. Success in community coalition building provides a model (Kaye & Wolff, 1995; Wolff, 1987), although at even larger and more inclusive levels.

To assist in that process, Table 9.1 offers suggestions by Ralph and Dwyer (1988) concerning the kind of documentation that will allow inferences to be made about preventive innovations as complex sociotechnical systems. These complement the praxis equation and other implementation considerations outlined throughout.

Action researchers/evaluators must accomplish a difficult task to make a clear and logical presentation of various types of data showing the operation and effects of various program elements that are incorporated into a systemwide preventive effort. It is a further and even more difficult step to relate these effects to long-term, large-scale outcomes. These criteria are rarely met by prevention programs in operation, even by well-funded university-based action research demonstration projects. Given these realities, it is noteworthy that the approach outlined in Table 9.1 is based on a legal model. That is, causal proof, strict experimental evidence, is not required; what must be presented is evidence that claims have been met, beyond a reasonable doubt. It is the accumulation of evidence, at any one point and over time, that is essential.

Pragmatically, those bringing programs into new settings must demonstrate that goals are better met after the inception of the program, that this continues to be the case for several years afterward, that there is implementation of the core principles, that there is receptivity and responsiveness among implementers and recipients, that quality is sustained despite changes in the configuration of initial implementers, that there have been no significant unintended negative effects, and that there is a process of renewal, linkage with other efforts, or MEF/MOD taking place to allow for generativity.

The steps in the process are summarized in Table 9.2, again derived from work of RMC Research with the National Diffusion Network. The tasks are listed from the perspective of a unit or entity whose goal is to bring a preventive effort to multiple settings. Thus, the final step—involving a network of implementing sites—is the one that distinguishes widespread from limited implementation. As we begin to look carefully and realistically at the widespread implementation of prevention activities, it is clear that an infrastructure is needed to foster connections among settings and relationships with the innovation developers or other centers of expertise. For example, RMC Research Corporation's (1995; Ralph & Dwyer, 1988) experience in monitoring the diffusion of programs suggests that in Year 1 of an effort to bring a program to other settings, 50% of the developer's activities are devoted to generating awareness of the innovation in many other sites. The

Table 9.1   Documenting the Impact of a Preventive Innovation on Schoolwide or Systemwide Change and Its Dissemination to Other
Settings: Considerations Before Declaring Success

If a baseline for comparison is used that is external to the focal setting, are the
preprogram similarities of the treatment and comparison schools or systems
documented for all educationally relevant variables in addition to those
directly addressed by the program (e.g., racial, ethnic, socioeconomic,
institution size, and resources)?

If the baseline is internal, are the pre- and postprogram conditions documented
by sufficient data to overcome normal fluctuations and demonstrate trends
convincingly?

If samples from the entire population are used, are they representative? Are they
large enough to generalize with confidence to the population as a whole?

What is the impact on core missions/goals? For example, in schools, what is the
impact on academics and/or behavior? What unintended positive and
negative effects might exist?

Are the students attaining program goals at better-than-predicted levels after
controlling for other student variables including socioeconomic status?

Are the effects sustained or do they represent gains in a single year that diminish
over time, or gains in a single grade that diminish in later grades?

Where are the changes taking place as expected? Where are changes not taking
place? What kinds of modifications need to be made?

Is there a plausible relationship between the nature of the changes made and
long-term or large-scale effects being claimed? Does the change represent
more than shifts in programmatic emphases and resources that were perhaps previously neglected? Have there been shifts in staff, professional
development, or allocated time?

---

other half of the work is split among defining the innovation,
developing materials targeting sites, and providing initial training.
By Year 4, the distribution of activities has shifted such that only
10% is devoted to awareness, with 30% in direct consultation, 25%
working with certified trainers, and the remaining time to
MEF/MOD and following up various implementation sites. Obviously, resources appropriate to the nature and quantity of work
required must be obtained, shifting as needed over time.

Relatedly, to learn more precisely about the diverse pathways that
define successful dissemination, it will be useful to differentiate and
study innovation implementation in first-, second-, and multi-

Table 9.1 Continued

Did the implementation coincide with other changes in the school's organization or resources that are not viewed as part of the systemwide reform program? Could these other changes have contributed to the observed effects?

Have there been changes in the population of the school or district? Is evidence presented to support the stability of conditions?

Do the changes or improvements compare favorably to standard practices in similar institutions? Is the demonstrated change worthwhile in terms of cost? Are the time savings worthwhile?

Have there been changes in measures or record keeping procedures over the course of the study that could affect the nature or size of outcomes? (This issue is a particularly important question when making use of school or district data collection not done specifically for the program evaluation; changes in report cards or standardized tests used by schools are not uncommon, for example.)

Is it possible that changes simply reflect developing trends in the larger educational milieu, for example, the influence of new state or federal requirements or changing social values?

How has the organization changed with regard to staff time, work demands, resource allocation, and other areas?

What is the pattern of the above findings across settings? What are the features of these settings? What differential effects are noted?

SOURCE: Information in this table is drawn from Ralph and Dwyer (1988).

generational contexts. Consider a model program as a "parent." From a generational perspective, there are numerous pathways that allow that parent to propagate with fidelity and integrity:

1. Pathways involving high levels of direct "parental" involvement
   a. In settings similar to the original
   b. In settings dissimilar to the original (similarity is defined in terms of target populations, implementation staff, and resources available)
2. Pathways involving low levels of direct parental involvement
3. Pathways involving high levels of involvement from primary assistants (trained directly by parents)
4. Pathways involving low levels of involvement from primary assistants

Table 9.2 Task Analysis for Single-Site and Widespread Prevention
Program Implementation

Project definition

    Determine key elements

    Decide range of acceptable variations

    Profile likely adopters

    Establish an adoption organization and what will be considered as adoptions

    Develop an overall diffusion plan and internal management system

    Specify diffusion elements of the project—key elements to be disseminated, core components/criteria for minimal adoption, note revisions available and/or needed to enhance replicability in adopter sites

    Identify target audiences

Marketing

    Generate awareness strategies and materials

    Identify related networks

    Target adopters

    Coordinate with other audiences—build effective working relationships with state education agencies, communication networks, professional associations

    Specify evaluation guidelines for adopters—documentation of implementation and impact

    Develop documentation and evaluation procedures for dissemination activities

    Develop overall awareness plan—design materials, presentations; organize project facilities for demonstration purposes, plan training sessions

    Conduct awareness activities

Installation

    Assess adopter readiness

    Negotiate adopter plans

    Review and finalize products

    Plan and conduct specialized consultation

---

5. Pathways involving high levels of involvement from second-generation trainees from the pilot

6. Pathways involving high levels of involvement from those experienced with one of the above levels of application but with no direct input from the model program

7. Pathways involving high levels of involvement from those who have seen a demonstration site, with relative degrees of connectedness with the model program/primary implementers

Table 9.2 Continued

Plan and conduct technical assistance

Develop adopter selection criteria

Negotiate with potential adopters—mutual expectations, availability and suitability of needed facilities, resources, materials, staff at adoption site, availability of consultation

Perform organizational assessment—identify key resources, personnel, subgroups; obtain commitments

Plan and conduct trainings

Develop support mechanisms within setting/district

Create an implementation plan, including evaluation design

Begin implementation plan

Follow-up

Evaluate use of key elements by adopters

Evaluate impact at selected sites

Provide additional follow-up to assure satisfactory replication

Monitor and conduct follow-up

Project network building

Maintain ongoing contact with adopters

Train trainers

Establish demonstration sites

Create information sharing networks of adopters, trainers, demonstration sites, site leaders

Create linkages with professional association training contexts

Extend project services through selection, training, management of certified trainers, satellite demonstration sites

Provide reports documenting diffusion activities, sharing ideas

SOURCE: Information in this table is drawn from Ralph and Dwyer (1988) and RMC Research Corporation (1995).

Successful widespread implementation of a "model" program requires it to traverse one or more of these pathways; furthermore, each specific instantiation of the model ideally will remain linked to the overall network of such implementations so that its experiences can inform others and so that it can contribute to further spreading the implementation of the model program.

An explication of the task and process issues involved in implementing a preventive effort in one and then many sites provides benchmarks useful both in an adoption site and in a "dissemination unit" for continuing their efforts. From accumulations of such documented examples, some of which may be more or less complete and address many or few of the concerns outlined in Tables 9.1 and 9.2 directly, inferences about the spread of a program can be sharpened with regard to contexts and conditions. Furthermore, much can be learned in general about the implementation of innovation in the prevention field.

Conclusions and Recommendations

Issues like violence, alcohol and other drug use, AIDS, academic failure, and school disaffection and dropout require public health solutions—bold, definitive, efficacious, widespread, and sustained efforts. What is at stake is the future health of our youth and what they will become when they are adults and in a position to take over the responsibilities of citizenship in our democracy. We cannot afford to have a situation in which the spread of preventive and competence-promoting innovations is approached naively, unrealistically, or misleadingly. The Emperor must be clothed, and the time for action is now. We must begin with the preparation of the key gatekeepers over preventive innovations in the schools. There are no shortcuts, inoculations, or preventive approaches that can succeed once "installed" in the absence of oversight and MEF/MOD.

The Social Decision Making and Problem Solving Project has been presented as an example of how conditions can be created so that health promotion and risk reduction programs can be brought into schools and implemented with integrity and skills acquisition. The kind of concerted, focused effort required needs to be incorporated into the formulation of public health policy documents such as *Healthy People 2010* so that the planning information they contain can reflect implementation realities.

What will it take, from an implementation perspective, to reach *Healthy People 2010* objectives for youth? First, all service objectives should include specific statements about high-quality implementation of programs. Such statements would then be matched by surveillance objectives that would examine the extent to which programs selected have a high likelihood of successful implementation, and the quality of the implementation effort.

Clearly, problems will persist in schools while efforts move forward to develop better models and procedures for developing the social and emotional skills of our youth. Nevertheless, we must ask what conditions make it most likely that programs for promoting the health of youth can be implemented. In brief, what is required is the development of a school-based infrastructure that will allow programs to be brought in thoughtfully, carried out carefully, and modified appropriately in light of feedback concerning their impact. Specifically, I recommend:

1. Educational administrators need to be prepared to be action researchers, considering the collective impact of prevention and competence-building programs and related innovations, working to combine them, and tracking their progress continually, until and even after goals appear to be attained.

2. Concomitant changes are needed in higher education, in teacher and administrator training and supervision, and in the preparation of pupil services staff. Institutions of educational preparation that are not willing and able to instill the necessary attitudes and skills to implement preventive and health promotive innovations in schools should not be accredited as places where educators are being prepared.

3. All schools should become centers for parenting support and education, to maximize the preventive impact of what takes place in schools and to help parents apply what is known about social and emotional development and problem prevention in their own homes.

Ultimately, there is no substitute for creating the infrastructure of widespread implementation of preventive innovation. The current emphasis on invention must be complemented with the realization that the challenges of implementing operator-dependent sociotechnical systems for prevention in nondemonstration contexts are both intellectual and practical and must be met if we are to reach our national health goals and improve our nation's standing among other countries with regard to the well-being of our youth.

References

Albee, G. W. (1982). Preventing psychopathology and promoting human potential. *American Psychologist, 37,* 1043-1050.

Baldridge, J. (1975). Organizational innovation: Individual, structural, and environmental impact. In J. Baldridge & T. Deal (Eds.), *Managing change in educational organizations* (pp. 151-175). Berkeley, CA: McCutchan.

Berman, P., & McLaughlin, M. (1980). Factors affecting the process of change. In M. M. Milstein (Ed.), *Schools, conflict, and change* (pp. 57-71). New York: Teachers College Press.

Blumberg, A. (1980). School organizations: A case of generic resistance to change. In M. M. Milstein (Ed.), *Schools, conflict, and change* (pp. 15-29). New York: Teachers College Press.

Bruene-Butler, L., Hampson, J., Elias, M. J., Clabby, J. F., & Schuyler, T. (1997). The Improving Social Awareness–Social Problem Solving Project. In G. W. Albee & T. P. Gullotta (Eds.), *Primary prevention works* (pp. 239-267). Thousand Oaks, CA: Sage.

Chavis, D. (1993). A future for community psychology practice. *American Journal of Community Psychology, 21,* 171-183.

Commins, W., & Elias, M. J. (1991). Institutionalization of mental health programs in organizational contexts: The case of elementary schools. *Journal of Community Psychology, 19,* 207-220.

Cowen, E. L. (1977). Baby steps toward primary prevention. *American Journal of Community Psychology, 5,* 1-22.

Elias, M. J. (1987). Establishing enduring prevention programs: Advancing the legacy of Swampscott. *American Journal of Community Psychology, 15,* 539-554.

Elias, M. J. (Ed.). (1993). *Social decision making and life skills development: Guidelines for middle school educators.* Gaithersburg, MD: Aspen.

Elias, M. J. (1994). Capturing excellence in applied settings: A participant conceptualizer and praxis explicator role for community psychologists. *American Journal of Community Psychology, 22,* 293-318.

Elias, M. J., & Bartz, K. (1995, June). *Talking with TJ: A corporate-led youth organization partnership for violence prevention and social competence promotion.* Presentation at the biennial meeting of the Society for Community Research and Action and APA Div. 27 (Community Psychology), Chicago.

Elias, M. J., & Clabby, J. F. (1992). *Building social problem solving skills: Guidelines from a school-based program.* San Francisco: Jossey-Bass.

Elias, M. J., Gager, P., & Hancock, M. (1993). *Prevention and social competence programs in use in New Jersey public schools: Findings from a statewide survey* (Working Paper No. 3, School Intervention Implementation Study). New Brunswick, NJ: Rutgers University, Department of Psychology.

Elias, M. J., Gager, P., & Leon, S. (in press). Spreading a warm blanket of prevention over all children: Guidelines for selecting substance abuse and related prevention curricula for use in the schools. *Journal of Primary Prevention.*

Elias, M. J., Hoover, H. V. A., & Poedubicky, V. (in press). Reaching at-risk students via computer-facilitated social problem solving lessons. *Elementary Guidance and Counseling Journal.*

Elias, M. J., & Tobias, S. E. (1996). *Social problem solving interventions in the schools.* New York: Guilford.

Elias, M. J., Tobias, S. E., & Friedlander, B. S. (1994). Enhancing skills for everyday problem solving, decision making, and conflict resolution in special needs students with the support of computer-based technology. *Special Services in the Schools, 8,* 33-52.

Elias, M. J., Weissberg, R., Zins, J., Kendall, P., Dodge, K., Jason, L., Rotheram-Borus, M., Perry, C., Hawkins, J., & Gottfredson, D. (1996). Transdisciplinary collaboration among school researchers: The Consortium on the School-Based Promotion of Social Competence. *Journal of Educational and Psychological Consultation, 8,* 25-44.

Erikson, E. (1982). *The life cycle completed: A review.* New York: Norton.

Federal Interagency Ad Hoc Committee on Health Promotion Through the Schools. (1992). *Healthy schools: A directory of federal programs and activities related to health promotion through the schools.* Washington, DC: U.S. Department of Health and Human Services.

Fleming, M. (1996). *Healthy youth 2000: A mid-decade review.* Chicago: American Medical Association, Department of Adolescent Health.

Fullan, M. (1994). *Change forces: Probing the depths of educational reform.* Bristol, PA: Falmer.

Hallmark Charitable Foundation. (1994). *Talking with TJ: A new educational resource to teach teamwork, cooperation, and conflict resolution.* Omaha, NE: Hallmark. (Available from Hallmark, Inc., 1002 N. 42nd Street, Omaha, NE 68131-9834)

Heller, M., & Firestone, W. (1995). Who's in charge here? Sources of leadership for change in eight schools. *Elementary School Journal, 96*(1), 65-86.

House, E. (1974). *The politics of educational innovation.* Berkeley, CA: McCutchan.

Johnston, J., Bauman, J., Milne, L., & Urdan, T. (1993). *Taking the measure of Talking With TJ: Series 1.* Ann Arbor: University of Michigan Institute for Social Research.

Kaye, G., & Wolff, T. (Eds.). (1995). *From the ground up: A workbook on coalition building and community development.* Amherst, MA: AHEC/Community Partners (Available from AHEC/Community Partners, 24 South Prospect Street, Amherst, MA 01002)

Kelly, J. G. (1979). 'Tain't what you do, it's the way you do it. *American Journal of Community Psychology, 7,* 244-258.

Kelly, J. G. (1984, March). *Seven criteria when doing community based prevention research.* Paper presented at the Prevention Research Methods Workshop, Center for Prevention Research, National Institute of Mental Health, Rockville, MD.

Kelly, J. G. (1990). Changing contexts and the field of community psychology, *American Journal of Community Psychology, 18,* 769-792.

Kids Count. (1995). *Kids Count, America: An annual national survey of the status of children.* Westport, CT: Annie Casey Foundation.

Lewin, K. (1951). *Field theory in social science.* New York: Harper & Row.

London, M., & MacDuffie, J. (1985). *Implementing managerial and technical innovations: Case examples and guidelines for practice.* Basking Ridge, NJ: AT&T Communications.

Lorion, R. (1993). Counting the stitches: Preventive intervention promises and public health. *American Journal of Community Psychology, 21,* 673-679.

Mrazek, P., & Haggerty, R. (Eds.). (1994). *Reducing risks for mental disorders: Frontiers for preventive intervention research.* Report of the Institute of Medicine Committee on Prevention of Mental Disorders, Division of Biobehavioral Sciences and Mental Disorders. Washington, DC: National Academy Press.

Nigro, L. (1995). *The Social Problem Solving Lab: Pre-referral intervention to enhance elementary students' critical thinking skills.* Unpublished dissertation, Rutgers University, Graduate School of Applied and Professional Psychology, New Brunswick, NJ.

O'Donnell, C., Tharp, R., & Wilson, K. (1993). Activity settings as the unit of analysis: A theoretical basis for community intervention and development. *American Journal of Community Psychology, 21,* 501-520.

Olson, L. (1994, November 2). Learning their lessons: Scaling up; bringing good schools to every community. *Education Week, 14*(9), 43-46.

Price, R. H., & Cherniss, C. (1977). Training for a new profession: Research as social action. *Professional Psychology, 8,* 222-231.

Price, R. H., Cowen, E. L., Lorion, R. P., & Ramos-McKay, J. (Eds.). (1988). *Fourteen ounces of prevention: A casebook for practitioners.* Washington, DC: American Psychological Association.

Price, R. H., & Lorion, R. (1989). Prevention programming as organizational reinvention: From research to implementation. In D. Shaffer, I. Phillips, & N. Enzer (Eds.), *Prevention of mental disorders, alcohol and other drug use in children and adolescents* (pp. 97-123). Office of Substance Abuse Prevention, Prevention Monograph No. 2 (DHHS Publication No. ADM 89-1646). Rockville, MD: U.S. Department of Health and Human Services.

Price, R. H, & Smith, S. (1985). *A guide to evaluating prevention programs in mental health* (DHHS Publication No. ADM 85-144). Washington, DC: U.S. Government Printing Office.

Psychological Enterprises Incorporated. (1993). *The student conflict manager/personal problem solving guide.* Morristown, NJ: Author.

Ralph, J., & Dwyer, M. C. (1988). *Making the case: Evidence of program effectiveness in schools and classrooms.* Washington, DC: U.S. Department of Education, Office of Educational Research and Improvement.

RMC Research Corporation. (1995). *National Diffusion Network schoolwide promising practices: Report of a pilot effort.* Portsmouth, NH: Author.

Rossi, P. H. (1978). Issues in the evaluation of human services delivery. *Evaluation Quarterly, 2,* 573-599.

Rothman, J., Erlich, J., & Teresa, J. (1976). *Promoting innovation and change in organizations and communities: A planning manual.* New York: John Wiley.

Rotter, J. B. (1954). *Social learning and clinical psychology.* Englewood Cliffs, NJ: Prentice Hall.

Sarason, S. B. (1983). *The culture of the school and the problem of change* (2nd ed.). Boston: Allyn & Bacon.

Schorr, L. (1988). *Within our reach: Breaking the cycle of disadvantage.* New York: Doubleday.

Stokols, D. (1986). The research psychologist as social change agent. *American Journal of Community Psychology, 14,* 595-599.

Stolz, S. B. (1984). Preventive models; Implications for a technology of practice. In M. Roberts & L. Peterson (Eds.), *Prevention of problems in childhood* (pp. 391-413). New York: John Wiley.

Tolan, P., Keys, C., Chertok, F., & Jason, L. (1990). (Eds.). *Researching community psychology: Issues of theory and methods.* Washington, DC: American Psychological Association.

Tornatzky, L., & Fleischer, M. (1986, October). *Dissemination and/or implementation: The problem of complex socio-technical systems.* Paper presented at the meeting of the American Evaluation Association, Kansas City, MO.

U.S. Department of Health and Human Services, Public Health Service. (1991). *Healthy people 2000: National health promotion and disease prevention objectives* (DHHS Publication No. PHS 91-50212). Washington, DC: U.S. Government Printing Office.

Van de Ven, A. (1986). Central problems in the management of innovation. *Management Science, 32,* 590-608.

Vincent, T., & Trickett, E. (1983). Preventive intervention and the human context: Ecological approaches to environmental assessment and change. In R. Felner, L. Jason, J. Moritsugu, & S. Farber (Eds.), *Preventive psychology: Theory, research, and practice* (pp. 67-86). New York: Pergamon.

Wolff, T. (1987). Community psychology and empowerment: An activist's insights. *American Journal of Community Psychology, 15,* 151-166.

Wolff, T. (1994). Keynote address given at the Fourth Biennial Conference. *Community Psychologist, 27*(3), 20-26.

Yin, R. (1979). *Changing urban bureaucracies: How new practices become routinized.* Lexington, MA: Lexington Books.

Index

About the Editors

Gerald R. Adams is Professor in the Department of Family Studies at the University of Guelph, Ontario, Canada. He is an associate editor for the series **Advances in Adolescent Development** and **Issues in Children's and Families' Lives**. He is a Fellow of the American Psychological Association, the American Psychological Society, and the American Association of Applied and Preventive Psychology. His research focuses on family psychology, adolescent development, family-school connections in predicting adjustment and academic success, and aspects of primary prevention and social interventions. He is the coauthor of five textbooks, more than a dozen books, and many research reports, chapters, and public journalist articles. He is on the editorial boards of journals in sociology, psychology, human development, family science, and education.

Thomas P. Gullotta is CEO of the Child and Family Agency in Connecticut. He currently is the editor of the *Journal of Primary Prevention*. He is a book editor for the **Advances in Adolescent Development** series and is the senior book series editor for **Issues in Children's and Families' Lives**. In addition, he serves on the editorial boards of the *Journal of Early Adolescence* and *Adolescence* and is an adjunct faculty member in the psychology and education departments of Eastern Connecticut State University. His published works focus on primary prevention and youth.

Robert L. Hampton, Ph.D., is Associate Provost for Academic Affairs, Dean for Undergraduate Studies, and Professor of Family Studies and Sociology at the University of Maryland, College Park. He has published extensively in the field of family violence and is editor of *Violence in the Black Family: Correlates and Consequences* (1987), *Black Family Violence: Current Research and Theory* (1991), *Family Violence: Prevention and Treatment* (1993), and *Preventing Violence in America* (1996). His research interests include interspousal violence, family abuse, male violence, community violence, resilience, and institutional responses to violence.

Bruce A. Ryan is Associate Professor in the Department of Family Studies at the University of Guelph, Ontario, Canada. He earned a doctorate in educational psychology from the University of Alberta and has served in numerous positions of responsibility at the University of Guelph and in child and family service associations and agencies in Ontario. His current research interests and most recent publications are focused on the relationship between family processes and school outcomes for children.

Roger P. Weissberg is Professor of Psychology at the University of Illinois at Chicago (UIC), where he is Director of Graduate Studies in Psychology and Executive Director of the Collaborative for the Advancement of Social and Emotional Learning (CASEL). He also directs the NIMH-funded Predoctoral and Postdoctoral Prevention Research Training Program in Urban Children's Mental Health and AIDS Prevention. He also holds an appointment with the Mid-Atlantic Laboratory for Student Success, funded by the Office of Educational Research and Improvement of the U.S. Department of Education. His research interests include school and community preventive interventions, urban children's mental health, and parent involvement in children's education. He has been President of the American Psychological Association's Society for Community Research and Action. He is a recipient of the William T. Grant Foundation's 5-year Faculty Scholars Award in Children's Mental Health, the Connecticut Psychological Association's 1992 Award for Distinguished Psychological Contribution in the Public Interest, and the National Mental Health Association's 1992 Lela Rowland Prevention Award.

About the Contributors

Richard D. Calvert, MSW, LCSW, is Director of Health and Social Services at the Child and Family Agency of S.E. Connecticut. He oversees the agency's 12 school-based health centers, which provide integrated primary medical and behavioral health care in elementary, middle, and high school settings. In 1990, he was honored by the Connecticut Youth Services Association for his advocacy efforts on behalf of Connecticut's youth.

Emory L. Cowen, Ph.D., is Professor of Psychology (and Psychiatry) and Director of the University of Rochester Center for Community Study. He was a founder of the Primary Mental Health Project (PMHP) and directed the project for its first 34 years. He is past president of Division 27 of the American Psychological Association (APA) and the recipient of its Distinguished Contributions and Seymour B. Sarason awards. He also received the APA Award for Distinguished Contributions to Psychology in the Public Interest. He has authored more than 300 journal articles, chapters, and books. His research activities and writing focus primarily on factors that relate to children's school adjustment and the development, evaluation, and dissemination of school-based prevention and well-ness enhancement programs for young children.

Lisa Davis, BSN, MBA, is a nurse consultant for the State of Connecticut, Department of Public Health, School and Adolescent Health Unit. She has 12 years of nursing experience, which include 3 years as a hospital staff nurse and 7 years of nursing administration in an urban community health center. Currently, she is responsible for the program administration of 17 school-based health centers in Connecticut.

Kenneth A. Dodge, Ph.D., Duke University, 1978, is Professor of Psychology and Director of the Clinical Training Program at Vanderbilt University. He has received the Distinguished Scientist Award for Early Career Contribution to Psychology from the American Psychological Association, the Boyd McCandless Award, and a Research Scientist Award from the National Institute of Mental Health. He has been a Fellow at the Center for Advanced Study in the Behavioral Sciences at Stanford, California. He is studying the development and prevention of antisocial behavior in children and adolescents.

Shauna L. Dowden is a graduate student in the clinical psychology program at the University of Connecticut. She serves as the editorial assistant for the *Journal of Primary Prevention* and as a research analyst for the University of Connecticut Health Center. Her research interests focus on physical punishment and psychological adjustment.

Maurice J. Elias, Ph.D., is Professor in the Department of Psychology at Rutgers University and Co-Developer of the Improving Social Awareness–Social Problem Solving Project. This project received the 1988 Lela Rowland Prevention Award from the NMHA, is approved by the Program Effectiveness Panel of the National Diffusion Network as a federally validated prevention program, and, most recently, has been named as a Model Program by the National Educational Goals Panel. In 1990, he was awarded the National Psychological Consultants to Management Award by the APA. In 1993, he received the Distinguished Contribution to the Practice of Community Psychology Award from the Society for Community Research and Action (APA, Division 27). Most recently, he is a member of the Leadership Team of the Collaborative for the Advancement of Social and Emotional Learning. His books include *Social Decision Making Skills: A Curriculum Guide for the Elementary Grades, Building Social Problem Solving Skills: Guidelines From a School-Based Program, Social Decision Making and Life Skills: Guidelines for Middle School Educators, Promoting Student Success Through Group Intervention,* and *Social Problem Solving Interventions in the Schools.*

Carolyn M. Fink is on the faculty at the University of Maryland Department of Special Education and the American University

Department of Education. She also directs religious education at Riverdale Presbyterian Church and raises three young sons. She received her doctorate from the University of Maryland studying school life histories of incarcerated women with learning problems. Her other research interests include strategies for teaching children with behavior disorders, qualitative methods of inquiry, and delinquency. In other professional activities, she has reviewed grant proposals for the U.S. Department of Education, taught a writing workshop for Baltimore City teachers, published a chapter on delinquency among learning disabled students, and written an ethnographic account of life in a juvenile training school. She has also published a study of the effect of grade retention on delinquent behavior.

Matia Finn-Stevenson earned her doctorate from Ohio State University. She is a research scientist at Yale University, with a joint appointment in the Department of Psychology and the Child Study Center of the School of Medicine. She is also Associate Director of the Bush Center in Child Development and Social Policy, where she is head of the School of the 21st Century. She has done extensive research in child development, children's services, parent training, and work-family life issues. In her current research, she focuses on the involvement of schools in child care and social support programs. She is author and coauthor of many scholarly publications, most recently related to child care and welfare, parental leave policies, and family support programs, including *Children: Development and Social Policies* and *Children in the Changing World*. She has been an adviser on domestic policy issues to the staff of the White House Office of Policy Development and a consultant to the Connecticut legislature's Committee on Work and Family, the Committee on Education and Labor, the U.S. House of Representatives, and the U.S. Senate Subcommittee on Children, Youth, Families, Alcohol, and Drug Abuse.

Denise C. Gottfredson is Professor in the Department of Criminology and Criminal Justice at the University of Maryland, College Park. She received her Ph.D. in social relations from Johns Hopkins University in 1980. She has directed numerous field experiments testing delinquency and drug abuse prevention programs and is committed to the development of productive collaborations between researchers and practitioners. She has written many journal articles, including several on researcher-practitioner collaboration to solve social problems, and is coauthor of *Victimization in Schools,* a study of school violence. She recently completed an evaluation of the effect of the closing of a juvenile correctional institution in Maryland, a study of a 3-year discipline management project that was implemented in six middle schools, and a study of cultural appropriateness in measurement instruments used to evaluate prevention programs. Currently, she is writing a book on schooling and delinquency, conducting an evaluation of Baltimore City's Drug Treatment Court, working on a report to Congress on Crime Prevention, and conducting a national study of school-based prevention practices.

Gary D. Gottfredson is President of Gottfredson Associates, Inc. He received his Ph.D. in psychology from Johns Hopkins University in 1976. He is author of a comprehensive theory-based approach to program development and evaluation known as PDE and author of several psychological assessment and evaluation tools, including the Position Classification Inventory for job analysis, the Career Attitudes and Strategies Inventory for assessing adult career status, and the Effective School Battery for school climate assessment. A licensed psychologist and Fellow of the APA and its division of Measurement, Evaluation, and Statistics, he is the recipient of an award for Outstanding Contributions to Personality and Career Research from the APA. He recently completed an evaluation of the Multicultural Education Program in the Pittsburgh Public Schools, has served as Consulting Editor for *Evaluation Review,* and is currently on the editorial boards of other journals. He is coauthor of *Victimization in Schools,* a scientific study of violence in America's schools and the ways schools can address it, and has authored dozens of journal articles, many on program evaluation.

Sharon L. Kagan, Ed.D., Senior Associate at Yale's Bush Center in Child Development and Social Policy, is recognized nationally and internationally for her work related to the care and education of young children and their families. She is a frequent consultant to the White House, Congress, the National Governor's Association, the Department of Education, and the U.S. Department of Health and Human Services, and numerous national foundations, corporations, and professional associations. Formerly Chair of the Family Resource Coalition Board of Directors, a member of the Governing Board of the National Association for the Education of Young

Children (NAEYC), President Clinton's education transition team, and National Commissions on Head Start and Chapter 1, she has received numerous awards, among them an honorary doctoral degree from Wheelock College and the Distinguished Alumna Award from Teachers College, Columbia University. Presently, she serves on more than 40 national boards and panels. She has written more than 100 publications. Augmenting her scholarship with work in the field, she has been a Head Start teacher and director, a fellow in the U.S. Senate, an administrator in the public schools, and Director of the New York City Mayor's Office of Early Childhood Education.

Carol Bartels Kuster is Associate Director for CASEL, the Collaborative for the Advancement of Social and Emotional Learning at the University of Illinois at Chicago. She received her Ph.D. in clinical/community psychology from the University of Maryland, College Park. Her research interests include social and emotional learning, family violence, parent training and education programs, and prevention of child abuse and neglect.

Michelle J. Neuman is a research assistant at the Yale Bush Center in Child Development and Social Policy. Her research has focused on policy areas related to children and families including early care and education policy, children's transitions to school, leadership in early care and education, family support, the education of homeless children and adolescents, and programs for children and families in France. She is a graduate of the Woodrow Wilson School of Public and International Affairs at Princeton University, where she also received a certificate in French language and culture.

Mary Jane Rotheram-Borus, Ph.D., is Professor of Clinical Psychology and Director, Clinical Research Center, in the Division of Social and Community Psychiatry, Neuropsychiatric Institute, University of California, Los Angeles. She received her Ph.D. in clinical psychology from the University of Southern California. Her research interests include HIV/AIDS prevention with adolescents, suicide among adolescents, homeless youths, assessment and modification of children's social skills, ethnic identity, group processes, and cross-ethnic interactions. She has received grants from the National Institute of Mental Health to study HIV prevention with adolescents, the chronically mentally ill, and persons with sexually transmitted diseases; to study interventions for children whose parents have AIDS and for HIV-positive adolescents; and to examine national patterns of use, costs, outcomes, and need for children's and adolescents' mental health service programs. Her research also has been funded by the National Science Foundation, National Institute on Drug Abuse, Society for Research in Child Development, and the W.T. Grant Foundation.

Stacy Skroban is a doctoral student and graduate research assistant in the Department of Criminology and Criminal Justice at the University of Maryland, College Park. Her primary research interests include delinquency prevention program evaluation, statistical methods, and criminal careers research. Recent publications include an evaluation of a school-based prevention demonstration.

Ernest Valente, Jr., Ph.D., University of North Carolina at Chapel Hill, 1992, is a Research Associate at the Association of American Medical Colleges in Washington, D.C., where he researches medical education and evaluates the functioning of Academic Medical Centers. His other research interests include conflict processing and the development of criminal and violent behavior in children.

Edward F. Zigler is Sterling Professor of Psychology, head of the psychology section of the Child Study Center, and Director of the Bush Center in Child Development and Social Policy at Yale University. He is author, coauthor, and editor of numerous scholarly publications and has conducted extensive investigations on normal child development and on psychopathology and mental retardation. He is founder of the School of the 21st Century, which has been adopted by more than 300 schools in 13 states across the country, and cofounder of CoZi, which is a combination of Dr. James P. Comer's School Development Program and Zigler's School of the 21st Century. He regularly testifies as an expert witness before congressional committees and has served as consultant to a number of cabinet-rank officers. He was one of the planners of Project Head Start; President Carter later named him Chair of the 15th anniversary of the project. From 1970 to 1972, he was the first Director of the U.S. Office of Child Development (now the Administration for Children, Youth, and Families) and chief of the Children's Bureau. Recently, he was a member of the advisory committee on Head Start Quality and Expansion and of the planning committee on Early Head Start.

Printed in the United States
By Bookmasters